# Myasthenia Gravis
## and Related Disorders

# CURRENT CLINICAL NEUROLOGY

Daniel Tarsy, MD, *Series Editor*

# MYASTHENIA GRAVIS AND RELATED DISORDERS

*Edited by*

## HENRY J. KAMINSKI, MD

*Departments of Neurology and Neurosciences*
*Case Western Reserve University*
*University Hospitals of Cleveland*
*Louis Stokes Cleveland Veterans Affairs Medical Center*
*Cleveland, OH*

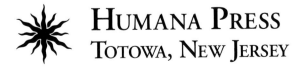

**HUMANA PRESS**
TOTOWA, NEW JERSEY

BS

Acquisitions Editor: Thomas H. Moore.

Cover design by Patricia F. Cleary.

Cover illustration: Electron micrographs of mouse diaphragm neuromuscular junction from a normal mouse and from a mouse with experimentally induced myasthenia gravis (Fig. 2, Chapter 1; *see* full caption and discussion on pp. 2–3).

For additional copies, pricing for bulk purchases, and/or information about other Humana titles, contact Humana at the above address or at any of the following numbers: Tel: 973-256-1699; Fax: 973-256-8341; E-mail: humana@humanapr.com or visit our website at http://humanapress.com

**Photocopy Authorization Policy:**

Printed in the United States of America.   10  9  8  7  6  5  4  3  2  1

**Library of Congress Cataloging-in-Publication Data**

Myasthenia gravis and related disorders / edited by Henry J. Kaminski
    p. ; cm.
  Includes bibliographical references and index.
  ISBN 1-58829-058-1 (alk. paper)
  1. Myasthenia gravis. 2. Neuromuscular diseases. 3. Myoneural junction. I. Kaminski, Henry J.
  [DNLM: 1. Myasthenia Gravis--physiopathology. 2. Myasthenia Gravis--therapy. 3. Neuromuscular Junction Diseases--diagnosis. 4. Neuromuscular Junction Disease--physiopathology. WE 555 M99427 2002] RC935.M8 M886 2002
  616.7'442--dc21
                                  2002017297

2/11/04

# Preface

From the first clear clinical descriptions in 1879 by Wilhelm Erb and in 1893 by Samuel Goldflam, myasthenia gravis has evolved to become the best understood autoimmune disorder, serving as a model for understanding not only autoimmunity, but also synaptic function. The objective of *Myasthenia Gravis and Related Disorders* is to provide the clinician and the scientist a common source for the understanding of this complex disorder.

*Myasthenia Gravis and Related Disorders* begins with a discussion of neuromuscular junction structure and function as well as a detailed description of the acetylcholine receptor, the central target of pathology in myasthenia gravis. The neuromuscular junction, as recently as the late 1980s, could only be depicted as a cartoon of a nerve terminal with synaptic vesicles as circles and an undulating muscle surface. Now unfolding is an intricate machinery that coordinates the release of synaptic vesicles upon depolarization of the nerve and a beautiful architecture of numerous specialized proteins that underlies the postsynaptic surface. Although it was appreciated in the 1970s that autoantibodies to the acetylcholine receptor were the primary cause of myasthenia gravis, investigations have led to the characterization of the intricate T cell dependence and cytokine influences on autoantibody production. With this understanding has come the possible categorization of myasthenia gravis patients based on demographic characteristics, autoantibody profiles, and thymic pathology. Definition of genetic susceptibility loci will certainly lead to further refinement in patient subgroups. The new century should see treatments that will specifically target the autoimmune defect, which are further specialized on the individual patient's genetic profile.

Despite the advances in the basic sciences, myasthenia gravis remains a challenging disorder to recognize and treat, with patients frequently complaining of delays in diagnosis, complications of treatment, and poor response to therapies. Chapters detail information regarding the clinical presentation, diagnostic evaluation, and treatment of myasthenia gravis. Although thymectomy is widely accepted, its benefit in the light of modern immunosuppressive therapies has come into question and a chapter discusses this controversy. The book concludes with a discussion of the most difficult to understand effects of myasthenia gravis, the psychological consequences of the disease. This subject is commonly neglected in myasthenia gravis texts but is becoming a focus of research. I include an appendix detailing recommendations of a Task Force of the Myasthenia Gravis Foundation of America for clinical research guidelines. These guidelines were a first step in knitting together the international community of investigators to adopt a common language to describe patients, treatments, and outcome. It is hoped that by the improvement of these recommendations, clinicians may study myasthenia gravis with the same rigor as their basic science colleagues.

Related to myasthenia gravis by clinical presentation or pathophysiology are the Lambert-Eaton syndrome, congenital myasthenias, and toxic neuromuscular junction disorders. A chapter discusses neuromyotonia because of its similarity in autoimmune pathology to myasthenia gravis and the occasional overlap of neuromyotonia with myasthenia gravis. Compared with myasthenia gravis, these diseases are only beginning to be defined at a molecular and immunologic level. Readers may be a bit surprised by the loss of "myasthenic" in referring to the Lambert-Eaton syndrome. This is done in deference to Vanda Lennon and Edward Lambert, who prefer this terminology.

All the authors have a personal relationship with myasthenia gravis, and this is appreciated in their writing, particularly that of Alfred Jaretzki and Robert Daroff. I hope this allows the reader to appreciate the human endeavor of not only medicine but scientific inquiry.

I thank all the contributing authors, in particular Robert Ruff and Robert Daroff, my long-time mentors, and I am indebted to Humana Press for making the book a reality. Appreciation is extended to the National Eye Institute at the National Institutes of Health, the Department of Veterans Affairs, and the Myasthenia Gravis Foundation of America for their support of my research as well as the research of many of the contributors. I also thank the Muscular Dystrophy Association for their support of neuromuscular research. To my patients who have given me more than I could ever return—thank you.

I dedicate this book to Janina Kaminski, my mother, and Linda Kusner, my wife.

*Henry J. Kaminski, MD*

# Contents

# Contributors

MARK A. AGIUS, MD • *Department of Neurology, University of California, Davis, CA*

BIANCA M. CONTI-FINE, MD • *Department of Biochemistry, Molecular Biology, and Biophysics, University of Minnesota, St. Paul, MN*

ROBERT B. DAROFF, MD • *Department of Neurology, University Hospitals of Cleveland and Case Western Reserve University, Cleveland, OH*

BRENDA DIETHELM-OKITA, BS • *Department of Biochemistry, Molecular Biology, and Biophysics, University of Minnesota, St. Paul, MN*

JOSE AMERICO M. FERNANDES FILHO, MD • *Department of Neurology, University Hospitals of Cleveland and Case Western Reserve University, Cleveland, OH*

JAMES M. GILCHRIST, MD • *Department of Clinical Neuroscience, Brown Medical School, Providence, RI*

CHRISTOPHER M. GOMEZ, MD, PhD • *Professor of Neurology, Department of Neurology and Neuroscience, University of Minnesota, Minneapolis, MN*

C. MICHEL HARPER, MD • *Departments of Neurology and Immunology, Mayo Clinic, Rochester, MN*

IAN HART, PhD, FRCP • *Department of Neurological Science, Walton Center for Neurology and Neurosurgery, Liverpool, United Kingdom*

JAMES F. HOWARD, JR., MD • *Department of Neurology, School of Medicine, University of North Carolina at Chapel Hill, NC*

ALFRED JARETZKI III, MD • *Department of Surgery, Columbia Presbyterian Medical Center and Columbia University, New York, NY*

HENRY J. KAMINSKI, MD • *Departments of Neurology and Neurosciences, Case Western Reserve University; University Hospitals of Cleveland; Louis Stokes Cleveland Veterans Affairs Medical Center, Cleveland, OH*

BASHAR KATIRJI, MD, FACP • *Department of Neurology, University Hospitals of Cleveland and Case Western Reserve University, Cleveland, OH*

JAN B.M. KUKS, MD • *Department of Neurology, State University Groningen, The Netherlands*

VANDA A. LENNON, MD, PhD • *Departments of Neurology and Immunology, Mayo Clinic, Rochester, MN*

JON M. LINDSTROM, PhD • *Department of Neuroscience, Medical School of the University of Pennsylvania, Philadelphia, PA*

ALEXANDER MARX, MD • *Institute of Pathology, University of Würzburg, Germany*

MONICA MILANI • *Department of Neuromuscular Diseases, Neurological Institute "C. Besta", Milan, Italy*

SURAJ A. MULEY, MB, BS • *Department of Neurology, Minneapolis VA Medical Center and University of Minnesota, Minneapolis, MN*

HANS J.G.H OOSTERHUIS, MD • *Department of Neurology, State University, Groningen, The Netherlands*

NORMA OSTLIE, MS • *Department of Biochemistry, Molecular Biology, and Biophysics, University of Minnesota, St. Paul, MN*

ROBERT H. PAUL, PhD • *Department of Psychiatry and Human Behavior, Miriam Hospital; Brown University Medical School, Providence, RI*

DAVID P. RICHMAN, MD • *Department of Neurology, University of California, Davis, CA*

ROBERT L. RUFF, MD, PhD • *Neurology Service, Louis Stokes Cleveland Veterans Affairs Medical Center; Departments of Neurology and Neurosciences, Case Western Reserve University, Cleveland, OH*

PHILIPP STROEBEL, MD • *Institute of Pathology, University of Würzburg, Würzburg, Germany*

JOSE I. SUAREZ, MD • *Departments of Neurology and Neurosurgery, Case Western Reserve University; University Hospitals of Cleveland, Cleveland, OH*

ANGELA VINCENT, MB, FRCPath • *Institute of Molecular Medicine, John Radcliffe Hospital and Oxford University, Oxford, United Kingdom*

WEI WANG, MD • *Department of Biochemistry, Molecular Biology, and Biophysics, University of Minnesota, St. Paul, MN*

# 1

# Neuromuscular Junction Physiology and Pathophysiology

## Robert L. Ruff

## INTRODUCTION

The aim of this chapter is to increase the reader's understanding of five factors: 1) the structure of the neuromuscular junction; 2) the mechanism triggering release of vesicles of acetylcholine from the nerve terminal; 3) the two ion channels on the postsynaptic membrane ($Na^+$ channels and acetylcholine receptors) that are critical for converting the chemical signal from the nerve terminal into a propagated action potential on the muscle fiber; 4) the safety factor for neuromuscular transmission and characteristics of the neuromuscular junction that contribute to the safety factor; and 5) the mechanism by which disease compromises the safety factor, leading to neuromuscular transmission failure.

## MOTOR NERVE PROPERTIES

Skeletal muscle fibers are innervated by large motor neurons of the anterior horn of the spinal cord (1). Each anterior horn cell gives rise to a single large myelinated motor nerve fiber or axon. Action potentials travel along motor axons by saltatory conduction, a process by which action potentials jump from node of Ranvier to node of Ranvier, with little current leaving the axon in the internodal region. The structure of the axons optimizes saltatory conduction in two ways:

1. The internodal regions of the axons are covered by insulating layers of myelin produced by Schwann cells. The myelin reduces the current loss across the internodal region by increasing the effective transmembrane resistance and decreasing the capacitance between the axon and the extracellular space (2,3).
2. The nodes of Ranvier have high concentrations of sodium ($Na^+$) channels, which produce the depolarizing current of the action potential. Vertebrate nodes of Ranvier contain about 2000 channels/$\mu m^2$ (4). The high density of $Na^+$ channels reduces

From: *Current Clinical Neurology: Myasthenia Gravis and Related Disorders*
Edited by: H. J. Kaminski © Humana Press Inc., Totowa, NJ

the threshold for generating an action potential *(4,5)*. In addition, nodes of Ranvier have few potassium (K[+]) channels *(5)*. Since outward K[+] currents counter the depolarizing action of Na[+] currents, the paucity of K[+] channels at the nodes of Ranvier minimizes inhibition of the action potential and allows the action potential to propagate rapidly along the axon at rates >50 m/s *(2)*.

## DISTAL MOTOR NERVE PROPERTIES

The distal portion of each motor nerve fiber branches into 20–100 thinner fibers. Each distal motor nerve fiber innervates a single muscle fiber with one nerve terminal. The muscle fibers innervated by a single motor nerve axon are called the motor unit. The terminal motor nerve branches are up to 100 μm long and are unmyelinated *(3)*. The unmyelinated terminal motor nerve branches contain delayed rectifier and inward rectifier K[+] channels as well as Na[+] channels *(5,6)*. Therefore, the amplitude and duration of the action potential in the terminal nerve fibers are controlled by K[+] channels as well as by Na[+] channels. The nerve terminal has few if any Na[+] channels; hence the action potential propagates passively into the nerve terminal. The lack of nerve terminal Na[+] channels and the presence of K[+] channels prevent action potentials from reverberating among the distal nerve branches. Neuromyotonia, also called Isaac's syndrome, is a disorder of neuromuscular transmission in which a single action potential propagating down a motor nerve produces repeated action potentials in the nerve terminals *(7)*. In many instances, neuromyotonia results from autoantibodies that interfere with the functioning of nerve terminal delayed rectifier K[+] channels *(7)*. Neuromyotonia demonstrates that the nerve terminal delayed rectifier K[+] channels regulate nerve terminal membrane excitability *(8)*.

## THE NERVE TERMINAL

Acetylcholine (ACh) is stored in vesicles within the nerve terminal (**Figs. 1 and 2**) *(3,9)*. The ACh-containing vesicles are aligned near release sites (called active zones) in the nerve terminal, where the vesicles will fuse with the presynaptic nerve terminal membrane *(3)*. The release sites are positioned over the clefts between the tops of the secondary synaptic folds of the postsynaptic muscle membrane *(3,10,11)*. Transmitter release requires Ca[2+] influx. Although the Ca[2+] channels responsible for ACh release are of the P/Q type *(12)*, N-type calcium channels are probably also present on mammalian motor nerve terminals *(13–15)*. The Ca[2+] channels that trigger ACh release are distributed as two parallel double rows with approximately five channels per row, a spacing of about 20 nm between rows, and a spacing of about 60 nm between the double rows of channels at the active zone *(16,17)*. A

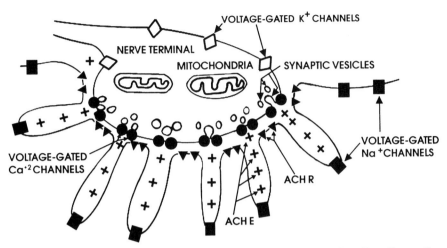

**Fig. 1.** Schematic representation of the neuromuscular junction. Details are discussed throughout the chapter.

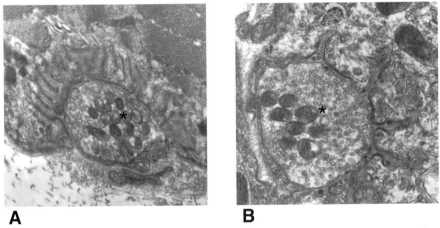

**A**   **B**

**Fig. 2.** Electron micrographs of (**A**) normal mouse diaphragm neuromuscular junction and (**B**) mouse diaphragm from a mouse with experimentally induced myasthenia gravis. The asterisks marks the nerve terminals. Note the small round structures in the nerve terminal, which are the synaptic vesicles. In B, there is a loss of synaptic folds, and within the synaptic cleft one can appreciate globular material, which probably represents degenerated junctional folds. (Courtesy of Dr. Henry Kaminski.)

high concentration of $Ca^{2+}$ channels at the active zones enables the $Ca^{2+}$ concentration to reach 100–1000 µM quickly in the nerve terminal regions where vesicle fusion occurs *(10,11)*. A normal nerve terminal action potential does not fully activate the nerve terminal $Ca^{2+}$ channels because the duration of the action potential is $\leq 1$ ms and the nerve terminal $Ca^{2+}$ channels are activated with a time constant of $\geq 1.3$ ms *(14)*. Increasing the duration of the nerve terminal action potential by blocking delayed rectifier potassium channels with tetraethylammonium (TEA) or 3,4-diaminopyridine (3,4-DAP) will increase calcium entry and increase ACh release *(14,18,19)*. In Lambert-Eaton syndrome (LES), antibodies directed against nerve terminal $Ca^{2+}$ channels reduce the $Ca^{2+}$ channel complement *(20–26)*. Neuromuscular transmission is impaired owing to a deficiency of vesicles released by the nerve terminal in response to an action potential. Treatment with 3,4-DAP improves neuromuscular transmission in LES by increasing the time that $Ca^{2+}$ channels are stimulated, resulting in increased $Ca^{2+}$ entry, which partially compensates for the deficiency of $Ca^{2+}$ channels *(27)*.

The approximation of synaptic vesicles and the presynaptic nerve terminal membrane may be opposed by electrostatic forces owing to the similar polarity of surface charges on the nerve terminal and vesicle membranes. $Ca^{2+}$ may bind to the membrane surfaces and neutralize the negative surface charges, thereby removing a restraint to membrane fusion *(28)*. Calcium may also open calcium-activated cationic channels, and the entry of cations may also reduce the negative surface charges on the synaptic vesicle and nerve terminal membranes *(29)*. Calcium also triggers conformation changes in large molecules that allow synaptic vesicles to detach from the cytoskeleton and that actively trigger membrane fusion *(30)*. Calcium entry may trigger phosphorylation of proteins including synaptotagmin *(31,32)*. Synexin and members of the synaptic vesicle-associated protein (SNAP) family of proteins are also modified by calcium *(33)*.

Synaptic vesicle fusion is a complex process that involves multiple proteins. The precise sequence of events leading to release of synaptic vesicle contents is not known. Prior to fusion the vesicles need to go through a process called docking, in which they are brought into proximity with the nerve terminal membrane. Next, the vesicles undergo priming, which makes them competent to respond to the calcium signal. Before docking occurs, syntaxin binds to munc18, and synaptobrevin binds to a synaptic vesicle protein, synaptophysin. The interaction of these proteins inhibits the formation of the docking complex. During docking, munc18 dissociates from the syntaxin and synaptophysin from synaptobrevin, allowing the synaptic core complex to form. Three proteins, two on the plasma membrane (syntaxin and SNAP 25) and one on the synaptic vesicle membrane (synaptobrevin) are thought to form a docking complex. *N*-ethylmaleimide-sensitive factor (NSF) and α-soluble NSF attachment protein (αSNAP) associate to form a fusion complex with the docking proteins. NSF, which is an ATPase, crosslinks multiple core complexes into a network, and ATP hydrolysis leads to hemifusion of the vesicle and presynaptic membranes. ATP hydrolysis appears to occur before calcium influx. Synaptotagmin probably acts as the calcium sensor.

How synaptotagmin serves to trigger the rapid discharge of synaptic vesicle contents is not known. The cytoplasmic portion of synaptotagmin includes two regions with high homology to the calcium- and phospholipid-binding domains of a protein kinase. Synaptotagmin probably binds phospholipid of the plasma membranes and syntaxin. Binding of calcium to synaptotagmin may alter interactions of synaptotagmin with membrane lipids and syntaxin transforming, allowing the membranes to fuse fully. Also, calcium may bind to the membrane surfaces and neutralize the negative surface charges, thereby removing a restraint to membrane fusion *(28)*. Exocytosis is somewhat inefficient in that only 1 in every 3–10 pulses of calcium leads to exocytosis, and only one of many docked vesicles fuses. After releasing its contents to the synaptic cleft, the synaptic vesicle membrane is recycled by a clathrin-mediated mechanism. After reuptake of the vesicles, the coated vesicles shed their coats and translocate into the interior. The synaptic vesicle membrane fuses with endosomes in the nerve terminal, and new vesicles bud from the endosome. The new vesicles accumulate ACh and other substances into the vesicles by active transport and translocate back to the active zone either by diffusion or by a cytoskeletal transport process. Several of the synaptic vesicle-associated proteins are targets for proteolytic cleavage by botulinum toxins.

## THE SYNAPTIC CLEFT

ACh diffuses across the synaptic cleft to activate ACh receptors (AChRs). Each synaptic vesicle fusion releases about 10,000 ACh molecules into the synaptic cleft *(34)*. ATP is also released by synaptic vesicle fusion, and the released ATP may modulate transmitter release of postsynaptic transmitter sensitivity *(35)*. An action potential propagating into the nerve terminal stimulates the fusion of 50–300 synaptic vesicles (i.e., the normal quantal content is between 50 and 300) *(36)*. Diffusion of ACh across the synaptic cleft is very rapid owing to the small distance to be traversed and the relatively high diffusion constant for ACh *(37)*. Acetylcholineesterase (AChE) in the basil lamina of the postsynaptic membrane accelerates the decline in concentration of ACh in the synaptic cleft, as does diffusion of ACh out of the cleft *(38)*. Inactivation of AChE prolongs the duration of action of ACh on the postsynaptic membrane and slows the decay of the ACh-induced endplate current *(39)*. The concentration of AChE is approximately 3000 molecules/

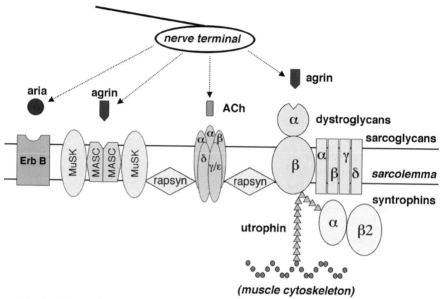

**Fig. 3.** Schematic representation of postsynaptic region of the neuromuscular junction. ACh = acetylcholine; aria = acetylcholine receptor-inducing activity; MASC = myotube-associated specificity component; MuSK = muscle-specific kinase.

$\mu m^2$ of postsynaptic membrane *(38)*, which is about five- to eightfold lower than the concentration of AChRs *(40)*. The concentration of AChE in the secondary synaptic folds is sufficiently high that most of the ACh entering a synaptic cleft is hydrolyzed. Consequently, the secondary synaptic folds act like sinks that terminate the action of ACh and prevent AChRs from being activated more than once in response to released ACh *(41)*. The space between the nerve terminal and the postsynaptic membrane is about 50 nm *(3)*.

The extracellular matrix in the neuromuscular junction is a complex collection of proteins that regulate the synthesis of postsynaptic proteins as well as the concentration of ACh. The endplate basement membrane is enriched with collagen IV ($\alpha$2-, $\alpha$4-, and $\alpha$5-chains) and contains several forms of laminin (laminin-4, laminin-9, and laminin-11), all of which bind to $\alpha$-dystroglycan in the endplate membrane (**Fig. 3**). Laminin-4 also binds to integrin. The laminin family of proteins forms a complex network in the synaptic space that anchors other extracellular matrix proteins including agrin, perlecan, and entactin. The collagen-tailed form of AChE in the synapse binds to perlecan, which in turn can bind to $\alpha$-dystroglycan. In addition to binding laminin and perlecan, $\alpha$-dystroglycan also binds agrin, integrin, and the myotube-associated specificity component/muscle-specific kinase (MASC/MUSK) complex. Agrin, MASC, and MuSK are associated with the formation and maintenance of AChR clustering *(30,42,43)*. Rapsyn is the molecule that specifically links AChRs *(44)*. The high synthesis of AChR component subunits at the neuromuscular junction is owing in part to AChR-inducing activity (ARIA), a molecule that is released by the nerve terminal. ARIAs activate ErbB receptor tyrosine kinases in the postsynaptic membrane. The ErbB receptors regulate the expression of AChR subunits by the subsynaptic nuclei. Acetylcholine binding protein (AChBP) is a recently described globular protein secreted by the specific subset of oligodendroglia and Schwann cells located around nerve terminals *(45)*. Production of AChBPs is regulated by synaptic activity and by binding ACh; AChBP may reduce the effective concentration of ACh in the synaptic cleft.

## POSTSYNAPTIC MEMBRANE SPECIALIZATION

The postsynaptic membrane area is increased by folding into secondary synaptic clefts or folds. AChRs are concentrated at the tops of the secondary synaptic folds *(46)*. The AChRs are concentrated at the tops of the secondary synaptic folds and firmly anchored to the dystrophin-related protein complex through rapsyn (**Fig. 3**) *(44,46)*. Rapsyn is important in clustering AChRs at the endplate during synaptogenesis, and rapsyn-deficient transgenic mice do not cluster AChRs, utrophin, and other dystrophin-related complex proteins *(46–49)*. Clusters of AChRs are connected to the cytoskeleton via associations with dystroglycan and sarcoglycan protein complexes *(30,42)*. The dystroglycan and sarcoglycan complexes connect to utrophin, which in turn connects to cytoskeleton by binding to actin (**Fig. 3**). Utrophin and dystrobrevin also connect to $\beta$1-syntrophin and $\beta$2-syntrophin, which in turn associates with nitric oxide synthase *(50,51)*, which produces the free radical gas nitric oxide that participates in signaling of many cellular processes. The presence of nitric oxide synthase at the neuromuscular junction suggests that nitric oxide could diffuse from its site of synthesis to affect target proteins in the nerve and muscle. $Na^+$ channels are concentrated in the depths of the secondary synaptic clefts (**Fig. 1**) *(46,52–57)*. Both the $Na^+$ channels and AChRs are rigidly located in the endplate membrane. $Na^+$ channels are locked in the membrane by their associations with ankyrin, the sarcoglycan complex, the dystroglycan complex, dystrobrevins, and dystrophin/utrophin.

Given the complex molecular composition of the nerve terminal, the extracellular matrix, and the endplate membrane and the precise alignment of the active zones on the nerve terminal with the clefts between the endplate synaptic folds, how does the neuromuscular junction accommodate to muscle fiber stretching and contracting? Surprisingly, the high efficiency of neuromuscular transmission is maintained during muscle stretch and contraction. The safety factor for neuromuscular transmission does not change for muscles at different lengths from 80 to 125% of the resting length *(58)*. The constancy of neuromuscular transmission is accomplished by the neuromuscular junction remaining rigid so that the endplate membrane does not deform when the muscle fiber changes length. The change in muscle fiber length is accomplished by folding and unfolding of the extrajunctional membrane while the endplate region remains rigid. The extreme stiffness of the endplate membrane adds mechanical and electrical stability to the neuromuscular junction, which enables the active zones on the nerve terminal to remain precisely aligned with the clefts of the synaptic folds and the safety factor for neuromuscular transmission to remain constant during muscle activity.

The concentration of AChRs at the endplate is about 15,000–20,000 receptors/$\mu m^2$ *(40)*. Away from the endplate, the concentration of AChRs is about 1000-fold lower, with a slight increase in AChR density at the tendon ends of the muscle fibers *(59)*. The relatively high concentration of AChRs at the endplate in part results because the muscle nuclei near the endplate preferentially express genes of the AChR subunits *(47,49)*. AChRs continually turn over, with old receptors internalized and degraded. The removed receptors are replaced with new receptors. The AChRs are not recycled. Early in development of skeletal muscle, the half-life of AChRs is short, about 13–24 h *(60)*. At a mature endplate, the half-life of AChRs is about 8–11 days. Crosslinking of receptors by AChR autoantibodies dramatically shortens AChR half-life by accelerating internalization of the receptors *(61,62)*. The AChRs are firmly anchored to the cytoskeleton *(46–49)*. $Na^+$ channels are also concentrated in the endplate region *(46,52–57)*. The increased density of $Na^+$ channels raises the safety factor for neuromuscular transmission *(54–57,63–65)*. In addition, a higher concentration of $Na^+$ channels may be needed because at the endplate two action potentials must be generated, one traveling toward each tendon end of the muscle fiber. The density of $Na^+$ channels varies with fiber type *(55–57)*. Fast twitch fibers have about 500–550 $Na^+$ channels/$\mu m^2$ on the endplate membrane, and slow twitch fibers have about 100–150 $Na^+$ channels/$\mu m^2$. In acquired autoimmune myasthenia gravis, antibodies directed at AChRs attack the endplate membrane. The antibodies fix complement, resulting in loss of endplate membrane. $Na^+$ channels as well as AChRs are lost from the endplate in myasthenia gravis, and the loss of endplate $Na^+$ channels reduces the safety factor for neuromuscular transmission *(65)*.

The size of the depolarization of the endplate membrane produced by a single motor nerve action potential (endplate potential) is determined by the product of the number of vesicles (or quanta) of ACh released (quantal content) and size of the endplate depolarization to a single vesicle (quantal size), with an adjustment for the AChR reversal potential *(2)*. Diseases that interfere with ACh release (such as LES) reduce the quantal content. Conditions that reduce the sensitivity of the postsynaptic membrane to ACh such myasthenia gravis reduce quantal size.

## SAFETY FACTOR
## FOR NEUROMUSCULAR TRANSMISSION

The safety factor *(SF)* for neuromuscular transmission can be defined as:

$$SF = \frac{EPP}{E_{AP} - E_M}$$

where EPP is the endplate potential amplitude, $E_M$ is the membrane potential, and $E_{AP}$ is the threshold potential for initiating an action potential *(66)*. Several factors contribute to increase the safety factor for neuromuscular transmission of fast-compared with slow-twitch mammalian skeletal muscle fibers *(67)*. The nerve terminal morphology and transmitter release properties of axons innervating fast- and slow-twitch fibers are different. The quantal contents of synapses on rodent fast-twitch fibers are larger than for slow-twitch fibers *(67,68)*. The postsynaptic sensitivities of fast-twitch fibers are also greater than those in slow-twitch fibers. Endplates on fast-twitch fibers depolarize more in response to quantitative iontophoresis of ACh *(69)*. Fast-twitch endplates have a higher concentration of $Na^+$ channels compared with slow-twitch endplates *(54–57,64,65)*. The increased $Na^+$ current on fast-twitch fibers may be also needed because fast-twitch fibers require larger depolarizations to initiate contraction compared with slow-twitch fibers *(70)*. The differences in synaptic transmission for fast- and slow-twitch fibers may be in response to the different functional properties of fast- and slow-twitch motor units. Slow-twitch motor units in mammals in vivo are tonically active at slow rates, whereas fast-twitch motor units are phasically active at high rates *(71)*. Under these conditions, transmitter depletion and other factors may not appreciably compromise neuromuscular transmission for slow-twitch fibers, whereas fast-twitch fibers may suffer from reduction in the endplate potential amplitude *(67,72–74)*. The effective safety factor for slow-twitch motor units from rat soleus muscle at a steady state firing rate of 10 Hz is about 1.8 *(67)*. The safety factor for neuromuscular transmission for fibers from the fast-twitch rat extensor digitorum longus muscle stimulated at 40 Hz drops from 3.7 for the first stimulation to 2.0 after 200 stimuli *(67)*. Differences in safety factor among muscles may contribute to the varied clinical manifestations

observed among patients with neuromuscular transmission disorders. The
compromise of safety factor underlies all neuromuscular transmission disorders, which are detailed in this text.

## REFERENCES

1. Burke RE. The structure and function of motor units. In: Karpati G, Hilton-Jones
   D, Griggs RC, eds. *Disorders of Voluntary Muscle*, 7th ed. Cambridge, Cambridge
   University Press, 2001, pp. 3–25.
2. Ruff RL. Ionic channels II. Voltage- and agonist-gated and agonist-modified channel properties and structure. *Muscle Nerve* 1986;9:767–786.
3. Salpeter MM. *The Vertebrate Neuromuscular Junction*. New York, Alan R. Liss,
   1987, pp. 1–439.
4. Ruff RL. Ionic channels: I. The biophysical basis for ion passage and channel gating. *Muscle Nerve* 1986;9:675–699.
5. Black JA, Kocsis JD, Waxman SG. Ion channel organization of the myelinated
   fiber. *Trends Neurosci* 1990;13:48–54.
6. Reid G, Scholz A, Bostock H, Vogel W. Human axons contain at least five types of
   voltage-dependent potassium channel. *J Physiol* 1999;518:681–696.
7. Shillito P, Molenaar PC, Vincent A, et al. Acquired neuromyotonia: evidence for
   autoantibodies directed against K+ channels of peripheral nerves. *Ann Neurol* 1995;
   38:714–722.
8. Nagado T, Arimura K, Sonoda Y, et al. Potassium current suppression in patients
   with peripheral nerve hyperexcitability. *Brain* 1999;122:2057–2066.
9. Katz B. *Nerve, Muscle and Synapse*. New York, McGraw-Hill, 1966.
10. Augustine GJ, Adler EM, Charlton MP. The calcium signal for transmitter secre-
    tion from presynaptic nerve terminals. *Ann NY Acad Sci* 1991;635:365–381.
11. Smith SJ, Augustine GJ. Calcium ions, active zones and synaptic transmitter release.
    *Trends Neurosci* 1988;10:458–464.
12. Protti DA, Sanchez VA, Cherksey BD, et al. Mammalian neuromuscular transmis-
    sion blocked by funnel web toxin. *Ann NY Acad Sci* 1993;681:405–407.
13. Catterall WA, De Jongh K, Rotman E, et al. Molecular properties of calcium chan-
    nels in skeletal muscle and neurons. *Ann NY Acad Sci* 1993;681:342–355.
14. Stanley EF. Presynaptic calcium channels and the transmitter release mechanism.
    *Ann NY Acad Sci* 1993;681:368–372.
15. Wray D, Porter V. Calcium channel types at the neuromuscular junction. *Ann NY
    Acad Sci* 1993;681:356–367.
16. Engel AG. Review of evidence for loss of motor nerve terminal calcium channels
    in Lambert-Eaton myasthenic syndrome. *Ann NY Acad Sci* 1991;635:246–258.
17. Pumplin DW, Reese TS, Llinas R. Are the presynaptic membrane particles calcium
    channels? *Proc Natl Acad Sci USA* 1981;78:7210–7213.
18. Lindgren CA, Moore JW. Calcium current in motor nerve endings of the lizard.
    *Ann NY Acad Sci* 1991;635:58–69.
19. Stanley EF, Cox C. Calcium channels in the presynaptic nerve terminal of the chick
    ciliary ganglion giant synapse. *Ann NY Acad Sci* 1991;635:70–79.
20. Leys K, Lang B, Johnston I, Newsom-Davis J. Calcium channel autoantibodies in
    the Lambert-Eaton myasthenic syndrome. *Ann Neurol* 1991;29:307–414.

21. Lambert EH, Eaton LM, Rooke ED. Defect of neuromuscular transmission associated with malignant neoplasm. *Am J Physiol* 1956;187:612–613.
22. Motomura M, Johnston I, Lang B, Vincent A, Newsom-Davis J. An improved diagnostic assay for Lambert-Eaton myasthenic syndrome. *J Neurol Neurosurg Psychiatry* 1995;58:85–87.
23. Nagel A, Engel AG, Lang B, Newsom-Davis J, Fukuoka T. Lambert-Eaton syndrome IgG depletes presynaptic membrane active zone particles by antigenic modulation. *Ann Neurol* 1988;24:552–558.
24. Lang B, Johnston I, Leys K, et al. Autoantibody specificities in Lambert-Eaton myasthenic syndrome. *Ann NY Acad Sci* 1993;681:382–391.
25. Viglione MP, Blandino JKW, Kim YI. Effects of Lambert-Eaton syndrome serum and IgG on calcium and sodium currents in small-cell lung cancer cells. *Ann NY Acad Sci* 1993;681:418–421.
26. Rosenfeld MR, Wong E, Dalmau J, et al. Sera from patients with Lambert-Eaton myasthenic syndrome recognize the $\beta$-subunit of $Ca^{2+}$ channel complexes. *Ann NY Acad Sci* 1993;681:408–411.
27. McEvoy KM, Windebank AJ, Daube JR, Low PA. 3,4-Diaminopyridine in the treatment of Lambert-Eaton myasthenic syndrome. *N Engl J Med* 1989;321:1567–1571.
28. Niles WD, Cohen FS. Video-microscopy studies of vesicle-planar membrane adhesion and fusion. *Ann NY Acad Sci* 1991;635:273–306.
29. Ehrenstein G, Stanley EF, Pocotte SL, et al. Evidence of a model of exocytosis that involves calcium-activated channels. *Ann NY Acad Sci* 1991;635:297–306.
30. Vincent A. The neuromuscular junction and neuromuscular transmission. In: Karpati G, Hilton-Jones D, Griggs RC, eds. *Disorders of Voluntary Muscle*, 7th ed. Cambridge, Cambridge University Press, 2001, pp. 142–167.
31. Perin MS, Fried VA, Mignery G, Jahn R, Südhof TC. Phospholipid binding by a synaptic vesicle protein homologous to the regulatory region of protein kinase C. *Nature* 1990;345:260–263.
32. Perin MS, Brose N, Jahn R, Südhof TC. Domain structure of synaptotagmin (p65). *J Biol Chem* 1991;266:623–629.
33. Zimmerberg J, Curran M, Cohen FS. A lipid/protein complex hypothesis for exocytotic fusion pore formation. *Ann NY Acad Sci* 1991;681:307–317.
34. Miledi R, Molenaar PC, Polak RL. Electrophysiological and chemical determination of acetylcholine release at the frog neuromuscular junction. *J Physiol (Lond)* 1983;334:245–254.
35. Etcheberrigaray R, Fielder JL, Pollard HB, Rojas E. Endoplasmic reticulum as a source of $Ca^{2+}$ in neurotransmitter secretion. *Ann NY Acad Sci* 1991;635:90–99.
36. Katz B, Miledi R. Estimates of quantal content during chemical potentiation of transmitter release. *Proc R Soc Lond* 1979;205:369–378.
37. Land BR, Harris WV, Salpeter EE, Salpeter MM. Diffusion and binding constants for acetylcholine derived from the falling phase of miniature endplate currents. *Proc Natl Acad Sci USA* 1984;81:1594–1598.
38. McMahan UJ, Sanes JR, Marshall LM. Cholinesterase is associated with the basal lamina at the neuromuscular junction. *Nature* 1978;271:172–174.
39. Katz B, Miledi R. The binding of acetylcholine to receptors and its removal from the synaptic cleft. *J Physiol (Lond)* 1973;231:549–574.
40. Land BR, Salpeter EE, Salpeter MM. Kinetic parameters for acetylcholine interaction in intact neuromuscular junction. *Proc Natl Acad Sci USA* 1981;78:7200–7204.

41. Colquhoun D, Sakmann B. Fast events in single-channel currents activated by ace-tylcholine and its analogues at the frog muscle end-plate. *J Physiol (Lond)* 1985; 369:501–557.

42. Holland PC, Carbonetto S. The extracellular matrix of skeletal muscle. In: Karpati G, Hilton-Jones D, Griggs RC, eds. *Disorders of Voluntary Muscle*, 7th ed. Cambridge, Cambridge University Press, 2001, pp. 103–121.

43. Gautam M, Noakes PG, Moscoso L. Defective neuromuscular synaptogenesis in agrin-deficient mutant mice. *Cell* 1996;85:525–535.

44. Gautam M, Noakes PG, Mudd J. Failure of postsynaptic specialization to neuro-muscular junctions of rapsyn-deficient mice. *Nature* 1995;377:232–236.

45. Smit AB, Syed NI, Schaap D, et al. A glia-derived acetylcholine-binding protein that modulates synaptic transmission. *Nature* 2001;411:261–267.

46. Flucher BE, Daniels MP. Distribution of Na+ channels and ankyrin in neuromus-cular junctions is complementary to that of acetylcholine receptors and the 43 kD protein. *Neuron* 1989;3:163–175.

47. Sanes JR, Johnson YR, Kotzbauer PT, et al. Selective expression of an acetylcho-line receptor-lacZ transgene in synaptic nuclei of adult muscle fibers. *Development* 1991;113:1181–1191.

48. Martinou JC, Falls DI, Fischback GD, Merlie JP. Acetylcholine receptor-inducing activity stimulates expression of the epsilon-subunit gene of the muscle acetylcho-line receptor. *Proc Natl Acad Sci USA* 1991;88:7669–7673.

49. Merlie JP, Sanes JR. Concentration of acetylcholine receptor mRNA in synaptic regions of adult muscle fibers. *Nature* 1985;317:66–68.

50. Brenman JE, Chao DS, Gee SH, et al. Interaction of nitric oxide synthase with the postsynaptic protein PSD-95 and $\alpha$1-synthophin mediated by PDZ domains. *Cell* 1996;84:757–767.

51. Kusner LL, Kaminski HJ. Nitric oxide synthase is concentrated at the skeletal mus-cle endplate. *Brain Res* 1996;730:238–242.

52. Haimovich B, Schotland DL, Fieles WE, Barchi RL. Localization of sodium chan-nel subtypes in rat skeletal muscle using channel-specific monoclonal antibodies. *J Neurosci* 1987;7:2957–2966.

53. Roberts WM. Sodium channels near end-plates and nuclei of snake skeletal muscle. *J Physiol (Lond)* 1987;388:213–232.

54. Ruff RL. Na current density at and away from end plates on rat fast- and slow-twitch skeletal muscle fibers. *Am J Physiol* 1992;262:C229–C234.

55. Ruff RL, Whittlesey D. Na$^+$ current densities and voltage dependence in human intercostal muscle fibres. *J Physiol (Lond)* 1992;458:85–97.

56. Ruff RL, Whittlesey D. Na$^+$ currents near and away from endplates on human fast and slow twitch muscle fibers. *Muscle Nerve* 1993;16:922–929.

57. Ruff RL, Whittlesey D. Comparison of Na$^+$ currents from type IIa and IIb human intercostal muscle fibers. *Am J Physiol* 1993;265:C171–C177.

58. Ruff RL. Effects of length changes on Na$^+$ current amplitude and excitability near and far from the end-plate. *Muscle Nerve* 1996;19:1084–1092.

59. Kuffler SW, Yoshikami D. The distribution of acetylcholine sensitivity at the post-synaptic membrane of vertebrate skeletal twitch muscles: iontophoretic mapping in the micron range. *J Physiol (Lond)* 1975;244:703–730.

60. Salpeter MM, Loring RH. Nicotinic acetylcholine receptors in vertebrate muscle: properties, distribution and neural control. *Prog Neurobiol* 1985;25:297–325.

61. Kao I, Drachman D. Myasthenic immunoglobulin accelerates acetylcholine receptor degradation. *Science* 1977;196:526–528.
62. Merlie JP, Heinemann S, Lindstrom JM. Acetylcholine receptor degradation in adult rat diaphragms in organ culture and the effect of anti-acetylcholine receptor antibodies. *J Biol Chem* 1979;254:6320–6327.
63. Caldwell JH, Campbell DT, Beam KG. Sodium channel distribution in vertebrate skeletal muscle. *J Gen Physiol* 1986;87:907–932.
64. Milton RL, Lupa MT, Caldwell JH. Fast and slow twitch skeletal muscle fibres differ in their distributions of Na channels near the endplate. *Neurosci Lett* 1992;135:41–44.
65. Ruff RL, Lennon VA. Endplate voltage-gated sodium channels are lost in clinical and experimental myasthenia gravis. *Ann Neurol* 1998;43:370–379.
66. Banker BQ, Kelly SS, Robbins N. Neuromuscular transmission and correlative morphology in young and old mice. *J Physiol (Lond)* 1983;339:355–375.
67. Gertler RA, Robbins N. Differences in neuromuscular transmission in red and white muscles. *Brain Res* 1978;142:255–284.
68. Tonge DA. Chronic effects of botulinum toxin on neuromuscular transmission and sensitivity to acetylcholine in slow and fast skeletal muscle of the mouse. *J Physiol (Lond)* 1974;241:127–139.
69. Sterz R, Pagala M, Peper K. Postjunctional characteristics of the endplates in mammalian fast and slow muscles. *Pflugers Arch* 1983;398:48–54.
70. Laszewski B, Ruff RL. The effects of glucocorticoid treatment on excitation-contraction coupling. *Am J Physiol* 1985;248:E363–E369.
71. Hennig R, Lømo T. Firing patterns of motor units in normal rats. *Nature* 1985;314:164–166.
72. Kelly SS, Robbins N. Sustained transmitter output by increased transmitter turnover in limb muscles of old mice. *J Neurosci* 1986;6:2900–2907.
73. Lev-Tov A. Junctional transmission in fast- and slow-twitch mammalian muscle units. *J Neurophysiol* 1987;57:660–671.
74. Lev-Tov A, Fishman R. The modulation of transmitter release in motor nerve endings varies with the type of muscle fiber innervated. *Brain Res* 1986;363:379–382.

# 2

# Acetylcholine Receptor Structure

## Jon M. Lindstrom

## INTRODUCTION

Nicotinic acetylcholine receptors (AChRs) are acetylcholine-gated cation channels. They play a critical postsynaptic role in transmission between motor nerves and skeletal muscles and in autonomic ganglia *(1,2)*. In the central nervous system, they also act presynaptically and extrasynaptically to modulate transmission by facilitating the release of many transmitters *(3,4)*. In the skin *(5)*, bronchial and vascular epithelia *(6,7)*, and other nonneuronal tissues *(8)*, they also mediate intercellular communication.

Abnormalities of AChRs are responsible for several human diseases. Mutations in AChRs are known to cause congenital myasthenic syndromes *(9)* and the rare autosomal dominant nocturnal frontal lobe form of epilepsy (ADNFLE) *(10–12)*. Autoimmune responses to AChRs are known to cause myasthenia gravis (MG) *(13)*, certain dysautonomias *(14)*, and some forms of pemphigus *(15)*. Nicotine acting on AChRs in the brain causes addiction to tobacco *(16,17)*. This is by far the largest medical problem in which AChRs play a direct role, and the largest preventable cause of disease, accounting for 430,000 premature deaths annually in the United States *(18)*.

Nicotine acting through AChRs has many physiologic effects, including beneficial ones such as inducing vascularization, neuroprotection, cognitive enhancement, anxiolysis, and antinociception. Thus, nicotinic agents are lead compounds for the development of drugs to treat many diseases including Alzheimer's disease, Parkinson's disease, chronic pain, and Tourette's syndrome *(19,20)*.

There are many known and potential subtypes of AChRs, each defined by the subunits that compose them *(1)*. All AChRs are formed by five homologous subunits organized around a central cation channel. There are 17 known AChR subunits: $\alpha 1$–10, $\beta 1$–4, $\gamma$, $\delta$, and $\epsilon$. In contrast to the many subtypes of neuronal AChRs, there are only two subtypes of muscle AChRs. These are a fetal subtype with an $(\alpha 1)_2 \beta 1 \gamma \delta$ stoichiometry and an adult subtype with an $(\alpha 1)_2 \beta 1 \epsilon \delta$ stoichiometry.

From: *Current Clinical Neurology: Myasthenia Gravis and Related Disorders*
Edited by: H. J. Kaminski © Humana Press Inc., Totowa, NJ

AChRs are part of a gene superfamily that includes the genes for subunits of ionotropic receptors for glycine, γ-aminobutyric acid (GABA), and serotonin *(21)*. The structural homologies of all of these receptors, and the sorts of evolutionary steps that produced this diversity of receptors, have been elegantly illustrated by experiments. One showed that changing only three amino acids in the channel lining part of an AChR subunit to amino acids found in receptors for GABA or glycine receptors resulted in AChRs with anion-selective channels like those of GABA or glycine receptors *(22)*. Another experiment showed that a chimera of the extracellular domain of an AChR subunit and the remainder of a serotonin receptor subunit produced an ACh-gated cation channel with the conductance properties of a serotonin receptor *(23)*.

Muscle AChRs are the best characterized of the AChRs *(21)*. The presence of a single type of synapse in skeletal muscle (with the exception of extraocular muscle; *see* Chap. 5) facilitated studies of AChR synthesis, developmental plasticity, and electrophysiologic function *(24–26)*. The presence of large amounts of muscle-like AChR in the electric organs of *Torpedo* species permitted the purification and characterization of AChRs, partial sequencing of their subunit proteins, cloning of the subunit cDNAs, and low-resolution electron crystallographic determination of their three-dimensional structure *(21,24,27,28)*. Low-stringency hybridization, starting with cDNAs for muscle AChR subunits, led to the cloning of subunits for neuronal AChRs *(24)*. Immunization with purified electric organ AChRs led to the discovery of experimental autoimmune myasthenia gravis (EAMG), the autoimmune nature of MG, and an immunodiagnostic assay for MG *(13,29)*. Monoclonal antibodies initially developed as model autoantibodies led not only to the discovery of the main immunogenic region (MIR) on α1-subunits and the molecular basis of the autoimmune impairment of neuromuscular transmission in MG *(13,30,31)*, but also to the immunoaffinity purification of neuronal nicotinic AChRs. mAbs have continued to provide useful tools for characterizing AChRs *(1)*.

This chapter reviews the basic structures of muscle and neuronal AChRs. It describes the antigenic structure of muscle AChRs and considers how this accounts for the pathologic mechanisms by which neuromuscular transmission is impaired in MG. This is briefly contrasted with the antigenic structure of a neuronal AChR involved in autoimmune dysautonomia. This chapter also considers the optimized functional structure of muscle AChRs, and how mutations impair AChR function in congenital myasthenic syndromes. The many AChR mutations identified in all the muscle AChR subunits in myasthenic syndromes is contrasted with the few disease-causing mutations discovered thus far in neuronal AChR subunits.

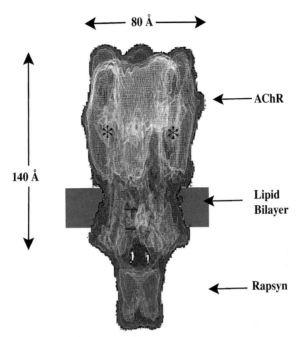

**Fig. 1.** *Torpedo* electric organ acetylcholine receptor (AChR) structure at 4.6 Å resolution determined by electron crystallography. The large extracellular domain contrasts with the smaller domain on the cytoplasmic surface. Rapsyn is a 43,000-dalton peripheral membrane protein through which muscle AChRs are linked to actin in the cytoskeleton to concentrate them at the tips of folds in the postsynaptic membrane adjacent to active zones in the presynaptic membrane at which ACh is released *(39)*. Proteins analogous to rapsyn may interact with neuronal AChRs, but have not yet been identified. (Modified with permission from Unwin N. Nicotinic acetylcholine receptor and the structural basis of fast synaptic transmission. *Philos Trans R Soc Lond B* 2000;1404:1813–1829.)

## SIZE AND SHAPE OF AChRs

Electron crystallography of two-dimensional helical crystalline arrays of AChRs in fragments of *Torpedo* electric organ membranes have revealed the basic size and shape of this muscle-type AChR to a resolution of 4.6 Å, as shown in **Fig. 1** *(28)*. Viewed from the side, a *Torpedo* AChR is roughly cylindrical, about 140 Å long and 80 Å wide. About 65 Å extend on the extracellular surface, 40 Å cross the lipid bilayer, and 35 Å extend below. Viewed from the top, the extracellular vestibule is a pentagonal tube with walls about 25 Å thick and a central pore about 20 Å in diameter. The channel across the membrane narrows to a close. Other evidence suggests that the open lumen of the channel becomes narrow (perhaps 7 Å across), sufficient only for rapid flow of hydrated cations like $Na^+$ or $K^+$. The five subunits are rod-like, oriented like barrel staves at a 10° angle around the central channel.

X-ray crystallography of a molluscan glial ACh binding protein recently revealed the structure of the extracellular domain of an AChR-like protein at atomic resolution *(32,33)*. Snail glia were found to release a water-soluble protein that modulated transmission by binding ACh. The cloned protein showed 24% sequence identity with the extracellular domain of human α7. α7 AChR subunits form homomeric AChRs. The extracellular domain cleaved by protein engineering from α7 assembles into water-soluble pentamers with the ligand binding properties of native α7 AChRs, but it does so very inefficiently *(34)*. Thus, the molluscan ACh binding protein probably contains sequence adaptations for efficient assembly and secretion as a water-soluble protein. Nonetheless, it is thought to provide a very good model for the basic structure of the extracellular domains of AChRs and other receptors in their superfamily. **Figure 2** shows that five ACh binding protein subunits assemble as the extracellular domains of AChR subunits would around the vestibule of the channel. A buffer component was found to occupy what was expected to be the ACh binding site, which is formed at the interface between subunits halfway up the side of the assembled protein. All the contact amino acids for this site corresponded to ones in AChRs that had been identified by affinity labeling or mutagenesis studies *(21,27,35)*. This and other features of the structure will be discussed in more detail in subsequent sections. Basically, most recognizable features were found about where they were expected to be from studies of native AChRs, providing confidence that the structure of the ACh binding protein has significant relevance to that of AChRs.

---

**Fig. 2.** Mollusc ACh binding protein structure at 2.7 Å resolution determined by X-ray crystallography. Atomic resolution structure of the ACh binding protein reveals the basic structure of AChR extracellular domains. It is a 62-Å-high cylinder that is 80 Å in diameter with an 18-Å diameter central hole. The structure is a homopentamer like α7 AChRs. There are five ACh binding sites at subunit interfaces, rather than the two ACh binding sites expected in a muscle AChR heteropentamer at interfaces between α1 and δ-, γ-, or ε-subunits. The ACh binding site is occupied by the buffer component $N$-2-hydroxyethylpiperazine-N'-2 ethanesulphonic acid (HEPES). The adjacent disulfide-linked cysteine pair corresponding to α1 192–193, which is characteristic of all AChR α-subunits, is on a projection of what can be defined as the "+" side of the subunit. It intercalates with the "−" side of the adjacent subunit to form the ACh binding site. As expected from studies of AChRs *(13,87)*, the sequence corresponding to the MIR of α1-subunits is located at the extracellular tip and oriented out away from the central axis of the subunit. The loop linked by a disul-

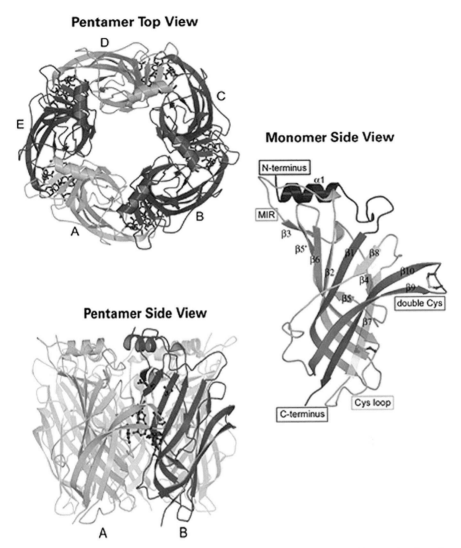

**Pentamer Top View**

**Monomer Side View**

**Pentamer Side View**

fide bond corresponding to that between cysteines 128 and 142 of α1-subunits, the signature loop characteristic of all subunits of the gene superfamily of which AChRs are a member, is located in the ACh binding protein at the base, near what would be the transmembrane portion of an AChR or the lipid bilayer. This loop sequence shows little homology with that of AChRs, especially at amino acids critical to subunit assembly, and is more hydrophilic than the sequences characteristic of AChRs. Thus, it may contain adaptations required for efficient assembly and water solubility of the binding protein, which give this loop a somewhat different structure or orientation than it would have in AChR subunits. (Modified with permission from Brejc K, van Dijk WJ, Klaassen, et al. Crystal structure of an ACh-binding protein reveals the ligand-binding domain of nicotinic receptors. *Nature* 2001;411:269–276.)

## STRUCTURES OF AChR SUBUNITS

All AChR subunits share several features *(1)*. **Figure 3** shows (diagrammatically) the transmembrane orientation of the mature polypeptide chain of a generic AChR subunit. To produce the mature polypeptide sequence, a signal sequence of about 20 amino acids is removed from the N-terminus of each subunit during translation as the N-terminal domain crosses the membrane into the lumen of the endoplasmic reticulum.

The large N-terminal extracellular domain of each subunit consists of about 210 amino acids containing a disulfide-linked loop that is characteristic of all receptors in this superfamily. In α1-subunits, it extends from cysteine 128 to cysteine 142. This sequence is among the most conserved of all AChR subunit sequences. In the ACh binding protein (**Fig. 2**), this loop is located near what would be the lipid bilayer or extracellular surface of the transmembrane regions *(33)*. Its conformation or orientation may differ

---

**Fig. 3.** Aspects of AChR structure. The transmembrane orientation of a generic AChR subunit is depicted in this diagram. The actual structure of the large extracellular domain of the ACh binding protein shown in **Fig. 2** provides a more detailed model for the extracellular domain. The transmembrane domains M1–4 are depicted as largely α-helical. The overall shape of the subunit is depicted as rod-like. Five of these rods assemble in a pentagonal array to form the AChR shown in **Fig. 1**. The subunits are organized around the ion channel so that the amphipathic M2 transmembrane domain from each subunit contributes to the lining of the channel. In muscle AChRs (e.g., with the subunit arrangement α1γα1δε), and in other heteromeric AChRs (e.g., with the subunit arrangement α4β2α4β2β2), there are only two ACh binding sites at interfaces between the + side of α subunits and complementary subunits, but small concerted conformation changes of all subunits are involved in activation and desensitization *(28,37)*. Thus, all subunits contribute to the conductance and gating of the channel, even if they are not part of an ACh binding site. The amino acids lining the ACh binding site have been identified by affinity labeling and mutagenesis studies *(21,35)* and have been found to correspond well to those identified in the crystal structure of the ACh binding protein *(33)*. Note the predominance of aromatic amino acids in this region. As in ACh esterase *(70)*, the quaternary amine group of ACh is thought to be bound through interactions with π electrons of these aromatic amino acids rather than ionic interactions with acidic amino acids. Note also that the ACh binding site is formed from amino acids from three different parts of the extracellular domain of the α-subunit interacting with three parts of the complementary subunit and that the interaction is at the interface between the + side and the α-subunit and the − side of the complementary subunit. Thus, the site is ideally positioned to trigger small concerted conformation changes between subunits, perhaps involving slight tilts in their orientation, thereby permit-

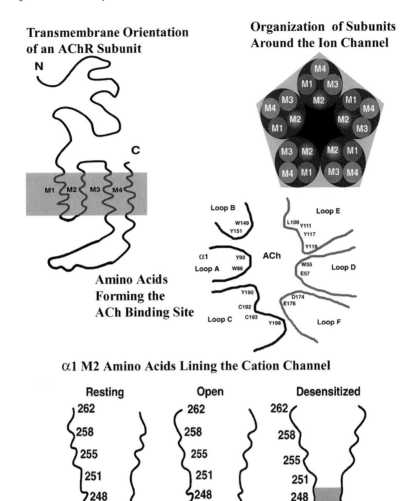

**Transmembrane Orientation
of an AChR Subunit**

**Organization of Subunits
Around the Ion Channel**

**Amino Acids
Forming the
ACh Binding Site**

**α1 M2 Amino Acids Lining the Cation Channel**

ting low-energy binding events in the extracellular domain to regulate opening, closing, and desensitization of the ion channel gate near the cytoplasmic vestibule of the channel. The amino acids lining the cation channel and accessible either from the extracellular or cytoplasmic surface have been determined largely by SCAM (37). The channel lining is thought to be formed by the extracellular third of M1 and M2. The figure depicts the M1–M2 linker at the cytoplasmic end of M1 and M2. In the closed, resting state of the channel, only a short region is occluded and inaccessible to labeling. In the closed desensitized state, a larger region is occluded.

somewhat in AChR subunits because the loop sequence in the ACh binding protein is not well conserved. It is hydrophobic in AChRs but hydrophilic in the binding protein. A proline in the loop, which is conserved in all AChR subunits, is missing in the binding protein. Mutating this proline to glycine disrupts assembly of AChR subunits and prevents transport to the surface of assembled AChRs *(36)*. The extracellular domains of AChR subunits contain one or more glycosylation sites, and in all but the $\alpha 7$–9 subunits, which can form homomeric AChRs, there is an N-glycosylation site at position 141 adjacent to the disulfide bond of the signature loop.

Three closely spaced, highly conserved, largely $\alpha$-helical transmembrane sequences (M1–M3) corresponding approximately to amino acids 220–310 extend between the large extracellular domain and the largest cytoplasmic domain. The N-terminal third of M1 and the hydrophilic side of M2 form each subunit's contribution to the lining of the channel *(21,37)*. This will be described in slightly more detail in a subsequent section on the channel and gate.

The large cytoplasmic domain between the transmembrane sequences M3 and M4 comprises 110–270 amino acids ($\alpha 4$ being by far the largest). This is the most variable region in sequence between subunits and between species. Consequently, many subunit-specific antibodies bind in this region *(38)*. The large cytoplasmic region of muscle AChRs interacts with rapsyn, a protein that links it to the cytoskeleton and thus helps to position it appropriately in the neuromuscular junction *(39)*. Proteins other than rapsyn are probably involved in interacting with the large cytoplasmic domain of neuronal AChRs to help transport them to and localize them at their various pre-, post-, and extrasynaptic sites of action, but these proteins have not yet been characterized *(40)*. The chaperone protein 14-3-3$\eta$ binds to $\alpha 4$ at serine 441 in the large cytoplasmic domain, especially when it is phosphorylated, helping to increase conformational maturation or assembly *(41)*. Several chaperone proteins are known to participate in the conformational maturation and assembly of muscle AChR subunits *(42–44)*. For example, COPI interacts at lysine 314 of $\alpha 1$-subunits. The large cytoplasmic domain contains phosphorylation sites and perhaps other sequences thought to be involved in regulating the rate of desensitization *(45,46)* and other properties such as intracellular transport *(47)*. Surprisingly, it even contains sequences that contribute to channel gating kinetics *(48)*.

A fourth transmembrane domain (M4), of about 20 amino acids, extends from the large cytoplasmic domain to the extracellular surface, leading to a 10–20-amino acid extracellular sequence. In the case of human $\alpha 4$-subunits, the C-terminal end of the $\alpha 4$ sequence has been found to form a site through which binding of estrogen enhances AChR function three- to sevenfold, while it inhibits the response of $\alpha3\beta2$ AChRs *(49,50)*. No functional role for the C-terminal sequence is yet known for other AChR subunits.

$\alpha$-subunits are defined by the presence of a disulfide-linked adjacent cysteine pair in the large extracellular domain homologous to $\alpha192$ and 193 of $\alpha1$-subunits. In all $\alpha$-subunits, other than $\alpha5$ and perhaps $\alpha10$, this is thought to contribute to the ACh binding site. These cysteines, after reduction of the disulfide bond between them, were the targets of the first affinity labels developed for AChRs *(21)*. In the ACh binding protein (**Fig. 2**), this cysteine pair is located at the tip of a protruding loop on what can be defined as the "+" side of the subunit. The ACh binding site is formed at the interface between the + side of an $\alpha$-subunit and the "–" side of an adjacent subunit, as will be discussed in somewhat more detail in a subsequent section.

## ORGANIZATION OF SUBUNITS IN AChR SUBTYPES

Homologous rod-like AChR subunits are organized in a pentagonal array around the central cation channel *(28)*. In the muscle type AChRs of *Torpedo* electric organ, the order of subunits around the channel is $\alpha1$, $\gamma$, $\alpha1$, $\delta$, and $\beta1$ *(21)*. In the adult muscle AChR subtype, $\epsilon$ substitutes for $\gamma$. Reflecting their similar functional roles and evolutionary origins *(51)* $\gamma$, $\delta$, and $\epsilon$ have especially similar sequences, as do $\beta1$, $\beta2$, and $\beta4$. In cDNA expression systems, $\beta2$ and $\beta4$ can substitute for $\beta1$ in muscle AChR *(52)*. The arrangement of subunits in major AChR subtypes is depicted in **Fig. 4**.

The primordial AChR was presumably homomeric, and heteromeric AChRs evolved subsequent to duplication of the primordial subunit *(51)*. AChR subunits are lettered in order of increasing molecular weight as they were discovered in the AChRs first purified from *Torpedo* electric organ, and they are numbered in the order in which their cDNAs were cloned *(24)*.

Homomeric AChRs can be formed by $\alpha7$-, $\alpha8$- and $\alpha9$-subunits *(1)*. In mammals, $\alpha7$ is the predominant homomeric AChR. Like muscle AChRs (although with much lower affinity) $\alpha7$, $\alpha8$, and $\alpha9$ AChRs bind $\alpha$-bungarotoxin ($\alpha$-BGT) and related snake venom peptide toxins to their ACh binding sites. Heteromeric neuronal AChRs containing $\alpha1$-6 in combination with $\beta2$–4 subunits do not bind $\alpha$-BGT. $\alpha8$ has been found only in chickens *(53)*. It can form heteromeric AChRs with $\alpha7$. $\alpha9$ can form heteromeric AChRs with $\alpha10$ *(54,55)*.

Heteromeric neuronal AChRs are formed from $\alpha$-subunits 2, 3, 4, or 6 in combination with $\beta2$ or $\beta4$ *(1)*. $\alpha5$ and $\beta3$ are present as additional subunits in AChRs in which ACh binding sites are formed by other $\alpha$- and $\beta$-subunits

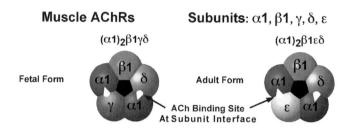

**Muscle AChRs**          **Subunits: α1, β1, γ, δ, ε**

$(\alpha1)_2\beta1\gamma\delta$                              $(\alpha1)_2\beta1\epsilon\delta$

Fetal Form                                           Adult Form

ACh Binding Site → At Subunit Interface

**Heteromeric
Neuronal AChRs**          **Subunits: α2-α6, β2-β4**

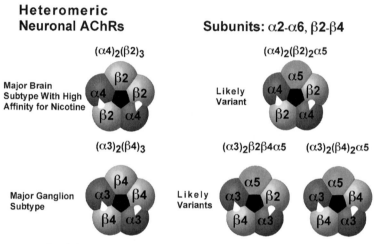

$(\alpha4)_2(\beta2)_3$                              $(\alpha4)_2(\beta2)_2\alpha5$

Major Brain Subtype With High Affinity for Nicotine                    Likely Variant

$(\alpha3)_2(\beta4)_3$            $(\alpha3)_2\beta2\beta4\alpha5$      $(\alpha3)_2(\beta4)_2\alpha5$

Major Ganglion Subtype                    Likely Variants

α5 and β3 may occupy only positions comparable to β1 in which they do not participate in forming ACh binding sites.
α6 can participate in forming ACh binding sites, but can also assemble in AChRs with, for example, α3 or α4 subunits.

**Homomeric
Neuronal AChRs**          **Subunits: α7-α10**

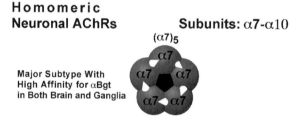

$(\alpha7)_5$

Major Subtype With High Affinity for αBgt in Both Brain and Ganglia

**Fig. 4.** Prominent acetylcholine receptor (AChR) subtypes. AChR subtypes are defined by their subunit compositions. The arrangement of AChR subunits around the channel is known for *Torpedo* electric organ muscle type AChRs *(21)* and is inferred for other types based on this example. The subunit stoichiometry of some neuronal AChR subtypes is known (196,197), and it is known that ACh binding sites can be formed at specific interfaces of α1-4- or α6- with β2- or β4-subunits

*(56–62)*. The AChR subunit pairs α2, α4; α3, α6; β2, β4; and α5, β3 are closely related in sequence, reflecting their origins by gene duplication and their similar functional roles *(51)*. The subunit compositions of these heteromeric neuronal AChRs can be as simple as α3β4α3β4β4 or α4β2α4β2β2, with two identical ACh binding sites. They can be more complex, involving three (e.g., α3β4α3β4α5) or more types of AChR subunits (α3β4α6β2β3). These can have two identical ACh binding sites (α4β2α4β2β2), two different ACh binding sites with one kind of α subunit (α3β2α3β4α5), as in muscle AChRs (α1εα1δβ1), or two different ACh binding sites with two different α subunits (α3β2α6β2β2). Many neurons express complex mixtures of ACh subunits *(63,64)*. Ganglionic neurons usually express α3, α5, α7, β2, and β4 subunits, which could potentially form many subtypes, but the function of α3β4 tends to predominate postsynaptically *(65,66)*. Adjacent neurons, within the same nucleus, can express different complex combinations of AChR subunits *(64,67)*. It remains to be determined which AChR subtypes are expressed from these subunit combinations, where they are located within the neurons, and what functional roles they play in postsynaptic transmission, presynaptic modulation, and extrasynaptic plasticity. What is clear is that AChRs can play many much more complex regulatory roles than their classic postsynaptic role in high safety factor neuromuscular transmission might suggest.

In muscle AChRs, ACh binding sites are formed at the interfaces of the + side of α1 with the – side of γ-, δ-, or ε-subunits, and β1-subunits do not participate in forming ACh binding sites *(21)*. In heteromeric neuronal AChRs, α5- and β3-subunits are thought to occupy positions comparable to those of β1 *(56,68)*. They contribute to both ion channel properties and agonist potency not only because they contribute to the lining of the channel but also because the ease with which the agonist-induced conformation changes of the whole AChR molecule take place in the course of activation or desensitization depends on the structures of all moving parts of the AChR *(69)*.

## ACETYLCHOLINE BINDING SITES

ACh binding sites are formed at the interfaces between subunits. This is shown in high resolution in the case of the ACh binding protein in **Fig. 2** and diagrammatically in **Fig. 3**. Both affinity labeling studies of native AChRs

---

but not with α5 or β3 *(50,60,62)*. All subunits are expected to participate in the structure of the channel and in conformation changes associated with activation and desensitization. (Modified with permission from Lindstrom J. Acetylcholine receptors and myasthenia. *Muscle Nerve* 2000;23:453–477.)

*(21,35)* and the structure of the ACh binding protein *(33)* reveal that the ACh binding site does not contain negatively charged amino acids to bind positively charged ACh. The ACh binding site contains many aromatic amino acids, and it is thought that interactions between the $\pi$ electrons of these amino acids and the quaternary amine play an important role in binding. The ACh binding site of ACh esterase also works this way *(70)*.

Tetramethylammonium is the simplest form of an agonist. The small movements initiated by the low-affinity binding at just this portion of the site must be sufficient to trigger channel opening.

The ACh binding sites are located half way up the extracellular domain *(33)*, far removed from the gate at the cytoplasmic end of the channel whose opening they regulate *(37)*. This regulation is thought to occur by means of small global conformation changes of the AChR protein, which may involve slight changes in the angles of the rod-like subunits to produce an iris-like regulation of channel opening *(28)*. Both the ACh binding site *(71)* and the cation channel *(37)* change conformation between the resting, open, and desensitized states. The amino acids lining the ACh binding site come from three parts of the + side of the $\alpha$-subunit and three parts of the − side of the complementary subunit *(21,33,35)*. It would seem that such an arrangement would be ideal for initiating and communicating small motions involved in ligand binding to motions along subunit interfaces throughout the molecule. The binding energies involved are small, as must be the differences between the resting and open conformations as the channel flickers open.

It is argued that the two ACh binding sites in muscle AChRs should differ in affinity for ACh ($K_D = \mu M$ vs mM) in order to ensure the rapid opening and closing of the channel *(25)*. The properties of the two ACh binding sites in muscle AChRs differ because they are formed at the interface of $\alpha$1 with $\gamma$-, $\delta$-, or $\varepsilon$-subunits *(72)*. The $\alpha$1$\gamma$ sites have higher affinity, producing longer channel opening at low ACh concentrations, as may be appropriate for fetal AChRs during synapse development (and may perhaps be useful when fetal AChRs help to compensate for AChR loss after autoimmune or genetic damage). The actual kinetics of gating, surprisingly, depend not just on properties of the ACh site or gate, but also on sequences in the large cytoplasmic domain *(48)*. During an endplate potential, ACh is present in the synaptic cleft at concentrations in the mM range for less than a millisecond *(73)*. Normally, this ensures a substantial safety factor for transmission because the ACh saturates the AChRs and the AChRs are in excess over what is needed to provide sufficient current to trigger an action potential (*see* Chap. 1). When the number of AChRs is reduced in autoimmune or congenital myasthenia, the current may be insufficient, or may become insufficient on successive stimuli, as fewer vesicles of ACh are released and AChRs accumulate in the desensitized state. Then some synthesis of the fetal form of AChR with higher affinity for ACh and consequent longer burst and channel open times may be critical for achieving sufficient current to more nearly ensure transmission.

Competitive antagonists ideally keep AChRs in the resting conformation. They are usually multivalent quaternary or tertiary amines thought to interact at both the ACh site and peripheral sites to stabilize the resting state. Some, like curare, may actually be very low-efficacy agonists *(74)*. α-BGT and related snake venom peptides of 8000–9000 daltons are large flat molecules that might cover 800–1200 Å of AChR surface *(75)*, corresponding perhaps to a 30 Å × 30 Å square centered on the ACh binding site. Only the tip of one finger of this structure might enter the actual ACh binding site *(75)*, but interactions formed slowly over a wide area on both sides of the subunit interface confer high affinity and stabilize the AChR in a resting state.

Exposure to ACh or other agonists for long periods causes desensitization, which is a conformation (or perhaps a set of conformations) characterized by a closed channel and higher affinity for agonists. In the normal course of neuromuscular transmission, desensitization is not a limiting factor. However, ACh esterase inhibitors given to treat MG (by increasing the concentration and duration of ACh to compensate for the loss of AChRs) can, at excessive doses, further impair transmission by causing accumulation of desensitized AChRs *(76)*. Nerve gases and insecticides that act as esterase inhibitors can have similar effects *(77)*. The depolarizing block surgical muscle relaxant succinylcholine should also have a similar component to its action in addition to producing a depolarizing blockade of action potential generation. Nicotine in tobacco users is present for many hours ($t_{1/2}$ for clearance = 2 h) at an average concentration of around 0.2 μ$M$, and it rises to nearly 1.0 μ$M$ briefly after inhalation of smoke *(78)*. The low affinity of muscle AChRs for nicotine normally prevents much effect on neuromuscular transmission. Nicotine, acting on several neuronal AChR subtypes with a wide range of affinities for nicotine, produces many behavioral effects (addiction, tolerance, anxiolysis, cognitive enhancement, antinociception) resulting from a complex mixture of activation, desensitization, and upregulation effects on the AChRs *(1,16)*.

Binding of agonists at two ACh binding sites is required for efficient activation of AChRs *(72)*. It is uncertain whether liganding of the sites stabilizes preexisting states of activation or induces conformation changes, although I find the latter model intuitively more appealing. Antagonist blockage of any one site is usually sufficient to prevent activation *(79)*. Homomeric AChRs, such as α7 AChRs, have five ACh binding sites. Desensitization at any one of these may be sufficient to prevent activation, probably accounting for the very rapid desensitization characteristic of such AChRs *(80)*.

## CATION CHANNEL AND ITS GATE

The cation channel is lined by amino acids from the M2 and N-terminal third of the M1 transmembrane domains, as depicted in **Fig. 3**. Much of the identification of amino acids lining the channel pore has been achieved using the substituted cysteine accessibility method (SCAM) *(21,37)*. In this method, successive amino acids along a putative transmembrane domain such as M1 or M2 are replaced by cysteine. This introduces a free thiol group, usually without greatly altering AChR function. Then a thiol alkylating agent that contains a positively charged amino group [e.g., aminoethyl methanethiosulfonate (MTSEA)] is applied from outside or inside the cell in which the mutated AChR is expressed. If MTSEA covalently reacts and blocks the channel, it is assumed that the substituted cysteine was exposed on the interior of the channel. From the periodicity at which cysteines are exposed, it can be inferred whether the domain has α-helical or another secondary conformation, and accessibility of the cysteine in the resting, open, or desensitized conformation determines the outer limits of the channel gate. Most of the M1 and M2 domains appear to be in an α-helical conformation. In the resting state, the open lumen of the channel extends to nearly the cytoplasmic surface, with only a small occluded region between α1 G240 and T244. The highly conserved sequence α1 G240, E241, K242, in the M1-M2 linker immediately preceding the cytoplasmic end of M2, lines the narrowest part of the channel in which the gate is located. Small motions in this region could open and close the channel. In the desensitized state, nearly half of the channel is occluded over a region extending from G240 to L251. Other mutagenesis studies have also helped define the structure of the channel *(27)*. Several polar or charged rings of amino acids lining the channel formed by homologous amino acids from each subunit form the selectivity filter.

## ANTIGENIC STRUCTURE
## AND THE MAIN IMMUNOGENIC REGION

Immunization with native α1 AChRs provokes antibodies directed primarily at the extracellular surface *(38,81)*. This is because more than half of the antibodies to AChR in an immunized animal or an MG patient are directed at the MIR *(30,31,82)*. This is a highly conformation-dependent epitope; thus immunization with denatured AChRs or subunits, by default, provokes antibodies to the cytoplasmic surface, whose epitopes are much less conformation-dependent *(38)*. Synthetic peptides can be used to induce antibodies to many parts of the AChR sequence, but many of the antibodies will not bind to AChRs in their native conformation *(38)*.

Monoclonal antibodies (MAbs) from rats and mice immunized with AChRs have provided excellent model autoantibodies and structural probes for AChRs *(1,31,82)*. Half or more of the mAbs to native α1 AChRs are directed at the main immunogenic region (MIR) *(30)*. Such antibodies compete with each other for binding and prevent the binding of more than half of the autoantibodies from MG patients *(31,82)*. Thus, the antibodies bind to overlapping regions but not necessarily to identical epitopes. The crystal structures of the binding sites of two MAbs to the MIR have been determined *(83,84)*. The two antibody binding sites differ because they recognize different aspects of the MIR and do not present a clear negative image of the whole structure. One is a crescent-shaped crevice and the other is relatively planar with a surface area of 2865 Å.

The structure of the MIR is being defined with increasing precision. Both absolutely conformation-dependent MAbs to the MIR and others that also bind to denatured α1 subunits with lower affinity depend critically on the same α1 amino acids (68 and 71), as shown by mutagenesis studies *(85)*. Several lines of evidence showed that the MIR is oriented so that an antibody bound to one α1-subunit cannot also bind the other α1-subunit in the same AChR but can efficiently crosslink adjacent AChRs *(86)*. Cryoelectron microscopy confirmed and extended these conclusions, showing that the MIR was located at the extracellular tip of α1-subunits and angled away from the central axis of the AChR *(87)*. In the ACh binding protein, the sequence that would form the MIR in an α1-subunit is located at the extracellular tip of the subunit near the N-terminus in a loop directed away from axis of the subunit, as shown in **Fig. 2** *(33)*. Because the sequence of this region in the ACh binding protein is not closely homologous to that of α1-subunits, the precise conformation of the MIR in α1-subunits must differ from that of this sequence of the binding protein. An antibody bound to the MIR would cover an even larger area of the α1 surface than is covered by a bound α-BGT molecule. The separation between the MIR at the tip of the subunit and the ACh binding site halfway down the side of the subunit reveals why antibodies to both the MIR and α-BGT can bind simultaneously to α1 AChRs. Few autoantibodies in MG are directed at the ACh binding site *(86)*. These facts form the structural basis of the basic immunodiagnostic assay for MG in which [125]I-labeled α-BGT is used to label detergent-solubilized human α1 AChRs specifically, to permit quantitation of MG patient autoantibodies in an immune precipitation assay *(88)*.

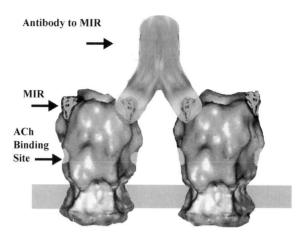

**Fig. 5.** Structural basis of the pathologic significance of the main immunogenetic region (MIR). The MIR is easily accessible on the extracellular surface. This permits binding of autoantibodies and complement. The MIR has a highly immunogenic conformation. There are two copies of the MIR, which contributes to its immunogenicity by permitting aggregation of receptor immunoglobulins on B-cells. It contributes to synaptic pathology by permitting crosslinking of acetylcholine receptors (AChRs) by antibodies to cause antigenic modulation. The MIR is oriented to facilitate crosslinking of adjacent AChRs by antibody while not permitting crosslinking of α1-subunits within an AChR. The MIR is away from the ACh binding site and subunit interfaces. Thus, antibodies to the MIR do not inhibit AChR function competitively or allosterically. Also, this permits binding of both antibodies and α-BGT simultaneously, so that immunodiagnostic assays can be done by indirect immunoprecipitation of detergent-solubilized AChRs labeled with $[^{125}I]\alpha$-BGT. AChRs are densely packed in a semicrystalline array at the tips of folds in the postsynaptic membrane. Thus, bound antibody and complement can cause focal lysis and shedding of AChR-rich membrane fragments, while the postsynaptic membrane can reseal. The result is loss of AChR and disrupted synaptic morphology, but not lethal lysis of the muscle fiber.

The fundamental pathologic significance of the MIR derives from its basic structure (represented diagramatically in **Fig. 5**). The MIR is highly immunogenic, perhaps because it has a novel shape, is easily accessible on the protein surface, and is present in two copies per AChR to permit multivalent binding and crosslinking of receptor immunoglobulins to stimulate B-cells efficiently. Because the MIR is easily accessible on the extracellular surface, antibodies can easily bind to it and fix complement. α1 AChRs are densely packed in a semicrystalline array at the tips of folds in the postsynaptic membrane, promoting high-avidity binding of antibodies and focal lysis of the postsynaptic membrane, but allowing the postsynaptic membrane to reseal after the membrane fragments containing antibodies, AChR, and complement are shed *(89)*. This process contributes to impairment of transmission both by destroying AChRs and by disrupting the morphology of the synapse in which presynaptic active zones of ACh release are normally located near postsynaptic patches of AChRs. The MIR is oriented at an angle that promotes crosslinking of AChR by antibodies. This triggers antigenic modulation, which is a crosslinking-induced increase in the rate of AChR internalization and lysosomal destruction *(90–92)*. MAbs to the MIR and most serum antibodies do not impair AChR function *(93)*. This is probably because the antibodies do not interfere with ACh binding and because antibodies bound to the MIR are far from the subunit interfaces where the subtle movements mediating activation and desensitization take place.

Some rat MAbs to the MIR on $\alpha 1$ bind very well to human $\alpha 1$-, as well as $\alpha 3$- and $\alpha 5$-subunits (which have similar MIR sequences) *(56)*. These MAbs do not recognize denatured $\alpha 3$, even though they do recognize denatured $\alpha 1$. MG patient antisera do not bind significantly to human $\alpha 3$ AChRs, and human autoantibodies to $\alpha 3$ do not bind to $\alpha 1$ *(14)*. Thus, the MIR epitopes recognized by rats and humans are not identical, even though they are close enough that antibodies to them compete for binding.

Prominent antibody epitopes on the cytoplasmic surfaces of $\alpha 1$-subunits and other subunits have been determined using antisera and antibodies *(31, 38)*. These epitopes are pathologically irrelevant because autoantibodies cannot bind to them in vivo.

The spectrum of autoantibodies to AChRs produced in MG patients is dominated by the MIR but includes other parts of the AChR and closely resembles the spectrum seen in animals with AChR or in dogs with idiopathic MG *(82,94)*. Many MG sera react better with extrajunctional AChRs *(95)*, possibly because the endogenous immunogen in MG has $\gamma$-subunits that may be more immunogenic because they are not normally expressed in adults. One unusual MG patient serum was found to be specific for $\gamma$ and occluded the $\alpha 1 \gamma$ ACh binding site, thereby inhibiting function *(96)*. Rare mothers have been found who make autoantibodies only to $\gamma$-subunits *(97)*. These have no effect on the mother (whose AChRs have only $\varepsilon$-subunits), but they paralyze or kill fetuses, causing arthrogryposis multiplex congenita.

$\alpha 1$-subunits also predominate in the T-cell response to AChRs, but epitopes have been found on all subunits *(98,99)*. Several $\alpha 1$ T-cell epitopes seem to predominate in MG, but there is disagreement between laboratories on which sequences comprise these epitopes. In Lewis rats, $\alpha 1$ 100–116 is a dominant T-cell epitope, but in brown Norway rats α172–205 predominates, as does α152–70 in buffalo rats *(100)*. There is probably similar diversity in human groups. Pathologically significant T-cell epitopes could derive from any part of an AChR subunit because the T-cells do not bind to native AChRs in vivo, but to peptide fragments digested by "professional" antigen-presenting cells like dendritic cells, or "interested amateurs" like AChR-reactive B-cells.

Before an AChR epitope can be recognized by the antigen receptor of a T-helper cell that will collaborate with an AChR-stimulated B-lymphocyte to produce plasma cells secreting autoantibodies to AChRs, the AChR peptide must first be bound by an MHC class II antigen-presenting protein *(101)*. The proteolytic processing mechanisms of the antigen-presenting cell and the binding properties of the various MHC class II proteins restrict the peptides that can be recognized by T-cells *(102)*. This is probably reflected in part in the higher incidence of HLA-A1, -B8, and -DR3 class II MHC determinants in young-onset Caucasian MG patients and different MHC determinants in other groups *(103)*. Inbred mice become resistant to EAMG subsequent to a single amino acid change in the I-$A_B$ protein *(104,105)*. The human α1 sequence 144–156 is recognized only when it is presented by HLA-DR4 class II protein variants with glycine at position 86 and not by a variant with valine at this position *(103)*. If humans were as inbred as these mouse strains, and if AChRs had only a few T-cell epitopes, MG would be much more genetically constrained than is actually the case.

## INDUCTION OF THE AUTOIMMUNE RESPONSE TO AChRs IN MG

The mechanisms that induce and sustain the autoimmune response to α1 AChRs in MG are not known. These mechanisms may differ in various forms of human MG, and mechanisms may differ between species. Human MG is a remitting and exacerbating disease in which the autoimmune response to α1 AChRs persists for years *(13,92)*. Canine MG is an acute disease in which the autoimmune response to AChRs and muscle weakness usually remit within 6 months, except when the MG is associated with a neoplastic growth *(106)*. This suggests that in humans a source of immunogen persists that does not in dogs. For example, a chronic occult infection in humans might involve a tissue that expresses α1 AChR in an unusual amount, place, or state of posttranslational modification, causing it to be immunogenic. In dogs, this infection might not persist. In either case, if chronic infection provided the immunogen, then appropriate antibiotic therapy might provide the cure.

MG in humans can be initiated and then terminated when the immunogen is removed. Rheumatoid arthritis patients treated with penicillamine sometimes develop autoimmune MG *(107,108)*. It is thought that, in these patients with a predisposition to autoimmune responses, a covalent reaction of penicillamine with thiol groups on α1 AChRs haptenizes them to produce new antigenic sites and provoke an autoimmune response *(109)*. Ending the penicillamine treatment ends the MG within a couple of months. Neonatal MG occurs in babies of mothers with MG as a result of passive transfer of auto-antibodies from the mother *(110,111)*. This also spontaneously remits within a couple of months. If passive or active EAMG is not sufficiently severe to be lethal, the animals recover as the response to the immunogen diminishes *(13)*. All four examples (penicillamine-induced MG, neonatal MG, passive and acute EAMG) illustrate that an autoimmune assault on neuromuscular junction AChRs sufficient to cause muscle weakness is not sufficient to present enough AChR to the immune system to sustain the autoimmune response. Something special must happen in human MG to chronically provide sufficient immunogen to sustain the autoimmune response.

A paraneoplastic autoimmune response may be present in some MG patients. Twelve percent of MG patients have thymoma, and 35% of thymoma patients have MG *(112)*. These patients characteristically make high levels of auto-antibodies to AChRs and to several structural proteins found within muscle cells, e.g., titin *(113–115)*. Thymic tumor cells do not usually express α1 AChRs *(99)*, but traces of AChRs have been detected in thymus myoid cells, thymic epithelia, and dendritic cells *(116,117)*. The autoantibodies to AChRs might result from a bystander adjuvant effect of the disruption caused by the tumor to an immune regulatory organ that contains traces of AChRs. Alternatively, viruses or other factors that cause the tumor might also cause disruption of AChR-expressing cells. In Lambert-Eaton syndrome (LES), tumor immunogens play a much more obvious role in provoking the autoimmune response. Sixty percent of these patients have small cell lung carcinomas *(118)* (as a result of addiction to tobacco through neuronal AChRs) *(1,16)*. These carcinomas express voltage-sensitive calcium channels, which are the target of the autoimmune response in LES. The muscular weakness that these patients exhibit due to autoantibody impairment of ACh release *(118)*, often for years before the tumor is discovered, is the tradeoff for development of a successful immune response to the tumor voltage-gated calcium channel that holds the otherwise rapidly fatal tumor in check.

In most MG patients, the immunogen is likely to be native muscle AChR or a closely related molecule, because the spectrum of autoantibody specificities in MG and EAMG is very similar *(82,94)*. It may often be a fetal muscle

AChR, given the selective reactivity for such AChRs by many MG patients *(95,119)*. Denatured AChR subunits or synthetic fragments of AChRs are extremely inefficient at inducing EAMG because they lack the MIR *(120–122)*. Thus, molecular mimicry of the AChR by a bacteria or virus expressing a protein with a short stretch of sequence similar to the AChR is unlikely to induce MG. However, bacterial DNA can be a potent adjuvant, and microbe-associated autoimmune responses have been found in connection with both relatively obvious *(123,124)* and more cryptic bacterial infections *(125)*.

## AUTOIMMUNE MECHANISMS THAT IMPAIR NEUROMUSCULAR TRANSMISSION IN MG AND EAMG

EAMG has been induced in many species by immunization with purified *Torpedo* electric organ AChR *(86)*. Native AChR is quite immunogenic, and EAMG has been induced with syngeneic AChR *(126)*, even in the absence of adjuvants *(127)*. The most detailed studies have been in Lewis rats *(86,89, 128)*. Some other rat strains produce high levels of antibodies to AChRs but are resistant to EAMG *(129)*. Some mouse strains are more resistant than others, but all are more resistant than are Lewis rats *(105)*.

Among MG patients, the absolute concentration of antibodies to AChR does not correlate closely with severity *(130,131)*, but, in general, patients with only ocular signs have lower concentrations than do patients with generalized MG, and changes in clinical state are usually paralleled by changes in antibody concentrations *(132)*.

The basic mechanisms by which autoantibodies to AChRs impair neuro-muscular transmission appear to be very similar in MG and chronic EAMG *(86,89)*.

There are forms of both MG and EAMG that are passively transferred by autoantibodies to AChRs. Passive transfer of EAMG is associated with an antibody and complement-dependent, transient phagocyte-mediated attack on the postsynaptic membrane that greatly amplifies the pathologic potency of the bound antibodies *(133,134)*. In neither chronic EAMG nor MG is anti-body-dependent phagocytic attack or cytotoxic T-lymphocyte attack on the postsynaptic membrane observed *(89)*. Repeated injection of mice with large amounts of MG patient IgG causes a mild form of muscular weakness *(135, 136)*. Mothers with MG can passively transfer MG to their babies *(110,111)*. Usually this is mild and transient, ending as maternal IgG is cleared from the baby.

Active immunization of Lewis rats with AChR in adjuvant results in chronic EAMG after about 30 days *(126)*. If sufficient AChR and adjuvants are used, this can be preceded by an acute phase of EAMG 8–11 days after immunization, which involves antibody and complement-dependent phagocytes, as in passive EAMG *(126,137–139)*. In both chronic EAMG and MG, ACh sensitivity is decreased, and decrementing electromyogram responses are observed, as transmission becomes more likely to fail on successive stimuli *(140,141)*. This is because decreased postsynaptic sensitivity to ACh reduces the safety factor for transmission, so failure becomes more likely as fewer vesicles of ACh are released on successive stimuli owing to depletion of docked vesicles. Serum autoantibody concentration is high, there is loss of more than half of muscle AChRs, and many of those that remain have antibodies bound *(126, 142)*. The structure of the postsynaptic membrane is disrupted: the folded structure is simplified, AChR content is reduced, antibodies and complement are bound, and focal lysis occurs with shedding of membrane fragments into the synaptic cleft *(137,143,144)*. In addition to AChR loss through complement-mediated lysis, loss occurs owing to antigenic modulation following crosslinking of AChRs by antibody *(90,91,145)*. Only a small fraction of antibodies to AChR are capable of inhibiting AChR function *(146–151)*. The lack of direct effect on AChR function by most antibodies to AChR is illustrated by the observation that, if rats are depleted by the C3 component of complement to prevent both lysis and phagocytic invasion, then passive transfer of IgG from rats with chronic EAMG can label at least 67% of the AChRs without causing weakness *(152)*.

## EFFECTS OF AChR MUTATIONS
## IN CONGENITAL MYASTHENIC SYNDROMES

The structure of muscle AChRs is optimized for this functional role *(25)*. Studies of congenital myasthenic syndromes due to mutations in AChR subunits *(89,153)* have clearly demonstrated that it is detrimental to either increase *(154)* or decrease *(155)* affinity for ACh, or increase *(156)* or decrease *(157)* the channel opening time. Such changes often result in large pleotropic changes in the number of AChRs and the morphology of the neuromuscular junction, further contributing to impairment of neuromuscular transmission. Below, some examples of the many congenital myasthenic syndromes elegantly characterized by Andrew Engel *(158,159)* and his coworkers will be described briefly with the intention of relating defects in aspects of the AChR structures previously described to specific functional defects and the resulting medical effects.

Synthesis of AChR subunits can be impaired or prevented by mutations in the promotor region *(160)* or frameshift mutations that result in truncation of the subunit *(160–163)*. These sorts of mutations are more frequent in ε-subunits than others because, in humans, expression of γ is induced, which partially compensates for the loss of ε. Expansion of the endplate area also helps to compensate for loss of AChRs. In mice, knockout of the ε-subunit is perinatally lethal *(164)*. Deletion mutants of α1-subunits are not seen, presumably because this would be lethal.

Mutations both within and outside the ACh binding region alter agonist potency and efficacy. Reciprocally, these mutations alter channel-opening kinetics. A mutation that replaces α1 glycine 153 with a serine (in loop B of the ACh binding site) decreases the rate of ACh dissociation, resulting in repeated channel opening during prolonged ACh binding and increased desensitization *(154)*. The resulting 100-fold increase in affinity prevents the normal rapid termination of transmission, resulting in excitotoxic damage, including reduced AChR amount, increased desensitization, and morphologic alterations of the postsynaptic region due to overloading with cations. ACh esterase inhibitors would not be beneficial therapy. This mutation was less disabling to the patient than were some mutations in the M2 channel lining region, which, by increasing the stability of the open state of the channel, prolonged channel opening fivefold longer than did this increase in affinity for ACh *(156)*.

A similar increase in agonist binding affinity, activation, and desensitization was also caused by a mutation in the α1 M2 domain V249F at a position that is not on the hydrophilic lining of the channel *(165)*. An ε P121L mutation near the E loop of the ACh binding site reduced the affinity for ACh in the open and desensitized states, resulting in infrequent and brief episodes of channel opening and, consequently, impaired transmission causing weakness *(155)*. The amount of AChR and synaptic morphology were normal owing to the absence of excitotoxicity in this mutation. An α1 N217K mutation in the M1 region was found to cause a 20-fold increase in the affinity of ACh for the resting state of the AChR *(166)*. This N is a conserved amino acid in the synaptic third of the M1 transmembrane domain, i.e., not a contact amino acid in the ACh binding site but part of the lumen of the channel, between the ACh binding site and the conserved P121 C122 in the middle of M1, a region known to move during the process of AChR activation *(167)*. Efficacy and potency of agonists are affected by mutations in the M2 channel-forming part of the AChR because some of the mutations so destabilize the resting conformation that even binding of choline (usually not an effective agonist) is sufficient to activate the AChR *(168)*. Thus, the levels of choline in serum are sufficient to cause "spontaneous" activation of AChRs and contribute to excitotoxic damage in these long channel congenital myasthenic syndromes. Experimental mutations in similar regions in M2 of α7 AChRs appear to stabilize a desensitized conformation in which some antagonists can behave as agonists *(169)*. Choline is selective as an agonist, although a weak one, for $\alpha 7$ AChRs *(170)*. This may be because the five ACh binding sites on $\alpha 7$ homomers permit the low-affinity binding of a sufficient number of choline molecules to trigger activation by this very weak agonist.

Mutations in the M2 channel-forming part of the AChR frequently affect the duration of channel opening, usually causing prolonged channel opening, resulting in excitotoxicity. For example, the T264P mutation in the $\varepsilon M2$ hydrophilic surface causes prolonged channel openings *(156)*. The $\alpha$ V249F mutation on the hydrophobic surface of M2 also causes an autosomal dominant slow channel myasthenic syndrome *(165)*. Agonist potency is increased and desensitization is enhanced sufficiently to impair function at physiologic rates of stimulation. Excitotoxic effects include loss of AChR, degeneration of junctional folds, cluttering of an enlarged synaptic cleft with bits of membranous debris, degeneration of synaptic mitochondria and other organelles, and apoptosis of some junctional nuclei. Mutations in the M2 regions of several AChR subunits cause slow channel syndromes *(163)*. Other mutations can cause excessively rapid closure of the channel, but also excessive conductance, so that the net effect is also excitotoxic *(157)*.

Myasthenic syndromes have also been identified in other parts of AChR subunits. One was found to involve two recessive mutations in $\varepsilon$ *(171)*. The C128S mutation at one end of the disulfide-linked signature loop in the extracellular domain inhibits AChR assembly. Then the $\varepsilon$ 1245ins 18 mutation, which duplicates 6 amino acids in the C-terminal half of the large cytoplasmic domain, surprisingly, forms AChRs with altered opening kinetics and reduced net openings. That mutations in and out of the ACh binding site affect agonist potency, and that mutations in and out of the channel affect gating, is all evidence that activation and desensitization of AChRs involves both local and global conformational changes and that mutations in distant parts of the AChR protein can affect the stability of various conformation states and the kinetics of transition between them. Clinically, it is interesting that the patient and her similarly affected siblings with these two mutations went through life exhibiting muscle weakness and fatigue, but the crisis that provoked detailed study was when the 36-year-old patient underwent surgery and was given a curariform muscle relaxant, which resulted in paralysis lasting for several hours owing to her low safety factor for transmission.

Another striking feature of mutations causing congenital myasthenic syndromes is that there are a lot of these mutations. Often a recessive mutation does not produce a phenotype until two occur simultaneously. Thus far, more than 60 such mutations have been found *(158,159)*. It seems likely that similar varieties of mutations will be found in other receptors and channels.

## NEURONAL AChR SUBTYPES AND FUNCTIONAL ROLES

There are many potential and a few known prominent neuronal AChR subtypes, as indicated in **Fig. 4** *(1)*. α4β2 AChRs account for most of the high-affinity nicotine binding in the brain. α2 AChRs in primate brain may assume some of the roles of α4 AChRs in rodent brains *(172)*. Some of these also have α5- or perhaps β3-subunits replacing the β2-subunit equivalent to β1 in muscle AChRs *(173)*. Autonomic ganglia postsynaptic AChRs are predominantly α3β4 AChRs, but α3β4α5 AChRs and subtypes containing β2 are also present. In brain aminergic neurons, α6 often in combination with β3 and β2 or β4 and sometimes α3 or α4 can potentially form a variety of complex subtypes *(60,64,73)*. α7 homomers are found both in autonomic ganglia and in brain. Neurons often contain complex mixtures of AChR subtypes *(63,64)*. In autonomic ganglia, α3 AChRs perform a postsynaptic role in transmission similar to that of muscle AChRs, but many brain AChRs are involved in pre- and extrasynaptic modulation of the release of many transmitters *(174)*, and some extrasynaptic α7 AChRs may play roles in trophic regulation *(65)*.

A good way to get an overview of the functional roles of neuronal AChRs is to examine the features of mice in which a particular subunit has been knocked out or replaced with a hyperactive mutant form. Knockout of α3-subunits is neonatally lethal *(175)*. Such mice lack autonomic transmission and die as a result of a distended and infected bladder. Knockout of α4-subunits causes loss of most high-affinity nicotine binding in brain, loss of nicotine-induced antinociception, and increased anxiety *(176,177)*. Replacement of α4 with excitotoxic M2 mutation was neonatally lethal, but a heterozygote survived that had reduced expression of the mutation owing to some expression of the neo cassette involved in making the mutant mouse *(178)*. These mice lost dopaminergic neurons in the substantia nigra, and exhibited altered motor behavior and learning as well as increased anxiety.

A problem in interpretation of knockout mice is that developmental compensation may minimize the apparent functional importance of the knockout subunit. The problem with knocking in a lethally excitotoxic mutant subunit is that any neuron that at any time in its development expresses some of the subunit risks dying, thus exaggerating the apparent functional importance of the subunit. Multinucleate muscle cells are large and rather resilient to the lethal excitotoxic effects of mutant AChRs, but smaller neurons may not be, especially early in development when their ability to buffer excess calcium ions entering through hyperactive AChRs is low *(179)*. Knockout of α7, surprisingly, produced few evident problems *(180,181)*. Knockin of an excitotoxic M2 mutant α7 was neonatally lethal *(182)*. Knockout of α9 prevented cochlear efferent stimulation *(183)*, as expected from its postsynaptic role there. Knockout of β2 altered some learning behaviors, caused increased neuronal death with aging, prevented nicotine-induced antinociception, and prevented nicotine reinforcement (i.e., addiction) *(184)*. Knockout of β4 produced viable mice, indicating that β2 expression must have compensated for loss of β4 in α3 AChRs in autonomic neurons *(185)*. When both β2 and β4 were knocked out, the effects were even more severe than knockout of the α3-subunit. Knockout of β3 altered motor activity and decreased anxiety *(186)*. β3 is usually found with α6 in aminergic neurons such as those in the substantia nigra, ventral tegmental area, and locus ceruleus involved in motor control and addiction to nicotine *(187)*.

Nicotinic AChRs are directly responsible for addiction to the nicotine in tobacco *(1,16)* and are more peripherally involved in many other neurologic problems *(1,19)*.

## AUTOIMMUNE IMPAIRMENT OF NEURONAL AChRs

Low levels of autoantibodies to α3 AChRs were found in 41% (19 of 46) of patients with idiopathic or paraneoplastic dysautonomias, and 9% (6 of 67) of patients with postural tachycardia syndrome, idiopathic gastrointestinal dysmotility, or diabetic autonomic neuropathy *(14)*. Antibody levels were higher in the more severely affected and decreased with improvement. Low levels of autoantibodies to α3 or α7 AChRs have also been found in a few patients with MG, LES, Guillain-Barré syndrome, or chronic inflammatory demyelinating polyneuropathy who also exhibited symptoms of autonomic dysfunction *(188)*. Unlike human MG, but like canine MG *(106)*, these autoimmune dysautonomias are often monophasic illnesses *(14)*. Details of the mechanisms by which the autoantibodies impair autonomic transmission are unknown, but they probably include some or all of the mechanisms observed in MG and EAMG.

It is interesting that rat MAbs to the MIR react well with human α3 AChRs *(56)*, yet MG patient antisera in general do not react with human α3AChRs *(14)*, and rats with EAMG do not exhibit obvious autonomic symptoms *(13)*. Thus, despite the similarities in primary sequences in the 66–76 regions of α1-, α3-, α5-, and β3-subunits, the conformation dependence of MIR antibody binding and the large areas of a protein occluded by a bound antibody can account for the apparent differences in MIR antibody specificity between rats and humans, despite mutual competition for binding to α1-subunits.

Low levels of AChR α3, α5, α7, α9, β2, and β4 AChR subunits have been reported in human keratinocytes, and ACh has been reported to modulate keratinocyte adhesion, proliferation, migration, and differentiation *(5)*. Autoantibodies in pemphigus patients have been found to be directed not only at des-moglien, but also at α9 AChRs and a novel keratinocyte ACh binding protein termed pemphaxin *(15)*. Pemphaxin is not the equivalent of the snail ACh binding protein *(33,189)*. Autoimmune responses to neuronal AChRs found in other nonneuronal tissues *(6-8)* have not yet been reported.

*A priori*, antibody-mediated autoimmune responses to receptors in brain would seem unlikely, owing to the presence of the blood-brain barrier. However, autoantibodies to glutamate receptors have been found in Rasmussen's encephalitis and certain forms of cerebellar degeneration *(190–192)*. Immunization of rabbits with bacterially expressed glutamate receptor protein causes lethal Rasmussen's-like seizures resulting from autoantibodies with agonist activity, which cause excitotoxic damage *(190)*. Thus, there is precedent for antibody-mediated autoimmune responses to brain neuronal AChRs, and it is possible that such responses could involve neuronal AChRs.

## EFFECTS OF HUMAN NEURONAL AChR MUTATIONS

Autosomal dominant nocturnal frontal lobe epilepsy (ADNFLE) is a rare form of epilepsy (resembling night terrors) caused by mutations in either α4- or β2-subunits in the M2 region *(10–12)*. A conundrum is that the α4 mutations involve loss of function, whereas the β2 mutations involve gain of function. There are two mutations known in α4 and two in β2. For example, replacement of α4 serine 247 in the M2 channel lining with a phenylalanine reduced channel function as a result of use-dependent functional upregulation, faster desensitization, slower recovery from desensitization, less inward rectification, and virtual elimination of $Ca^{2+}$ permeability *(193)*. Although many functions of α4β2 AChRs in brain are unknown, α4β2 AChRs have been shown to promote the release of the inhibitory transmitter GABA *(194)*. Thus, reduced function of α4β2 AChRs might produce the excessive activation characteristic of epilepsy, if, under the right circumstances in the wake/ sleep cycle, reduced AChR function caused reduced inhibition. However, the two most recently discovered ADNFLE mutations were both in β2 subunits and were found to cause excessive function when expressed with α4 *(11,12)*. As an example, a V287M mutation in a conserved valine near the C-terminal end of M2 causes a 10-fold increase in ACh potency and reduced desensitization *(11)*. Since β2 can also function in combinations with α2, α3, and α6, it is possible that one of these combinations or α4β2 AChRs in a different circuit could account for ADNFLE. Clearly, it is much more difficult to study neuronal AChR mutations than muscle AChRs because the many complex functions of neuronal AChRs in many overlapping circuits are not well known and because biopsy material is not usually available or easy to study.

The autonomic dysfunction and neonatal lethality of α3 or β2 plus β4 knockouts in mice *(175,185)* resemble the human disease megacystic micro-colon hypoperistalsis syndrome. No AChR mutations have yet been found to account for this disease *(195)*.

The large number of mutations found in muscle AChRs *(153,159)* make it seem likely that there are many neuronal AChR mutation syndromes to be discovered. Instead of affecting a single subtype of AChR, and producing symptoms of one basic type, with varying degrees or features of myasthenia, congenital neuronal AChR mutation syndromes will probably be discovered that affect a wide range of AChR subtypes. These mutations might produce hyper- and hypofunction, and result in a wide range of pleotropic phenotypes affecting both the central and peripheral nervous systems as well as the non-neuronal tissues in which these AChRs are expressed.

## ACKNOWLEDGMENTS

The Lindstrom laboratory is supported by a grant from the NIH.

## REFERENCES

1. Lindstrom J. The structures of neuronal nicotinic receptors. In: Clementi F, Gotti C, Fornasari D, eds. *Neuronal Nicotinic Receptors Handbook*. Experimental Pharmacology, vol. 144. New York, Springer, 2000, pp. 101–162.
2. Berg D, Shoop R, Chang K, et al. Nicotinic acetylcholine receptors in ganglionic transmission. In: Clementi F, Gotti C, Fornasari D, eds. *Neuronal Nicotinic Receptors Handbook*. Experimental Pharmacology, vol. 144. New York, Springer, 2000, pp. 247–270.
3. Zoli M. Distribution of cholinergic neurons in the mammalian brain with special reference to their relationship with neuronal nicotinic receptors. In: Clementi F, Gotti C, Fornasari D, eds. *Neuronal Nicotinic Receptors Handbook*. Experimental Pharmacology, vol. 144. New York, Springer, 2000, pp. 13–30.
4. Kaiser S, Soliokov L, Wonnacott S. Presynaptic neuronal nicotinic receptors: pharmacology, heterogeneity, and cellular mechanisms. In: Clementi F, Gotti C, Fornasari D, eds. *Neuronal Nicotinic Receptors Handbook*. Experimental Pharmacology, vol. 144. New York, Springer, 2000, pp. 193–212.
5. Grando S, Horton R. The keratinocyte cholinergic system with acetylcholine as an epidermal cytotransmitter. *Curr Opin Dermatol* 1997;4:262–268.
6. Maus A, Pereira E, Karachunski P, et al. Human and rodent bronchial epithelial cells express functional nicotinic acetylcholine receptors. *Mol Pharmacol* 1998; 54:779–788.
7. Macklin K, Maus A, Pereira E, et al. Human vascular endothelial cells express functional nicotinic acetylcholine receptors. *J Pharmacol Exp Ther* 1998;287: 435–439.
8. Sekhon HS, Jia YB, Raab R, et al. Prenatal nicotine increases pulmonary alpha 7 nicotinic receptor expression and alters fetal lung development in monkeys. *J Clin Invest* 1999;103:637–647.

9. Engel AG, Ohno K, Sine SM. Congenital myasthenic syndromes—recent advances. *Arch Neurol* 1999;56:163–157.

10. Steinlein OK. Neuronal nicotinic receptors in human epilepsy. *Eur J Pharmacol* 2000;393:243–247.

11. Phillips HA, Favre I, Kirkpatrick M, et al. CHRNB2 is the second acetylcholine receptor subunit associated with autosomal dominant nocturnal frontal lobe epilepsy. *Am J Hum Genet* 2001;68:225–231.

12. De Fusco M, Becchetti A, Patrignani A, et al. The nicotinic receptor beta 2 subunit is mutant in nocturnal frontal lobe epilepsy. *Nat Genet* 2000;26:275–276.

13. Lindstrom J. Acetylcholine receptors and myasthenia. *Muscle Nerve* 2000;23:453–477.

14. Vernino S, Low PA, Fealey RD, et al. Autoantibodies to ganglionic acetylcholine receptors in autoimmune autonomic neuropathies. *N Engl J Med* 2000;343:847–855.

15. Grando SA. Autoimmunity to keratinocyte acetylcholine receptors in pemphigus. *Dermatology* 2000;201:290–295.

16. Dani J, Ji D, Zhou F-M. Synaptic plasticity and nicotine addiction. *Neuron* 2001;31:349–352.

17. Epping-Jordan M, Watkins S, Koob G, et al. Dramatic decreases in brain reward function during nicotine withdrawal. *Nature* 1998;393:76–79.

18. Peto R, Lopez AD, Boreham J, et al. Mortality from tobacco in developed countries—indirect estimation from national vital statistics. *Lancet* 1992;339:1268–1278.

19. Lloyd GK, Williams M. Neuronal nicotinic acetylcholine receptors as novel drug targets. *J Pharmacol Exp Ther* 2000;292:461–467.

20. Heeschen C, Jang J, Weis M, et al. Nicotine stimulates angiogenesis and promotes tumor growth and atherosclerosis. *Nat Med* 2001;7:833–839.

21. Karlin A, Akabas MH. Toward a structural basis for the function of nicotinic acetylcholine receptors and their cousins. *Neuron* 1995;15:1231–1244.

22. Galzi J-L, Devillers-Thiery A, Hussy N, et al. Mutations in the channel domain of a neuronal nicotinic receptor convert ion selectivity from cationic to anionic. *Nature* 1992;359:500–505.

23. Eisele JL, Bertrand S, Galzi J-L, et al. Chimeric nicotinic serotonergic receptor combines distinct ligand-binding and channel specificities. *Nature* 1993;366:479–483.

24. Lindstrom J. Purification and cloning of nicotinic acetylcholine receptors. In: Arneric S, Brioni D, eds. *Neuronal Nicotinic Receptors: Pharmacology and Therapeutic Opportunities.* New York, John Wiley & Sons, 1999, pp. 3–23.

25. Jackson MB. Perfection of a synaptic receptor—kinetics and energetics of the acetylcholine-receptor. *Proc Natl Acad Sci USA* 1989;86:2199–2203.

26. Sanes JR, Lichtman JW. Development of the vertebrate neuromuscular junction. *Annu Rev Neurosci* 1999;22:389–442.

27. Corringer PJ, LeNovere N, Changeux J-P. Nicotinic receptors at the amino acid level. *Annu Rev Pharmacol Toxicol* 2000;40;431–458.

28. Unwin N. Nicotinic acetylcholine receptor and the structural basis of fast synaptic transmission. *Philos Tran R Soc Lond B* 2000;1404:1813–1829.

29. Patrick J, Lindstrom J. Autoimmune response to acetylcholine receptor. *Science* 1973;180:871–872.

30. Tzartos SJ. Lindstrom JM. Monoclonal antibodies used to probe acetylcholine receptor structure: localization of the main immunogenic region and detection of similarities between subunits. *Proc Natl Acad Sci USA* 1980;77:755–759.

31. Tzartos SJ, Barkas T, Cung MT, et al. Anatomy of the antigenic structure of a large membrane autoantigen, the muscle-type nicotinic acetylcholine receptor. *Immunol Rev* 1998;163:89–120.

32. Smit AB, Syed NI, Schaap D, et al. A glia-derived acetylcholine-binding protein that modulates synaptic transmission. *Nature* 2001;411:261–268.

33. Brejc K, van Dijk WJ, Klaassen, et al. Crystal structure of an ACh-binding protein reveals the ligand-binding domain of nicotinic receptors. *Nature* 2001;411: 269–276.

34. Wells GB, Anand R, Wang F, Lindstrom J. Water-soluble nicotinic acetylcholine receptor formed by α7 subunit extracellular domains. *J Biol Chem* 1998;273:964–973.

35. Grutter T, Changeux J-P. Nicotinic receptors in wonderland. *Trends Biochem Sci* 2001;26:459–463.

36. Fu DX, Sine SM. Asymmetric contribution of the conserved disulfide loop to subunit oligomerization and assembly of the nicotinic acetylcholine receptor. *J Biol Chem* 1996;271:31,479–31,484.

37. Wilson GG, Karlin A. Acetylcholine receptor channel structure in the resting, open, and desensitized states probed with the substituted-cysteine-accessibility method. *Proc Natl Acad Sci USA* 2001;98:1241–1248.

38. Das MK, Lindstrom J. Epitope mapping of antibodies to acetylcholine receptor-alpha subunits using peptides synthesized on polypropylene pegs. *Biochemistry* 1991;30:2470–2477.

39. Maimone MM, Merlie JP. Interaction of the 43 kd postsynaptic protein with all subunits of the muscle nicotinic acetylcholine-receptor. *Neuron* 1993;11:53–66.

40. Conroy WG, Berg DK. Rapsyn variants in ciliary ganglia and their possible effects on clustering of nicotinic receptors. *J Neurochem* 1999;73:1399–1408.

41. Jeanclos E, Lin L, Trevel M, Rao J, DeCoster M, Anand R. The chaperone protein 14-3-3 η interacts with the nicotinic receptor α4 subunit. *J Biol Chem* 2001;276: 28,281–28,290.

42. Keller S, Lindstrom J, Taylor P. Involvement of the chaperone protein calnexin and the acetylcholine receptor β subunit in the assembly and cell surface expression of the receptor. *J Biol Chem* 1996;271:22,871–22,877.

43. Keller D, Taylor P. Determinants responsible for assembly of the nicotinic acetylcholine receptor. *J Gen Physiol* 1999;113:171–176.

44. Keller SH, Lindstrom J, Taylor P. Adjacent basic amino acid residues recognized by the COPI complex and ubiquitination govern endoplasmic reticulum to cell surface trafficking of the nicotinic acetylcholine receptor alpha-subunit. *J Biol Chem* 2001;276:18,384–18,391.

45. Miles K, Huganir RL. Regulation of nicotinic acetylcholine-receptors by protein-phosphorylation. *Mol Neurobiol* 1988;2:91–124.

46. Fenster CP, Beckman ML, Parker JC, et al. Regulation of alpha 4 beta 2 nicotinic receptor desensitization by calcium and protein kinase C. *Mol Pharmacol* 1999; 55:432–443.

47. Williams BM, Temburni MK, Levy MS, et al. The long internal loop of the α3 subunit targets nAChRs to subdomains within individual synapses on neurons in vivo. *Nat Neurosci* 1998;1:557–562.
48. Bougat C, Bren N, Sine SM. Structural basis of the different gating kinetics of fetal and adult acetylcholine receptors. *Neuron* 1994;13:1395–1402.
49. Paradiso K, Zhang J, Steinbach J. The C terminus of the human nicotinic α4β2 receptor forms a binding site required for potentiation by an estrogenic steroid. *J Neurosci* 2001;21:6561–6568.
50. Curtis L, Buisson B, Bertrand S, Bertrand D. Allosteric potentiation of the α4β2 neuronal nicotinic acetylcholine receptor by estradiol. *Neurosciences Society Meeting* 2000; abstract 235.13.
51. LeNovere N, Changeux JP. Molecular evolution of the nicotinic acetylcholine-receptor—an example of a multigene family in excitable cells. *J Mol Evol* 1995; 40:155–172.
52. Duvoisin R, Deneris E, Patrick J, Heinemann S. The functional diversity of the neu-ronal nicotinic receptors is increased by a novel subunit: β4. *Neuron* 1989;3: 487–496.
53. Schoepfer R, Conroy W, Whiting P, Gore M, Lindstrom J. Brain α-bungarotoxin binding-protein cDNAs and mAbs reveal subtypes of this branch of the ligand-gated ion channel gene superfamily. *Neuron* 1990;5:35–48.
54. Elgoyhen A, Vetter D, Katz E, et al. Alpha 10: a determinant of nicotinic cholinergic receptor function in mammalian vestibular and cochlear mechanosensory hair cells. *Proc Natl Acad Sci USA* 2001;98:3501–3506.
55. Lustig LR, Peng H, Hiel H, Yamamoto T, Fuchs P. Molecular cloning and mapping of the human nicotinic acetylcholine receptor alpha 10 (CHRNA10). *Genomics* 2001;73:272–283.
56. Wang F, Gerzanich V, Wells GB, et al. Assembly of human neuronal nicotinic receptor α5 subunits with α3, β2, and β4 subunits. *J Biol Chem* 1996;271:17,656–17,665.
57. Forsayeth JR, Kobrin E. Formation of oligomers containing the β3 and β4 subunits of the rat nicotinic receptor. *J Neurosci* 1997;17:1531–1538.
58. Fucile S, Barabino B, Palma E, et al. α5 subunit forms functional α3β4α5 nAChRs in transfected human cells. *Neuroreport* 1997;8:2433–2436.
59. Vailati S, Hanke W, Bejan A, et al. Functional α6-containing nicotinic receptors are present in chick retina. *Mol Pharmacol* 1999;56:11–19.
60. Kuryatov A, Olale F, Cooper J, Choi C, Lindstrom J. Human α6 AChR subtypes: subunit composition, assembly, and pharmacological responses. *Neuropharmacology* 2000;39:2570–2590.
61. Groot-Kormelink P, Luyten W, Colquhoun D, Silviotti L. A reporter mutation approach shows incorporation of the "orphan" subunit β3 into a functional nicotinic receptor. *J Biol Chem* 1998;273:15,317–15,320.
62. Boorman J, Groot-Kormelink P, Silviotti L. Stoichiometry of human recombinant neuronal nicotinic receptors containing the β3 subunit expressed in *Xenopus* oocytes. *J Physiol* 2000;529:565–577.
63. Conroy WG, Berg DK. Neurons can maintain multiple classes of nicotinic acetylcholine-receptors distinguished by different subunit compositions. *J Biol Chem* 1995;270:4424–4431.

64. Lena C, deKerchove d'Exaerde AD, et al. Diversity and distribution of nicotinic acetylcholine receptors in the locus ceruleus neurons. *Proc Natl Acad Sci USA* 1999;96:12,126–12,131.

65. Shoop RD, Chang KT, Ellisman MH, Berg D. Synaptically driven calcium transients via nicotinic receptors on somatic spines. *J Neurosci* 2001;21:771–781.

66. Nelson M, Wang F, Kuryatov A, et al. Functional properties of human nicotinic AChRs expressed in IMR-32 neuroblastoma cells resemble those of α3β4 AChRs expressed in permanently transfected HEK cells. *J Gen Physiol* 2001;118: 563–582.

67. Klink R, deKerchove d'Exaerde A, Zoli M, Changeux J-P. Molecular and physiological diversity of nicotinic acetylcholine receptors in the midbrain dopaminergic nuclei. *J Neurosci* 2001;21:1452–1463.

68. Ramirez-Latorre J, Yu C, Qu X, et al. Functional contributions of α5 subunit to neuronal acetylcholine receptor channels. *Nature* 1996;380:347–351.

69. Gerzanich V, Wang F, Kuryatov, A, Lindstrom J. α5 subunit alters desensitization, pharmacology, Ca++ permeability and Ca++ modulation of human neuronal α3 nicotinic receptors. *J Pharmacol Exp Ther* 1998;286:311–320.

70. Sussman JL, Harel M, Frolow F, et al. Atomic-structure of acetylcholinesterase from *Torpedo californica*—a prototypic acetylcholine-binding protein. *Science* 1991;253:872–879.

71. Bohler S, Gay S, Bertrand S, et al. Desensitization of neuronal nicotinic receptors conferred by N-terminal segments of the β2 subunit. *Biochemistry* 2001;40:2066–2074.

72. Prince RJ, Sine SM. Acetylcholine and epibatidine binding to muscle acetylcholine receptors distinguish between concerted and uncoupled models. *J Biol Chem* 1999;274:19,623–19,629.

73. Kuffler S, Yoshikami D. The number of transmitter molecules in a quantum. *J Physiol* 1975;251:465–482.

74. Steinbach J, Chen Q. Antagonist and partial agonist actions of d-tubocurarine at mammalian muscle acetylcholine-receptors. *J Neurosci* 1995;15:230–240.

75. Malany S, Osaka H, Sine SM, Taylor P. Orientation of αneurotoxin at the subunit interfaces of the nicotinic acetylcholine receptor. *Biochemistry* 2000;39:15,388–15,398.

76. Magleby K. Neuromuscular transmission. In: Engel A, Franzini-Armstrong C, eds. *Myology: Basic and Clinical*, 2nd ed, vol. 1. New York, McGraw Hill, 1994, pp. 442–463.

77. Gunderson CH, Lehmann CR, Sidell FR, Gabbari B. Nerve agents—a review. *Neurology* 1992;42:946–950.

78. Benowitz N. Pharmacology of nicotine: addiction and therapeutics. *Annu Rev Pharmacol Toxicol* 1996;36:597–613.

79. Kopta C, Steinbach J. Comparison of mammalian adult and fetal nicotinic acetylcholine receptors stably expressed in fibroblasts. *J Neurosci* 1994;14:3922–3933.

80. Papke RL, Meyer E, Nutter T, Uteshev V. α7 receptor-selective agonists and modes of α7 receptor activation. *Eur J Pharmacol* 2000;393:179–195.

81. Froehner SC. Identification of exposed and buried determinants of the membrane-bound acetylcholine receptor from *Torpedo californica*. *Biochemistry* 1981;20: 4905–4915.

82. Tzartos SJ, Seybold ME, Lindstrom JM. Specificities of antibodies to acetylcholine receptors in sera from myasthenia gravis patients measured by monoclonal antibodies. *Proc Natl Acad Sci USA* 1982;79:188–192.

83. Kontou M, Leonidas D, Vatzaki E, et al. The crystal structure of the Fab fragment of a rat monoclonal antibody against the main immunogenic region of the human muscle acetylcholine receptor. *Eur J Biochem* 2000;267:2389–2396.

84. Poulas K, Eliopoulas E, Vatzoki E, et al. Crystal structure of Fab 198, an efficient protector of the acetylcholine receptor agonist myasthenogenic antibodies. *Eur J Biochem* 2001;268:3685–3693.

85. Saedi MS, Anand R, Conroy WG, Lindstrom J. Determination of amino-acids critical to the main immunogenic region of intact acetylcholine-receptors by in vitro mutagenesis. *FEBS Lett* 1990;267:55–59.

86. Lindstrom J, Shelton GD, Fujii Y. Myasthenia gravis. *Adv Immunol* 1988;42:233–284.

87. Beroukhim R, Unwin N. 3-Dimensional location of the main immunogenic region of the acetylcholine receptor. *Neuron* 1995;15:323–331.

88. Lindstrom J. An assay for antibodies to human acetylcholine receptor in serum from patients with myasthenia gravis. *Clin Immunol Immunopathol* 1977;7:36–43.

89. Engel A, ed. *Myasthenia Gravis and Myasthenic Disorders*. Contemporary Neurology Series. New York, Oxford University Press, 1999.

90. Heinemann S, Bevan S, Kullberg R, Lindstrom J, Rice J. Modulation of the acetylcholine receptor by anti-receptor antibody. *Proc Natl Acad Sci USA* 1977;74: 3090–3094.

91. Drachman DB, Angus CW, Adams RN, Michelson J, Hoffman G. Myasthenic antibodies cross-link acetylcholine receptors to accelerate degradation. *N Engl J Med* 1978;298:1116–1122.

92. Drachman D. The biology of myasthenia gravis. *Annu Rev Neurosci* 1981;4:195–225.

93. Blatt Y, Montal MS, Lindstrom J, Montal M. Monoclonal antibodies specific to the β-subunit and γ-subunit of the *Torpedo* acetylcholine receptor inhibit single-channel activity. *J Neurosci* 1986;6:481–486.

94. Shelton GD, Cardinet GH, Lindstrom JM. Canine and human myasthenia gravis autoantibodies recognize similar regions on the acetylcholine receptor. *Neurology* 1988;38:1417–1423.

95. Weinberg CB, Hall ZW. Antibodies from patients with myasthenia gravis recognize determinants unique to extrajunctional acetylcholine receptors. *Proc Natl Acad Sci USA* 1979;76:504–508.

96. Burges J, Wray DW, Pizzighella S, Hall Z, Vincent A. A myasthenia gravis plasma immunoglobulin reduces miniature endplate potentials at human endplates in vitro. *Muscle Nerve* 1990;13:407–413.

97. Vincent A, Newland C, Brueton L, et al. Arthrogryposis multiplex congenita with maternal autoantibodies specific for a fetal antigen. *Lancet* 1995;346:24–25.

98. Conti-Fine BM, Navaneetham D, Karachunski PI, et al. T cell recognition of the acetylcholine receptor in myasthenia gravis. *Ann NY Acad Sci* 1998;841:283–308.

99. Beeson D, Bond AP, Corlett L, et al. Thymus, thymoma, and specific T cells in myasthenia gravis. *Ann NY Acad Sci* 1998;841:371–387.

100. Fujii Y, Lindstrom J. Specificity of the T-cell immune response to acetylcholine receptor in experimental autoimmune myasthenia gravis—response to subunits and synthetic peptides. *J Immunol* 1988;140:1830–1837.
101. Hohlfeld R, Wekerle H. The immunopathogenesis of myasthenia gravis. In: Engel A, ed. *Myasthenia Gravis and Myasthenic Disorders.* Contemporary Neurology Series, vol. 56. New York, Oxford University Press, 1999, pp. 87–110.
102. Raju R, Spack E, David C. Acetylcholine receptor peptide recognition in HLA DR3-transgenic mice: in vivo responses correlate with MHC-peptide binding. *J Immunol* 2001;167:1118–1124.
103. Ong B, Willcox N, Wordsworth P, et al. Critical role for the val/gly[86] HLA-DR-β dimorphism in autoantigen presentation to human T-cells. *Proc Natl Acad Sci USA* 1991;88:7343–7347.
104. Christadoss P, Lindstrom JM, Melvold RW, Talal N. IA subregion mutation prevents experimental autoimmune myasthenia gravis. *Immunogenetics* 1985;21:33–38.
105. Christadoss P, Poussin M, Deng CS. Animal models of myasthenia gravis. *Clin Immunol* 2000;94:75–87.
106. Shelton D, Lindstrom J. Spontaneous remission in canine myasthenia gravis: implications for assessing human therapies. *Neurology* 2001;57:2139–2141.
107. Russell A, Lindstrom J. Penicillamine induced myasthenia gravis associated with antibodies to the acetylcholine receptor. *Neurology* 1989;28:847–849.
108. Vincent A, Newsom-Davis J, Martin V. Anti-acetylcholine receptor antibodies in D-penicillamine associated myasthenia gravis. *Lancet* 1978;I:1254.
109. Penn AS, Low BW, Jaffe IA, Luo L, Jacques J. Drug-induced autoimmune myasthenia gravis. *Ann NY Acad Sci* 1998;841:433–449.
110. Keesey J, Lindstrom J, Cokely A. Anti-acetylcholine receptor antibody in neonatal myasthenia gravis. *N Engl J Med* 1977;296:55.
111. Vernet der Garabedian B, Lacokova M, Eymard B, et al. Association of neonatal myasthenia gravis with antibodies against the fetal acetylcholine receptor. *J Clin Invest* 1994;94:555–559.
112. Willcox H. Thymic tumors with myasthenia gravis or bone marrow dyscrasias. In: Peckham M, ed. *Oxford Textbook of Oncology.* New York, Oxford University Press, 1995, pp. 1562–1568.
113. Vincent A, Newsom-Davis J. Acetylcholine receptor antibody characteristics in myasthenia gravis. I: patients with generalized myasthenia or disease restricted to ocular muscles. *Clin Exp Immunol* 1982;49:257–265.
114. Baggi F, Andreetta F, Antozzi C, et al. Anti-titin and antiryanodine receptor antibodies in myasthenia gravis patients with thymoma. *Ann NY Acad Sci* 1998;841: 538–541.
115. Cikes N, Momoi M, Williams C, et al. Striational autoantibodies: quantitative detection by enzyme immunoassay in myasthenia gravis, thymoma and recipients of D-penicillamine or allogenic bone marrow. *Mayo Clin Proc* 1998;63:474–481.
116. Wakkach A, Guyon T, Bruand C, et al. Expression of acetylcholine receptor genes in human thymic epithelial cells. Implications for myasthenia gravis. *J Immunol* 1996;157:3752–3760.
117. Zheng Y, Whatly L, Liu T, Levinson A. Acetylcholine receptor α subunit in mRNA expression in human thymus: augmented expression in myasthenia gravis and upregulation by interferon-δ. *Clin Immunol* 1999;91:170–177.

118. Vincent A, Lang B, Newsom-Davis. Autoimmunity to the voltage-gated calcium channel underlies the Lambert-Eaton myasthenic syndrome, a paraneoplastic disorder. *TINS* 1989;12:496–502.
119. Vincent A, Willcox N, Hill M, et al. Determinant spreading and immunoresponses to acetylcholine receptors in myasthenia gravis. *Immunol Rev* 1998;164:157–168.
120. Bartfeld D, Fuchs S. Specific immunosuppression of experimental autoimmune myasthenia gravis by denatured acetylcholine receptor. *Proc Natl Acad Sci USA* 1978;75:4006–4010.
121. Lindstrom J, Einarson B, Merlie J. Immunization of rats with polypeptide chains from *Torpedo* acetylcholine receptor causes an autoimmune response to receptors in rat muscle. *Proc Natl Acad Sci USA* 1978;75:769–773.
122. Lindstrom J, Peng X, Kuryatov A, et al. Molecular and antigenic structure of nicotinic acetylcholine receptors. *Ann NY Acad Sci* 1998;841:71–86.
123. Bachmaier K, Nen N, de la Maza L, et al. *Chlamydia* infections and heart disease linked through antigenic mimicry. *Science* 1999;283:1335–1339.
124. Nachamkin I, Allos B, Ho T. *Campylobacter* species and Guillain Barré syndrome. *Clin Microbiol Rev* 1998;11:555–567.
125. Faller G, Steininger H, Kranzlein J, et al. Antigastric autoantibodies in *Helicobacter pylori* infection: implications of histological and clinical parameters of gastritis. *Gut* 1997;41:619–623.
126. Lindstrom J, Einarson B, Lennon V, Seybold M. Pathological mechanisms in EAMG. I: Immunogenicity of syngeneic muscle acetylcholine receptor and quantitative extraction of receptor and antibody-receptor complexes from muscles of rats with experimental autoimmune myasthenia gravis. *J Exp Med* 1976;144: 726–738.
127. Jermy A, Beeson D, Vincent A. Pathogenic autoimmunity to affinity-purified mouse acetylcholine receptor induced without adjuvant in BALB/c mice. *Eur J Immunol* 1993;23:973–976.
128. Lindstrom J. Experimental induction and treatment of myasthenia gravis. In: Engel A, ed. *Myasthenia Gravis and Myasthenic Disorders.* Contemporary Neurology Series, New York, Oxford University Press, 1999, pp. 111–130.
129. Zoda T, Krolick K. Antigen presentation and T cell specificity repertoire in determining responsiveness to an epitope important in experimental autoimmune myasthenia gravis. *J Neuroimmunol* 1993;43:131–138.
130. Lindstrom J, Seybold M, Lennon V, Whittingham S, Duane D. Antibody to acetylcholine receptor in myasthenia gravis: prevalence, clinical correlates, and diagnostic value. *Neurology* 1976;26:1054–1059.
131. Vincent A, Newsom-Davis J. Acetylcholine receptor antibody as a diagnostic test for myasthenia gravis: results in 153 validated cases and 2,967 diagnostic assays. *J Neurol Neurosurg Psychiatry* 1985;48:1246–1252.
132. Seybold M, Lindstrom J. Patterns of acetylcholine receptor antibody fluctuation in myasthenia gravis. *Ann NY Acad Sci* 1981;377:292–306.
133. Lindstrom J, Engel A, Seybold M, Lennon V, Lambert E. Pathological mechanisms in EAMG. II: Passive transfer of experimental autoimmune myasthenia gravis in rats with anti-acetylcholine receptor antibodies. *J Exp Med* 1976;144:739–753.
134. Tzartos S, Hochschwender S, Vasquez P, Lindstrom J. Passive transfer of experimental autoimmune myasthenia gravis by monoclonal antibodies to the main

immunogenic region of the acetylcholine receptor. *J Neuroimmunol* 1987;15: 185–194.

135. Toyka KV, Drachman DB, Pestronk A, Kao I. Myasthenia gravis: passive transfer from man to mouse. *Science* 1975;190:397–399.

136. Toyka KV, Birmberger KL, Anzil AP, et al. Myasthenia gravis: further electrophysiological and ultrastructural analysis of transmission failure in the mouse passive transfer model. *J Neurol Neurosurg Psychiatry* 1978;41:746–753.

137. Engel A, Tsujihata M, Lambert E, Lindstrom J, Lennon V. Experimental autoimmune myasthenia gravis: a sequential and quantitative study of the neuromuscular junction ultrastructure and electrophysiologic correlation. *J Neuropathol Exp Neurol* 1976;35:569–587.

138. Engel A, Tsujihata M, Lindstrom J, Lennon V. End-plate fine structure in myasthenia gravis and in experimental autoimmune myasthenia gravis. *Ann NY Acad Sci* 1976;274:60–79.

139. Engel A, Sakakibara H, Sahashi K, et al. Passively transferred experimental autoimmune myasthenia gravis. *Neurology* 1979;29:179–188.

140. Bevan S, Heinemann S, Lennon V, Lindstrom J. Reduced muscle acetylcholine sensitivity in rats immunized with acetylcholine receptor. *Nature* 1976;260:438–439.

141. Lambert E, Lindstrom J, Lennon V. End-plate potentials in experimental autoimmune myasthenia gravis in rats. *Ann NY Acad Sci* 1976;274:300–318.

142. Lindstrom J, Lambert E. Content of acetylcholine receptor and antibodies bound to receptor in myasthenia gravis, experimental autoimmune myasthenia gravis, and in Eaton-Lambert syndrome. *Neurology* 1978;28:130–138.

143. Sahashi K, Engel A, Lindstrom J, Lambert EH, Lennon V. Ultrastructural localization of immune complexes (IgG and C3) at the end-plate in experimental autoimmune myasthenia gravis. *J Neuropathol Exp Neurol* 1978;37:212–223.

144. Sahashi K, Engel A, Lambert E, Howard F. Ultrastructural localization of the terminal and lytic ninth complement component (C9) at the motor end-plate in myasthenia gravis. *J Neuropathol Exp Neurol* 1980;39:160–172.

145. Appel S, Anwyl R, McAdams M, Elias S. Accelerated degradation of acetylcholine receptor from cultured rat myotubes with myasthenia gravis sera and globulins. *Proc Natl Acad Sci USA* 1977;74:2130–2134.

146. Bufler J, Pitz R, Czep M, Wick M, Franke C. Purified IgG from seropositive and seronegative patients with myasthenia gravis reversibly blocks currents through nicotinic acetylcholine receptor channels. *Ann Neurol* 1998;43:458–464.

147. Burges J, Vincent A, Molenaar P, et al. Passive transfer of seronegative myasthenia gravis to mice. *Muscle Nerve* 1994;17:1393–1400.

148. Donnelly D, Mihovilovic M, Gonzalez-Ros J, et al. A noncholinergic site-directed monoclonal antibody can impair agonist-induced ion flux in *Torpedo californica* acetylcholine receptor. *Proc Natl Acad Sci USA* 1984;81:7999–8003.

149. Fels G, Plumer-Wilk R, Schreiber M, Maelicke A. A monoclonal antibody interfering with binding and response of the acetylcholine receptor. *J Biol Chem* 1986; 261:15,746–15,754.

150. Gomez G, Richman D. Anti-acetylcholine receptor antibodies directed against the α bungarotoxin binding site induce a unique form of experimental myasthenia. *Proc Natl Acad Sci USA* 1983;80:4089–4093.

151. Lang B, Richardson G, Rees J, Vincent A, Newsom-Davis J. Plasma from myasthenia gravis patients reduces acetylcholine receptor agonist-induced $Na^+$ flux into TE671 cell line. *J Neuroimmunol* 1988;19:141–148.

152. Lennon V, Seybold M, Lindstrom J, Cochrane C, Yulevitch R. Role of complement in pathogenesis of experimental autoimmune myasthenia gravis. *J Exp Med* 1978;147:973–983.

153. Engel A, Ohno K, Sine S. Congenital myasthenic syndromes. *Arch Neurol* 1999; 56:163–167.

154. Sine SM, Ohno K, Bougat C, et al. Mutation of the acetylcholine-receptor alpha-subunit causes a slow-channel myasthenic syndrome by enhancing agonist binding-affinity. *Neuron* 1995;15:229–239.

155. Ohno K, Wang HL, Milone M, et al. Congenital myasthenic syndrome caused by decreased agonist binding affinity due to a mutation in the acetylcholine receptor epsilon subunit. *Neuron* 1996;17:157–170.

156. Ohno K, Hutchinson DO, Milone M, et al. Congenital myasthenic syndrome caused by prolonged acetylcholine-receptor channel openings due to a mutation in the M2 domain of the epsilon-subunit. *Proc Natl Acad Sci USA* 1995;92:758–762.

157. Engel A, Uchitel O, Walls T, et al. Newly recognized congenital myasthenic syndrome associated with high conductance and fast closure of the acetylcholine receptor channel. *Ann Neurol* 1993;34:38–47.

158. Engel A, Ohno K, Milone M, Sine S. Congenital myasthenic syndromes caused by mutations in acetylcholine receptor genes. *Neurology* 1997;48(Suppl 5):S28–S35.

159. Engel A, Ohno K, Wang H-L, Milone M, Sine S. The molecular basis of congenital myasthenic syndromes: mutations in the acetylcholine receptor. *Neuroscientist* 1998;4:185–194.

160. Ohno K, Anlar B, Engel A. Congenital myasthenic syndrome caused by a mutation in the Ets-binding site of the promoter region of the acetylcholine receptor ε subunit gene. *Neuromusc Dis* 1999;9:131–135.

161. Ohno K, Anlar B, Ozdirim E, et al. Myasthenic syndromes in Turkish kinships due to mutations in the acetylcholine receptor. *Ann Neurol* 1998;44:234–241.

162. Ohno K, Quiram P, Milone M, et al. Congenital myasthenic syndromes due to heteroallelic nonsense/missence mutations in the acetylcholine receptor ε subunit gene: identification and functional characterization of six new mutations. *Hum Mol Gene* 1997;6:753–766.

163. Engel A, Ohno K, Milone M, et al. New mutations in acetylcholine receptor subunit genes reveal heterogeneity in the slow channel congenital myasthenic syndrome. *Hum Mol Genet* 1996;5:1217–1227.

164. Missias A, Mudd J, Cunningham J, et al. Deficient development and maintenance of postsynaptic specializations in mutant mice locking an "adult" acetylcholine receptor subunit. *Development* 1997;124:5075–5086.

165. Milone M, Wang H-L, Ohno, et al. Slow channel syndrome caused by enhanced activation, desensitization, and agonist binding affinity due to mutation in the M2 domain of the acetylcholine receptor α subunit. *J Neurosci* 1997;17:5651–5665.

166. Wang H-L, Auerbach A, Bren N, et al. Mutation in the M1 domain of the acetylcholine receptor α subunit decreases the rate of agonist dissociation. *J Gen Physiol* 1997;109:757–766.

167. Lo D, Pinkham J, Stevens C. Role of a key cystein residue in the gating of the acetylcholine receptor. *Neuron* 1991;6:31–40.
168. Zhou M, Engel A, Auerbach A. Serum choline activates mutant acetylcholine receptors that cause slow channel congenital myasthenic syndromes. *Proc Natl Acad Sci USA* 1999;96:10,466–10,471.
169. Bertrand D, Devillers-Thiery A, Revah F, et al. Unconventional pharmacology of a neuronal nicotinic receptor mutated in the channel domain. *Proc Natl Acad Sci USA* 1992;89:1261–1265.
170. Alkondon M, Pereira E, Eisenberg H, Albuquerque E. Choline and selective antagonists identify two subtypes of nicotinic acetylcholine receptors that modulate GABA release from CAI interneurons in rat hippocampal slices. *J Neurosci* 1999; 19:2693–2705.
171. Milone M, Wang H-L, Ohno K, et al. Mode switching kinetics produced by a naturally occurring mutation in the cytoplasmic loop of the human acetylcholine receptor ε subunit. *Neuron* 1998;20:575–588.
172. Han Z-Y, LeNovere N, Zoli M, et al. Localization of nAChR subunit mRNAs in the brain of *Macaca mulatta*. *Eur J Neurosci* 2000;12:3664–3674.
173. Vailati S, Moretti M, Balestra B, et al. β3 subunit is present in different nicotinic receptor subtypes in chick retina. *Eur J Pharmacol* 2000;393:23–30.
174. Wonnacott S. Presynaptic nicotinic ACh receptors. *Trends Neurosci* 1997;20:92–98.
175. Xu W, Gelber S, Orr-Urtreger A, et al. Megacystis, mydriasis, and ion channel defect in mice lacking the α3 neuronal nicotinic receptor. *Proc Natl Acad Sci USA* 1999;96:5746–5751.
176. Marubio L, del Mar Arroyo-Jiminez M, Cordero-Erausquin M, et al. Reduced antinociception in mice lacking neuronal nicotinic receptor subunits. *Nature* 1999; 398:805–810.
177. Ross S, Wong J, Clifford J, et al. Phenotypic characterization of an α4 neuronal nicotinic acetylcholine receptor subunit knockout mouse. *J Neurosci* 2000;20:6431–6441.
178. Labarca C, Schwarz J, Deshpande P, et al. Point mutant mice with hypersensitive α4 nicotinic receptors show dopaminergic defects and increased anxiety. *Proc Natl Acad Sci USA* 2001;98:2786–2791.
179. Berger F, Gage F, Vijayaraghavan S. Nicotinic receptor-induced apoptotic cell death of hippocampal progenitor cells. *J Neurosci* 1998;18:6871–6881.
180. Orr-Urtreger A, Göldner F, Saeki M, et al. Mice deficient in the α7 neuronal nicotinic acetylcholine receptor lack α bungarotoxin binding sites and hippocampal fast nicotinic currents. *J Neurosci* 1997;17:9165–9171.
181. Franceschine D, Orr-Urtreger A, Yu W, et al. Altered baroreflex responses in α7 deficient mice. *Behav Brain Res* 2000;113:3–10.
182. Orr-Urtreger A, Broide R, Kasten M, et al. Mice homozygous for the L250T mutation in the α7 nicotinic acetylcholine receptor show increased neuronal apoptosis and die within 1 day of birth. *J Neurochem* 2000;74:2154–2166.
183. Vetter D, Liberman M, Mann J, et al. Role of α9 nicotinic ACh receptor subunits in the development and function of cochlear efferent innervation. *Neuron* 1999; 23:91–103.
184. Picciotto M, Caldarone B, King S, Zachariou V. Nicotinic receptors in the brain: links between molecular biology and behavior. *Neuropsychopharmacology* 2000; 22:451–465.

185. Xu W, Orr-Urtreger A, Nigro F, et al. Multiorgan autonomic dysfunction in mice lacking the β2 and β4 subunits of neuronal nicotinic acetylcholine receptors. *J Neurosci* 1999;19:9298–9305.
186. Allen R, Cui C, Heinemann S. Gene targeted knockout of the β3 neuronal nicotinic acetylcholine receptor subunit. *Soc Neurosci Abstr* 1998;24:1341.
187. Vailati S, Moretti M, Balestra M, et al. β3 subunit is present in different nicotinic receptor subtypes in chick retina. *Eur J Pharmacol* 2000;393:23–30.
188. Balestra B, Moretti M, Longhi R, et al. Antibodies against neuronal nicotinic receptor subtypes in neurological disorders. *J Neuroimmunol* 2000;102:89–97.
189. Nguyen V, Ndoye A, Grando S. *Pemphigus vulgaris* antibody identifies pemphaxin—a novel keratinocyte annexin-like molecule binding acetylcholine. *J Biol Chem* 2000;275:29,466–29,476.
190. Rogers S, Andrews J, Gahring L, et al. Autoantibodies to glutamate receptor in GluR3 in Rasmussen's encephalitis. *Science* 1994;265:648–651.
191. Rogers S, Twyman R, Gahring L. The role of autoimmunity to glutamate receptors in neurological disease. *Mod Med Today* 1996;2:76–81.
192. Gahring L, Rogers S. Autoimmunity to glutamate receptors in Rasmussen's encephalitis: a rare finding or the tip of an iceberg? *Neuroscientist* 1998;4:373–379.
193. Kuryatov A, Gerzanich V, Nelson M, Olale F, Lindstrom J. Mutation causing autosomal dominant nocturnal frontal lobe epilepsy alters $Ca^{++}$ permeability, conductance, and gating of human α4β2 nicotinic acetylcholine receptors. *J Neurosci* 1997;17:9035–9047.
194. Alkondon M, Periera E, Eisenberg H, Albuquerque E. Nicotinic receptor activation in human cerebral cortical interneurons: a mechanism for inhibition and disinhibition of neuronal networks. *J Neurosci* 2000;20:66–75.
195. Lev-Lehman E, Bercovich D, Xu W, Stockton D, Beaudit A. Characterization of the human β4 nAChR gene and polymorphisms in CHRNA3 and CHRNB4. *J Hum Genet* 2001;46:362–366.
196. Anand R, Conroy WG, Schoepfer R, Whiting P, Lindstrom J. Chicken neuronal nicotinic acetylcholine receptors expressed in *Xenopus* oocytes have a pentameric quaternary structure. *J Biol Chem* 1991;266:11,192–11,198.
197. Cooper E, Couturier S, Ballivet M. Pentameric structure and subunit stoichiometry of a neuronal nicotinic acetylcholine receptor. *Nature* 1991;350:235–238.

# 3

# Immunopathogenesis of Myasthenia Gravis

## Bianca M. Conti-Fine, Brenda Diethelm-Okita, Norma Ostlie, Wei Wang, and Monica Milani

## INTRODUCTION

Myasthenia gravis (MG) is a prototypic antibody-mediated autoimmune disease and also the best characterized such disease: autoantibodies against the nicotinic acetylcholine receptor (AChR) at the neuromuscular junction (NMJ) cause the myasthenic manifestations *(1–4)*. Anti-AChR T-cells play a crucial role in the pathogenesis of MG, because they permit and modulate the synthesis of the high-affinity antibodies that cause AChR loss, damage of the NMJ, and failure of neuromuscular transmission. T-cells may even be the prime movers in MG pathogenesis, because activation of potentially self-reactive CD4$^+$ T-cells, commonly present in healthy people, may trigger autoimmune responses. This might occur because of crossreactivity of self-reactive CD4$^+$ T-cells with microbial antigens, or because of the action of microbial superantigens *(5,6)*.

In this chapter we briefly review the characteristics and pathogenic mechanisms of anti-AChR antibodies. We then describe the characteristics of the CD4$^+$ T-cell responses in MG and how specific immunosuppressive treatments of MG could target the anti-AChR CD4$^+$ T-cells. We also discuss the role that the thymus might play in the development of the anti-AChR autoimmune response. Finally, we present different models of the possible pathogenic mechanisms of MG.

## ANTIACETYLCHOLINE ANTIBODIES IN MYASTHENIA GRAVIS AND EXPERIMENTAL AUTOIMMUNE MYASTHENIA GRAVIS

Antimuscle AChR antibodies are the only direct cause of the neuromuscular transmission failure in MG. MG patients do not have detectable AChR-

From: *Current Clinical Neurology: Myasthenia Gravis and Related Disorders*
Edited by: H. J. Kaminski © Humana Press Inc., Totowa, NJ

specific cytotoxic phenomena mediated by T-cells *(7)*, and treatment of experimental animal with purified IgG from MG patients, or with anti-AChR antibodies, induces the symptoms of MG *(8–11)*. Also, procedures that reduce the concentration of anti-AChR antibodies, such as plasmapheresis, improve myasthenic weakness *(12)*.

Most (90%) of MG patients have anti-AChR antibodies in their serum, and IgG is detected bound at their NMJ *(1–4)*. About 10% of MG patients do not have detectable serum anti-AChR antibodies *(13)*. Some "seronegative" MG patients may synthesize small amounts of highly pathogenic antibodies, which quickly disappear from the serum because they bind to the NMJ *(14)*. However, other seronegative MG patients make autoantibodies that disrupt the neuromuscular transmission and are directed to muscle antigens other than the AChR *(15; see below)*.

The AChR is a large protein that can form many potential antibodies epitopes and accommodate simultaneous binding of several different antibodies *(16)*. The anti-AChR antibodies in MG patients recognize a complex epitope repertoire that is different in individual subjects *(1–4,16)*. Even the anti-AChR antibodies that recognize an individual AChR epitope region are polyclonal and do not share a dominant idiotype *(17)*. Furthermore, the anti-AChR antibodies of MG patients include different subclasses of the IgG heavy chain and different types of light chains *(1,16)*. Thus, many B-cell clones contribute to the anti-AChR antibody response in MG.

The epitope recognized and the type of heavy chain used by the anti-AChR antibodies influence their ability to cause failure of neuromuscular transmission and myasthenic weakness. Pathogenic antibodies need to recognize accessible areas of the AChR, or they could not bind to the intact postsynaptic membrane of the NMJ. Furthermore, certain surface areas of the AChR, like the main immunogenic region (MIR), are ideally situated to permit crosslinking of nearby AChR molecules *(16–18)*. Antibodies against those epitopes may be especially pathogenic for two reasons. First, they can accelerate AChR degradation *(19–21)* by a mechanism termed antigenic modulation *(22)*. Second, binding of several of these antibodies to the closely packed AChR molecules on the NMJ postsynaptic membrane would provide an ideal geometry for binding of complement and activation of the complement cascade *(16)*. The action of complement on the NMJ is an important pathogenic mechanism of anti-AChR antibodies *(23,24)*: anti-AChR antibodies of subclasses that bind complement effectively probably have a high pathogenic potential *(25)*.

Immunization of experimental animals with AChR from different sources causes experimentally acquired MG (EAMG), which reproduces the clinical and electrophysiologic features of MG *(1,16)*. Because of the strong structural similarity of muscle-type AChR from even distant species *(26)*, EAMG can be induced by immunization with the easily purified AChR from the electric organ of *Torpedo* and *Electrophorus* fish. Fish electric tissue is embryologically a modified muscle, and it is exceedingly rich in AChR *(26)*. Also, immunization with syngeneic AChR causes EAMG *(27,28)*: this indicates that self-reactive T- and B-cells specific for muscle AChR survive clonal deletion and persist in healthy adult animals.

Patrick and Lindstrom *(29)* first demonstrated the induction of EAMG in rabbits. Later studies described the induction of EAMG in a variety of species *(30–32)*. The most commonly used and the most useful animals for studying EAMG are Lewis rats, which are highly susceptible to EAMG *(31,33,34)*, and different mouse strains *(32,35,36)*. Mice have a lot of "spare" AChR at their NMJ, and they develop myasthenic weakness only when most of the AChR has been destroyed *(16)*. Different strains of mice have different susceptibilities to EAMG *(32,35–37)*. Even the most susceptible strains are relatively resistant to EAMG, and myasthenic weakness is usually subclinical *(1,16)*. Still, mice are quite useful for studying the mechanisms of EAMG, because their immune system is well characterized and there are abundant reagents to identify the different types and states of activation of mouse immune cells. Furthermore, a variety of congenic mouse strains carry null mutations of genes for cytokines or other molecules important in the immune response; other strains carry transgenes encoding important immune receptors or mediators. The C57Bl/6 strain is susceptible to EAMG, and it is the best studied mouse strain *(1,3,16)*. As in MG, high-affinity anti-AChR antibodies, whose synthesis is modulated by anti-AChR CD4$^+$ T-cells, cause the failure of neuromuscular transmission in EAMG *(1,3,16)*.

Anti-AChR antibodies cause the weakness, and in a given patient fluctuations in their serum concentration loosely correlate with disease severity *(38)*. However, there is little correlation between the serum anti-AChR antibody concentration among patients and the severity of their symptoms *(39)*. Some MG patients have high serum anti-AChR antibodies and minimal weakness. Conversely, severely ill MG patients may have few serum anti-AChR antibodies. Also, in EAMG the serum concentration of anti-AChR antibodies correlates poorly with the severity of myasthenic manifestations: EAMG-resistant and -susceptible rodent strains usually develop serum anti-AChR antibodies in comparable concentrations *(25,32,35,40–41)*. These findings suggest that only particular subpopulations of anti-AChR antibodies are pathogenic, whereas others are unable (or less able) to cause NMJ damage. The pathogenic antibodies may be made in different amounts in individual MG patients and rodent strains.

# EPITOPES RECOGNIZED
# BY ANTIACETYLCHOLINE RECEPTOR ANTIBODIES

Although the epitope repertoire of anti-AChR antibodies in MG patients and EAMG animals is heterogeneous and individual *(1)*, most of them recognize epitopes formed by the α-subunit *(1,16)*. This might occur because the muscle AChR has two α-subunits and one copy of the other subunits *(26)*: the α-subunit may be twice as effective as the others in activating T- and B-cells.

## The Main Immunogenic Region

Many of the anti-α-subunit antibodies recognize a set of largely overlapping epitopes, termed MIR *(16,17)*. Anti-MIR antibodies are highly pathogenic: they cause AChR loss in muscle cell cultures *(20)*, induce myasthenic weakness when injected into rodents *(42)*, and mediate the AChR loss in muscle cell cultures exposed to sera of MG patients *(21)*. Because of their abundance and pathogenicity, they are especially important in the development of MG.

The two MIRs of each AChR molecule are located on well-defined bumps at the tip of each of the domains formed by an α-subunit *(18)*. Residues within the sequence segment 67–76 of the α-subunit contribute to formation of the MIR: Asp68, Pro69, Asp71, and Tyr72 are especially important for binding of anti-MIR antibodies *(43–45)*.

Some structural characteristics of the MIR may contribute to its immunodominance, as discussed elsewhere. Also, most of the antibodies to a protein antigen may recognize just a few epitopes: the dominance of the MIR may reflect an especially focused antibody response. Molecular mimicry between the MIR and epitopes on unrelated but common antigens might also cause the immunodominance of the MIR. A sequence region of the AChR involved in forming the MIR is similar to a region of the pol-polyprotein of several human retroviruses (**Fig. 1**), and to a sequence region of the U1 small nuclear ribonucleoprotein—an autoantigen in systemic lupus erythematosus *(46)*. Crossreactivity of the MIR with epitopes on microbial or autologous antigens might facilitate the antibody response to the MIR and contribute to the MIR immunodominance.

## The Cholinergic Site

MG patients may have small amounts of anti-AChR antibodies that recognize the cholinergic binding site *(1,16)*. These may be important in certain presentations of MG, because antibodies to the cholinergic site cause an acute form of EAMG, without inflammation or necrosis at the NMJ *(47)*. Anti-

**A**

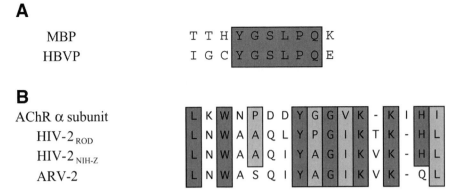

**Fig. 1.** Homology of self-epitopes and viral protein sequences may prove important in the pathogenesis of multiple sclerosis and myasthenia gravis. (**A**) Homology between the 66–75 sequence of human myelin basic protein and the 589–598 sequence of the hepatitis B virus polymerase. (**B**) Homology between the α56–80 sequence segment of human AChR and the polyprotein from three different human retroviruses (ARV-2 pol polyprotein segment 419–434, HIV-2$_{ROD}$ pol polyprotein segment 448–463, and HIV-2$_{NIH-Z}$ pol polyprotein segment 447–462).

bodies that recognize the cholinergic site and block the AChR function might contribute to the myasthenic weakness, in spite of their low concentration in the patients' sera. They might cause acute myasthenic crises and are probably responsible for the *Mary Walker phenomenon (48)*.

The Mary Walker phenomenon bears the name of the English physician who first realized that cholinesterase inhibitors could relieve the symptoms of MG *(49)*. This sobriquet refers to the increasing weakness that occurring in muscles that were not exercised, after vigorous exercise of other muscle groups. The Mary Walker phenomenon is consistent with the presence of soluble factors bound to muscle, released after exercise, and able to block neuromuscular transmission. Anti-AChR antibodies attached to the cholinergic binding sites at the NMJ may well be among those factors. The large concentrations of ACh in the synaptic cleft of the NMJ after strenuous exercise, especially in the presence of cholinesterase inhibitors, might cause the detachment of anti-AChR antibodies bound to the cholinergic site by competitive binding. The detached antibodies could diffuse away, to reach and block the AChR of other muscles.

## Non-AChR Antigens

Some MG patients do not have detectable anti-AChR antibodies *(13,22)*, yet the disease improves after removal of the blood antibodies by plasmapheresis

*(12,13)*, and their serum causes AChR dysfunctions in vitro *(50)*. These findings suggested that antibodies to the AChR, or to other proteins involved in neuromuscular transmission, cause myasthenic weakness. About 70% of the AChR-seronegative patients have autoantibodies against a protein important in neuromuscular transmission, the receptor tyrosine kinase MuSK *(15)*. Anti-MuSK antibodies interfere with the agrin/MuSK/AChR/ clustering in myotubes and alter MuSK function at the adult NMJ *(15)*.

Other AChR-seronegative patients make small amounts of pathogenic antibodies that bind the muscle AChR with high affinity *(14)*. Such antibodies are continuously removed from the bloodstream and may be undetectable in the serum.

MG patients may also have serum antibodies against other muscle or synaptic proteins (e.g., a presynaptic membrane protein that binds β-bungaro-toxin, and the $Ca^{2+}$-releasing sarcoplasmic membrane), whose block or destruction may contribute to the weakness *(51,52)*. MG patients without thymomas frequently have serum antibodies to myofibrillar muscle proteins (myo-sin, tropomyosin, troponin, α-actinin, and actin) *(53)*. The presence of anti-myosin antibodies in the serum correlates with the severity of the disease *(54)*. Some antibodies against myosin and fast troponin-1 crossreact with muscle AChRs, and specifically with the MIR, suggesting that these proteins bear epitopes structurally reminiscent of AChR epitopes *(55)*. MG patients with thymoma make antibodies that recognize contractile proteins of striated muscle in amounts correlating with that of anti-AChR antibodies *(56)*. Most of these antibodies bind to titin *(57)*, a giant myofibrillar protein, which may play a role in the elastic recoil of muscle fibers *(58)*. MG patients with thymoma may also have antibodies against the ryanodine receptor, the calcium channel of the sarcoplasmic reticulum *(59)*. It is not known whether the non-anti-AChR antibodies play a role in the pathogenesis of weakness in thymoma patients.

## ANTIACETYLCHOLINE RECEPTOR CD4+ T-HELPER CELLS

Most of the anti-AChR antibodies in the sera of MG patients are high-affinity IgGs, which are synthesized only after cytokines secreted by CD4+ T-helper cells activate the B-cells *(1–4)*. Anti-AChR CD4+ T-cells are common in the blood and thymi of MG patients *(1,3)*, and they have T-helper function *(60)*.

Several lines of evidence suggest that the CD4+ T-helper cells play a critical role in MG pathogenesis. Treatment of MG patients with anti-CD4 antibodies causes clinical and electrophysiologic improvement, which correlates with a disappearance of the AChR-induced T-cell responses in vitro *(61)*. Also, a decrease in the anti-AChR activity of blood T-cells is the only consistent and early effect of thymectomy *(62)*, a common treatment in the management of MG *(63)*. Previous studies used an in vivo cell transfer model to demonstrate the pivotal role of AChR-specific CD4$^+$ T-cells in rat EAMG: adoptive transfer into sublethally irradiated, thymectomized rats of a mixture of B-cells and CD4$^+$ T-cells from rats immunized with AChR caused synthesis of anti-AChR antibodies and EAMG weakness, whereas transfer of B-cells alone did not *(64)*. Other studies confirmed the essential role of CD4$^+$ T-cells for EAMG induction in rodents *(65,66)*. The findings obtained in EAMG support an important role of anti-AChR CD4$^+$ T-cells also in human MG.

Experiments in severe combined immunodeficient (SCID) mice grafted with immune cells from the blood of MG patients have proved that synthesis of pathogenic anti-AChR antibodies, and development of myasthenic manifestations, require CD4$^+$ T-cells, specifically anti-AChR CD4$^+$ T-cells *(14)*. SCID mice do not have functional B- and T-cells, and they tolerate xenografts *(67)*. When transplanted with fragments of thymus or with blood mononuclear cells (BMCs) from MG patients, but not from healthy controls, SCID mice develop human anti-AChR antibodies in the blood and at the NMJ and are weak *(13,68,69)*. The use of SCID mice engrafted with mixtures of blood immune cells from MG patients demonstrated that development of myasthenic weakness (and of human anti-AChR antibodies in the serum and bound to the AChR at the NMJ) required the presence of CD4$^+$ T-cells *(14)*. Furthermore, the inclusion, as CD4$^+$ T-cells, of anti-AChR CD4$^+$ T-cells induced synthesis of human anti-AChR antibodies and myasthenic signs, whereas CD4$^+$-depleted BMCs supplemented with CD4$^+$ T-cells specific for irrelevant antigens did not *(14)*. These findings directly demonstrate that anti-AChR CD4$^+$ T-cells are necessary for production of pathogenic anti-AChR antibodies.

Healthy individuals usually have blood CD4$^+$ T-cells specific for autoantigens, including the muscle AChR *(70–73)*, yet the presence of potentially autoreactive CD4$^+$ T-cells seldom leads to autoimmune diseases. Autoreactive T-cells may survive clonal deletion during their maturation in the thymus because their T-cell receptors (TCRs) bind the self-epitope/MHC complex with low affinity *(74)* (**Fig. 2**). T-cell activation requires effective binding of the TCR to the T-epitope/MHC complex: thus, low-affinity autoreactive T-cells may never be activated during adult life. The common presence of autoreactive CD4$^+$ T-cells in healthy people also suggests that mechanisms of peripheral tolerance keep the activity of potentially self-reactive CD4$^+$ T-cells in check. Failure of those mechanisms is a likely cause of autoimmune diseases, including MG.

The epitopes recognized by the anti-AChR CD4$^+$ T-cells of MG patients, the structure of their TCRs, and the functional effects of the cytokines they

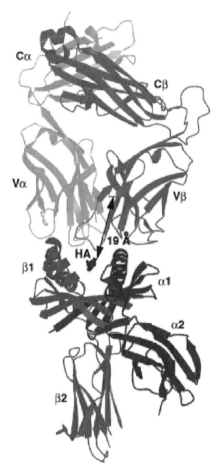

**Fig. 2.** Example of the complex T-cell receptor (TCR) MHC class II peptide. The figure shows the interaction of an αβTCR, the influenza HA peptide 306–318, and HLA-DR1. The TCR is represented on the top of the figure; C and V refer respectively to the constant and variable domains of the α- and β-chains. The peptide is indicated as HA, and HLA-DR1 is on the bottom of the figure. The arrow indicates the distance between the C-terminus of the peptide and residue 3 of the TCR Vβ domain. (Reproduced with permission of Oxford University Press from Hennecke J, Carfi A, Wiley DC. Structure of a covalently stabilized complex of a human alphabet T-cell receptor, influenza HA peptide and MHC class II molecule, HLA-DR1. *EMBO J* 2000;19:5611–5624.)

secrete are important to understand the pathogenesis of MG. The first two characteristics may give clues about the mechanisms that trigger and maintain the anti-AChR response. The third may help in understanding the mechanisms that cause the intermittent progress of MG and the different clinical presentations among MG patients.

## Epitope Repertoire

The epitope repertoire of the autoimmune CD4[+] T-cells in MG patients has been characterized extensively *(1)*. CD4[+] T-cells recognize denatured sequence segments of the antigen: thus, biosynthetic and synthetic sequences of the human AChR could be used to identify sequence regions and even individual residues forming epitopes recognized by the CD4[+] T-cells of MG patients *(1,75,76* and references therein).

Studies in experimental autoimmune diseases, including EAMG, have examined the characteristics and evolution in time of the epitope repertoire of self-reactive CD4[+] T-cells. In rodent EAMG, most of the anti-AChR CD4[+] T-cells recognize a limited number of epitopes, all formed by the α-subunit *(77–79)*. In C57Bl/6 mice, prolonged immunization with AChR leads to a focusing of the CD4[+] repertoire onto a single short segment of the α-subunit, recognized by highly pathogenic CD4[+] T-cells *(80* and references therein). Also, in rat EAMG most pathogenic anti-AChR CD4[+] T-cells recognize one epitope sequence of the AChR α-subunit *(77)*. The characteristics of the epitope repertoire of rodent anti-AChR CD4[+] T-cells are in contrast with what occurs in other experimental autoimmune diseases, in which the autoimmune CD4[+] T-cells recognize one or very few epitopes initially, but their recognition of the autoantigen spreads in time to many other epitopes, and even to other proteins of the target tissues *(81)*.

The finding that many anti-AChR antibodies of MG patients recognize epitopes on the α-subunit was consistent with the possibility that in MG the anti-AChR CD4[+] T-cell response also focuses on a few immunodominant epitopes: there may be preferential collaboration between T-helper and B-cells that recognize epitopes with the same antigen domain *(1)*. Since in both MG and rodent EAMG the anti-AChR antibody response is focused on the α-subunits (and on the MIR), the anti-AChR CD4[+] T-cells of MG patients might also recognize primarily one or more α-subunit epitopes. Early studies found that CD4[+] T-cell lines propagated from the blood of MG patients, using stimulation with *Torpedo* AChR, recognized the α-subunits almost exclusively *(82)*, bolstering the hypothesis that the α-subunit dominates sensitization of CD4[+] T-cells in MG. However, those early findings were probably due to the higher level of sequence identity among α-subunits from different species than among the other AChR subunits *(16,26)*: the use of an AChR from a distant species favored propagation of CD4[+] T-cells that recognized the highly conserved α-subunit. MG patients have blood CD4[+] T-cells that recognize each of the AChR subunits, including the adult muscle AChR ε-subunit and the embryonic γ-subunit *(83–87).** CD4$^+$ T-cell lines specific for any of the AChR subunits could be propagated from the blood of MG patients *(92–97).* Those anti-AChR CD4$^+$ T-cells lines responded vigorously when challenged with purified mammalian muscle AChR: thus, they recognized epitopes that derived from processing of the AChR molecule.

MG patients who had generalized weakness for several years usually had CD4$^+$ T-cells that recognized all AChR subunits, whereas patients who had generalized weakness for short times usually recognized only a few subunits *(85).* In generalized MG patients, the CD4$^+$ T-cell recognition of AChR subunits, once established, appears to persist in time, and the intensity of the CD4$^+$ T-cell response to the AChR subunits increases with disease duration *(85).* These findings were consistent with spread of the CD4$^+$ T-cell repertoire in MG, because they suggest that the number of CD4$^+$ T-cells that become sensitized to the AChR (and possibly the number of AChR epitopes they recognize) increased with time. Longitudinal studies of the same MG patients verified that both the number of AChR-specific CD4$^+$ T-cells and the number of epitopes they recognized increased as the disease progressed *(87).* Comparison of the epitope repertoire of anti-AChR CD4$^+$ T-cell lines propagated from the same generalized MG patients, at time intervals of up to 10 years *(76;* Diethelm-Okita, Howard, and Conti-Fine, unpublished data) confirmed that the epitope repertoire of the anti-AChR CD4$^+$ T-cells spreads to an increasing number of epitopes and demonstrated that CD4$^+$ T-cells sensitized to an epitope persisted for many years.

In summary, the results of several studies indicate that, unlike rodent EAMG, in generalized MG the CD4$^+$ T-cells recognize complex repertoires of epitopes formed by all the AChR subunits. Spread of CD4$^+$ T-cell sensitization to increasingly larger parts of the AChR molecule during MG progression is the likely cause of the numerous CD4$^+$ epitopes on the AChR. The different evolution of the epitope repertoire of the anti-AChR CD4$^+$ T-cells in MG and EAMG underlines the different pathogenic mechanisms of spontaneous autoimmune diseases and their experimental models, induced by immunization with autoantigens in adjuvants.

Administration of synthetic peptide analogs of epitopes recognized by autoimmune CD4$^+$ T-cells [altered peptide ligands (APLs)] may prevent and even cure certain experimental autoimmune diseases *(98).* The APLs bind to the

---

*After innervation of the skeletal muscles, the γ-subunit is substituted for by the ε-subunit *(16,26).* However, the extraocular muscles (EOMs) of adult mammals still express the embryonic γ-subunit *(88,89),* which is also expressed in the adult thymus *(90,91).* We will discuss the implications of these findings for models of MG pathogenesis later.

MHC class II molecules and compete with the peptide epitopes derived from the autoantigen, without stimulating the epitope-specific CD4$^+$ T-cells. By this mechanism, treatment with APLs may shut off an autoimmune response, at least temporarily. APLs might also anergize the pathogenic CD4$^+$ T-cells, or stimulate modulatory antiinflammatory CD4$^+$ T-cells, or both *(98–100)*. APL-based approaches may not be effective for MG management, because the anti-AChR CD4$^+$ T-cells recognize many epitopes presented by different class II isotypes and alleles. Furthermore, the therapeutic effects of APLs are ephemeral: they disappear when administration of APLs is discontinued.

### CD4$^+$ T-Cells of MG Patients Recognize "Universal," Immunodominant AChR Epitopes

A few short sequence regions of the AChR are recognized by most or all MG patients, regardless of their MHC type *(83,84,93,94,96,97,101)*. MG patients have abundant CD4$^+$ T-cells sensitized to epitopes within those AChR sequences *(85,101)*. Thus, the AChR forms universal, immunodominant epitopes for sensitization of self-reactive human CD4$^+$ T-cells. Studies that used SCID mice engrafted with immune cells from MG patients demonstrated that CD4$^+$ T-cells specific for universal AChR epitopes induced synthesis of pathogenic anti-AChR antibodies and myasthenic manifestations *(14)*. This finding suggests that the CD4$^+$ T-cells recognizing universal AChR epitope sequences are important in the pathogenesis of MG.

Exogenous protein antigens, such as tetanus and diphtheria toxoids, also bear universal epitopes that sensitize CD4$^+$ T-cells in most or all humans *(102)*. Universal epitope sequences are all flanked by relatively unstructured, highly mobile sequence loops, exposed to the solvent: these structural features probably facilitate their release during antigen processing *(102* and references therein)*. Solvent-exposed loops would be easily accessible to the processing proteases. Human antigen-presenting cells (APCs) express a variety of MHC class II molecules, especially if they are heterozygous at the MHC locus. Furthermore, most human class II molecules do not have stringent sequence requirements for their peptide ligands. Thus, most peptide sequences released upon antigen processing will probably encounter a human class II molecule able to bind and present them to CD4$^+$ T-cells.

### Unstable Recognition of AChR Epitopes by CD4$^+$ T-Cells of Ocular MG Patients

The first symptoms of MG usually include, or are limited to, weakness of the ocular muscles. In most patients the myasthenic weakness spreads over time to the skeletal muscles, but in about 15% of the patients it remains limited to the muscles that move the eye [the extraocular muscles (EOMs)] or lift the eyelid (the levator palpebrae) *(4,103)*. The causes of the preferential involvement of the ocular muscles in MG are unknown *(104)*. Physiologic properties of the EOM synapses may contribute to their preferential involvement in MG. The EOMs are especially susceptible to the development of myasthenic weakness when a reduction of the AChR function occurs *(104,105)*. EOM weakness is also the most common and earliest manifestation in congenital MG, in which genetic defects of the AChR expression or structure affect the AChR of all muscles to a similar extent *(106)*. The motor neurons that innervate the EOM have high firing frequencies, which may make their synapses especially susceptible to myasthenic fatigue *(104,105)*. Furthermore, the EOMs include tonic fibers, whose force of contraction is a function of the size of the depolarization at their endplates: any AChR loss (and the resulting reduction in endplate potential) would cause decreased strength of those tonic fibers.

Patients with ocular MG have lower concentrations of serum anti-AChR antibodies than generalized MG patients, and 50% of them do not have detectable antibodies *(1,22,103)*. In ocular MG, the clinical symptoms may remain localized to the EOMs because their modest anti-AChR antibody synthesis is insufficient to affect the function of muscles other than the EOMs. Unique antigenic properties of the AChR expressed by the EOM might also contribute to the selective involvement of the EOM in ocular MG. The EOM express both embryonic and adult AChR isotypes, whereas skeletal muscles express only adult AChR *(88,107)*. Furthermore, some ocular MG patients have antibodies that specifically recognize EOM synapses containing AChR with fetal properties *(105)*. These findings suggested that the antibodies and the CD4[+] T-cells of ocular MG patients may preferentially recognize the embryonic AChR and cause preferential weakness of the EOMs *(85,104)*. However, other studies have contradicted that hypothesis *(87,108,109)*.

Several investigations examined T-cell recognition of the AChR in small groups of ocular MG patients. One study found that their CD4[+] T-cells consistently recognized the embryonic γ-subunit, and had minimal and sporadic responses to the adult ε-subunit *(85)*. In contrast, another study found that some ocular MG patients had CD4[+] T-cells and antibodies specific for the adult AChR *(109)*. Either a stable heterogeneity in the characteristics of the CD4[+] response in ocular MG patients, or an unstable recognition of the AChR, with changes over time of the subunits recognized by the CD4[+] T-cells, might have caused those discrepancies. A later study *(87)* supported the second possibility. That study found that CD4[+] T-cells from ocular MG patients may recognize any AChR subunit: however, they seldom recognized all AChR subunits, even when the disease had lasted for many years. Also, ocular MG patients had lower CD4$^+$ T-cell responses to the AChR subunits than generalized weakness MG patients, and the repertoire of their anti-AChR CD4$^+$ T-cells was unstable over time: CD4$^+$ T-cells that recognized a given subunit appeared and disappeared over a few weeks or months.

The low and unstable responses of the anti-AChR CD4$^+$ T-cells agree with the sporadic and scarce serum anti-AChR antibodies of ocular MG patients *(1,22)*. It is likely that in ocular MG the symptoms are limited to the EOMs because of the modest anti-AChR immune response, as well as the high susceptibility of the EOMs to myasthenic weakness. Ocular MG patients might still have regulatory immunosuppressive circuits that counteract the activated pathogenic CD4$^+$ T-cells and make them ineffective in driving a pathogenic antibody response. In generalized weakness MG patients, the persistence and spreading of the anti-AChR CD4$^+$ T-cell response as the disease progresses suggest a more substantial failure of the normal mechanisms of downregulation of the self-reactive CD4$^+$ T-cells.

## T-CELL Vβ AND Vα USAGE BY ANTI-AChR CD4$^+$ T-CELLS

The TCR, which confers antigen specificity to the CD4$^+$ T-cells, is a membrane protein that binds the complex between a class II MHC molecule and an epitope sequence of the antigen.

Anti-AChR CD4$^+$ T-cells of MG patients express TCRs, which are usually αβ heterodimers *(110,111)*. The TCR β-subunit is especially interesting because its variable region forms important structural elements of the binding sites for both the epitope/MHC complex and superantigens *(112–114)*.

The variable region genes of the β-subunit result from somatic rearrangement of germline-encoded V (variable), D (diversity), and J (joining) segments *(112,113)*. There are more than 100 different human TCR Vβ genes, which can be grouped into 24 families based on the extent of their sequence similarity *(115)*. The Vβ gene family used by a TCR determines the ability of the resulting TCR to interact with different superantigens *(114,116)*.

Superantigens bind and link the antigen-binding domain of a TCR and a class II molecule on the surface of a APC *(116)*. Similar to what occurs after engagement of the TCR with the specific epitope/MHC molecule complex on the APC surface, crosslinking by a superantigen permits costimulation, and therefore activation, of the CD4$^+$ T-cell *(114,116)*. Each superantigen is specific for particular Vβ gene families *(114,116)*, and it activates all CD4$^+$ T-cells expressing TCR that utilize the preferred Vβ family or families. A superantigen may initiate an autoimmune response by activating self-reactive T-cells that express the preferred Vβ family *(117,118)*.

The TCR antigen-binding site is formed by two sets of three sequence segments, termed complementarity-determining regions (CDR) 1, 2, and 3; they are within the variable domains of each of the two TCR subunits (112–114). The CDR1 and the CDR2 are formed by the V segment, whereas the CDR3 is formed by the sequence at the joining of the V, D, and J segments of the β-subunit, or the V and J segments of the α-subunit, with the constant (C) region segment (112–114). The V(D)J/C joining may be inaccurate, thus increasing the potential variability of the CDR3. The CDR sequences, especially CDR3, may give clues as to whether an antigen drove the selection of CDR displaying a similar sequence motif, compatible with epitope binding. On the other hand, clonal expansion in most patients of autoimmune CD4[+] T-cells bearing TCRs formed by the products of certain Vβ gene families, without any common CDR3 sequence motif, suggests the action of a superantigen. Also, the Vα gene family used by a TCR may influence the binding of certain superantigens (119). Determination of the Vα gene family used by autoimmune TCRs (and of the sequence of their CDR3 regions) may yield further clues about the presence of antigen-driven clonal expansion, and perhaps also about the action of a superantigen.

The search for clues supporting one or the other model is complicated by the evolution in time of the autoimmune CD4[+] T-cells responses, with spreading of the T-cell repertoire. Recruitment of CD4[+] T-clones that recognize new epitopes and use different TCR genes may obscure the characteristics of the T-cells whose activation triggered the autoimmune response.

Several studies have examined the TCR Vβ and Vα usage in MG patients. Some studies investigated the overall Vβ usage in the thymus and blood of MG patients, and others examined the Vβ and Vα usage by AChR-specific CD4[+] T-cell lines propagated from MG patients (110,111,120–124).

Investigation of Vβ usage in unselected T-cells from the thymus or blood yielded conflicting results. Some studies did not find evidence of clonal expansion of T-cells or of preferential Vβ usage in myasthenic thymi (120, 124). In contrast, other studies (121–123) found evidence of clonal expansion and preferential Vβ usage in MG patients, although their results did not always agree on the Vβ families that seemed to be expanded. These studies investigated a limited number of patients and used different assays of TCR Vβ usage; a biased representation in small samples and different shortcomings of the methods used may explain the discrepancies.

Studies that examined AChR-specific CD4[+] T-cells from MG patients (110, 111,123) all concluded that the Vα and Vβ repertoire of anti-AChR CD4[+] T-cells was diverse and characteristic of the individual patient. For each patient, the CD4[+] T-cells specific for a given AChR epitope had relatively restricted

Vα and Vβ usage. Still, in each patient the overall Vα and Vβ usage of the anti-AChR CD4⁺ T-cells was heterogeneous, because the anti-AChR CD4⁺ T-cells could recognize a number of different epitopes. Even CD4⁺ T-cells that recognized universal AChR epitopes used different Vβ families in different patients *(110)*.

In spite of the heterogeneity of their epitope repertoire and the Vβ and Vα usage, the anti-AChR CD4⁺ T-cells used the Vβ4 and Vβ6 families frequently, even when they recognized different AChR epitopes *(110)*. Even unselected blood CD4⁺ T-cells of MG patients used Vβ4 and Vβ6 to a significantly higher extent than the blood CD4⁺ T-cells of normal subjects *(124)*. These findings are consistent with the possibility that a superantigen might have triggered the anti-AChR CD4⁺ response. Also, some Vα families were used with unexpected high frequency by anti-AChR CD4⁺ T-cells of MG patients *(125)*, perhaps reflecting the action of a superantigen in triggering the anti-AChR response *(119)*.

Experimental treatments with the aim of suppressing a specific undesirable immune response include attempts to interfere with the ability of a TCR to bind the specific peptide epitope/MHC molecule complex, by administration or induction of antibodies that recognized the antigen-binding site of the TCR *(126,127)*. This sort of treatment was successful in rodent experimental autoimmune encephalitis (EAE). In rodent EAE, the pathogenic CD4⁺ T-cells initially recognize only one epitope of myelin basic protein and preferentially use a single TCR Vβ family *(128)*. The diverse epitope repertoire and TCR Vβ and Vα usage of the anti-AChR CD4⁺ T-cells in MG makes it unlikely that this approach will be useful for the treatment of MG.

## ROLES OF CYTOKINES
## SECRETED BY DIFFERENT CD4⁺ SUBSETS

A network of cytokines modulates the development and course of normal and pathologic immune responses *(129–131)*. Cells that mediate acquired or innate immune (as well as nonimmune) cells can secrete cytokines and express cytokine receptors, which make them responsive to the action of these chemical messengers. Identification of the cytokines produced by the anti-AChR T- and B-cells and of the cytokines that modulate their activity is a necessary step in the elucidation of the pathogenic mechanisms of MG. Also, future treatments of MG aimed at restoring a state of tolerance to the AChR will probably include interventions in the cytokine network.

Some cytokines [e.g., interleukin (IL)-2] augment the activity of immune cells; other cytokines [e.g., the transforming growth factor (TGF)-β family] downregulate immune responses. Because of their ability to influence the activity of a variety of cells, many cytokines may have complex and contrasting effects on the immune system: they might augment or decrease an immune response, depending on the phase of the immune response when they exerted their action and the cellular types on which they acted.

In antibody-mediated diseases like MG, cytokines, which induce proliferation and differentiation of B-cells, may cause an increase in the mature B-cells that secrete high-affinity, pathogenic anti-AChR antibodies. Other cytokines may increase the antibody synthesis indirectly, by increasing the activity of CD4[+] T-helper cells and APCs. Cytokines with antiinflammatory activity, like IL-4, IL-10, and TGF-β, downregulate activated APCs and Th1 CD4[+] T-cells and therefore may protect from autoimmune diseases. However, IL-4 and IL-10 are also growth and differentiation factors for B-cells: thus their effects on antibody-mediated autoimmune diseases appear to be complex.

Activated CD4[+] T-cells can differentiate into subtypes that secrete different cytokines *(129–131)*. The simplest classification of differentiated CD4[+] T-cells discriminates between Th1 and Th2 cells. Th1 cells secrete proinflammatory cytokines, such as interferon (IFN)-γ and IL-2. Th2 cells secrete antiinflammatory cytokines, such as IL-4 and IL-10. IL-4 is a growth factor for a third subset of differentiated CD4[+] T-cells, sometimes referred to as Th3 cells, that secrete TGF-β. Both Th1 and Th2 cells secrete cytokines that are proliferation and differentiation factors for B-cells and therefore induce antibody synthesis. Th1 cytokines induce synthesis of antibodies that fix complement and are most effective at causing tissue damage, whereas Th2 cytokines induce synthesis of antibodies that do not bind complement *(132)*.

Anti-AChR Th1 cells, and the cytokines they secrete, are probably important in the pathogenesis of MG. MG patients usually have abundant anti-AChR Th1 cells, which recognize many AChR epitopes, including several universal epitopes *(101)*. Experiments in SCID mice engrafted with immune cells from MG patients suggest that anti-AChR Th1 cells induce synthesis of pathogenic antibodies: SCID mice grafted with B-cells and macrophages from MG patients, supplemented with AChR-specific CD4[+] T-cell lines propagated with IL-2 (a growth factor for Th1 cells) developed human anti-AChR antibodies and weakness, whereas control mice that received the same blood B-cells and macrophages, without anti-AChR CD4[+] T-cells, did not develop anti-AChR antibodies or myasthenic weakness *(14)*.

Studies that examined the presence of anti-AChR Th2 and Th3 cells in MG patients have yielded inconclusive results. Some studies determined the cytokines secreted by blood lymphocytes of MG patients after challenge in vitro with AChR. They concluded that AChR challenge induced expression of a variety of cytokines, consistent with a response of both Th1 and Th2 cells, or of Th0 cells (the precursor to both Th1 and Th2 subsets, which can secrete small amounts of both Th1 and Th2 cytokines), or of all three CD4$^+$ T-cell types *(133–135)*. Most anti-AChR CD4$^+$ T-cell lines propagated from the blood of MG patients secreted IL-2, but not IL-4, indicating that they comprised only Th1 cells *(97)*. This result was not surprising, since those CD4$^+$ T-cell lines had been propagated by cycles of stimulation with purified AChR and IL-2, which preferentially expands Th1 cells. Rarely, AChR-specific polyclonal CD4$^+$ T-cell lines from MG patients secreted both IL-2 and IL-4, suggesting that they comprised both Th1 and Th2 cells *(136)*. It is unlikely that those lines included Th0 cells because they were obtained by multiple cycles of exposure to AChR antigens, which should have caused antigen-induced differentiation of all Th0 cells.

Several studies have examined the role or roles of cytokines in rodent EAMG. Some studies determined the susceptibility to EAMG of mice strains genetically deficient in a cytokine or a cytokine receptor *(25,41,137–140)*, or hyper-producing a cytokine because of the presence of a transgene *(141)*. Other studies examined the effect on EAMG development of manipulating the concentration of different cytokines during immunization with the AChR: administration of a cytokine increased its concentration, whereas administration of an anticytokine antibody neutralized the endogenous cytokine *(137, 142)*. Other studies determined the pattern of secretion of different cytokines after treatments that induced tolerance to the AChR and protection from EAMG *(143–146)*. Those studies consistently suggested that CD4$^+$ Th1 cells are involved in the synthesis of pathogenic anti-AChR antibodies and development of EAMG, whereas IL-4 and TGF-β may play a protective role. Mice genetically deficient in IL-12, which is essential for development of Th1 cells, were resistant to induction of EAMG: they synthesized Th2-induced anti-AChR antibodies that bound to the AChR at the NMJ but did not bind and activate complement and were ineffective at causing NMJ destruction *(25,137)*. Mice genetically deficient in IFN-γ or in its receptor had increased resistance to EAMG compared with wild-type mice *(138,140)*. IL-4 does not seem to play a pathogenic role, because mice genetically deficient in IL-4 developed EAMG with even higher frequency and severity than normal mice *(41)*. Thus, IL-4 may have a protective role in EAMG, either because of its antiinflammatory action on Th1 cells and APCs, or indirectly, as a growth factor for TGF-β-secreting modulatory cells.

Oral, nasal, or subcutaneous administration of AChR or AChR peptides recognized by CD4$^+$ T-cells induced AChR-specific CD4$^+$ T-cells that secreted

IL-4 and TGF-β, protected from induction of EAMG, and even reversed established myasthenic manifestations *(143,145–148)*. These treatments were ineffective in mice genetically deficient in IL-4 *(41)*. Furthermore, protection from EAMG could be passively transferred into the IL-4-deficient mice by the use of CD4$^+$ T-cells of wild-type mice treated nasally with CD4$^+$ epitope peptides of the AChR *(149)*. These studies suggest a protective role of Th2 and/or Th3 cells in EAMG. However, Th2 cytokines might also facilitate synthesis of anti-AChR antibodies, and development of EAMG because of their stimulating action on B-cell proliferation and differentiation.

The results of a study that examined the susceptibility to EAMG of C57Bl/6 mice that carried an IL-10 transgene controlled by the IL-2 promoter support this possibility *(141)*. In these mice the T-cells that synthesize transgenic IL-10 include activated Th1 cells, which produce IL-10 only at the time of their activation *(150)*. Because of the transient expression of the transgene, the immune system of these mice is not significantly different from that of control littermates: the serum IgG levels and the numbers and phenotypes of T- and B-cells are normal *(150)*. Moreover, although IL-10 is a potent downregulator of Th1 cells *(129–131)*, IFN-γ synthesis in these transgenic mice is reduced but not abrogated *(150)*. Transgenic expression of IL-10 in the T-cells of the mice facilitated development of EAMG after immunization *(140)*: the mice developed EAMG with greater frequency and severity than wild-type C57Bl/6 mice. Also, immunization with small amounts of AChR, insufficient to induce EAMG in wild-type mice, caused EAMG in the IL-10 transgenic animals. The IL-10 transgenic mice had an increased anti-AChR antibody response, compared with nontransgenic animals, which probably caused their increased susceptibility to EAMG.

Thus, in this transgenic system, the action of IL-10 as a proliferation and differentiation factor for B-cells overshadows the many actions of IL-10 as a downregulator of Th1 responses and antigen presentation. In support of a facilitatory role of IL-10 in the pathogenesis of EAMG, another study found that mutant C57Bl/6 mice genetically deficient in IL-10 and immunized with *Torpedo* AChR developed less severe myasthenic weakness than wild-type mice, although they appeared to synthesize comparable amounts of anti-AChR antibody *(151)*.

IL-10 reduces the expression of costimulatory molecules and cytokines by APCs *(152–155)* and inhibits the transcription of IL-12 genes during the primary antigen stimulus *(156)*, thus reducing activation of Th1 cells. Also, IL-10 affects CD4$^+$ T-cells and resting T-cells by inhibiting IL-2 production and T-cell growth *(157,158)*, inducing a long-term antigen-specific anergic state of CD4$^+$ T-cells when present during antigen challenge *(159–160)*, and increasing activation-induced T-cell death mediated by Fas/Fas ligand *(161)*. Because of its ability to downregulate Th1 cells and the synthesis of a variety of cytokines, IL-10 is considered possible for therapy of undesirable immune responses *(162,163)*.

However, the enhanced susceptibility to EAMG of IL-10 transgenic mice, the resistance to EAMG of mice genetically deficient in IL-10, and the pathogenic role of IL-10 in systemic lupus erythematosus, another antibody-mediated autoimmune disease *(164,165)*, raise concerns about the suitability of IL-10 to curb antibody-mediated autoimmune diseases and suggest that IL-10 might be a target, rather than a tool, in the suppression of undesirable antibody responses. MG patients have increased blood levels of AChR-specific cells that secrete IL-10 *(166)*, a finding consistent with a pathogenic role of this cytokine in MG. Also, the effects of IL-10 on T-cell-mediated experimental autoimmune responses are complex and conflicting *(167–170)*.

In summary, the consistent presence in MG patients of anti-AChR Th1 cells that can induce synthesis of anti-AChR antibodies and the findings that in rodents Th1 cytokines facilitate or even permit EAMG development suggest that Th1 cells may have a preeminent pathogenic role in MG. This probably reflects the ability of Th1 cells to drive the synthesis of anti-AChR antibodies that bind and activate complement, and therefore can cause effective destruction of the NMJ. Anti-AChR Th1 and anti-AChR Th2 cells secreting IL-4 and IL-10, as well as TGF-β-secreting "Th3" cells, may also be present. By analogy with the protective function in rodent EAMG of Th2 and Th3 cytokines, in MG regulatory circuits that include IL-4 and TGF-β as mediators or effectors might also downregulate the anti-AChR response. If so, favoring the differentiation of anti-AChR CD4$^+$ T-cells toward the Th2 and Th3 phenotypes may be a useful approach to turn off the anti-AChR immune response specifically.

The findings that a Th2 cytokine, IL-10, facilitates synthesis of pathogenic anti-AChR antibodies and appearance of myasthenic weakness indicate that approaches attempting to potentiate anti-AChR Th2 cells may be fraught with dangers. Elucidation of the intricacies of the cytokine networks in MG and EMG will be necessary to make interventions in such networks a viable option for MG treatment.

## CD8$^+$ CELLS IN MYASTHENIA GRAVIS AND EXPERIMENTAL AUTOIMMUNE MYASTHENIA GRAVIS

CD8$^+$ T-cells may be effectors of immune and autoimmune responses, by virtue of their cytotoxic activity. They play an important role in a variety of experimental autoimmune diseases, which cannot be induced in animals depleted of CD8$^+$ T-cells *(171,172)*. This also holds true for a mouse anti-body-mediated disease, a lupus-like disease induced by anti-DNA antibodies: MHC class I-deficient mice, which do not have functional CD8$^+$ T-cells, are resistant to developing this syndrome *(173)*. CD8$^+$ T-cells may have also immunomodulatory functions and may downregulate immune responses. For example, in Theiler's murine encephalomyelitis, a virus-induced demyelinating disease reminiscent of multiple sclerosis, CD8$^+$ T-cells have a regulatory function *(174)*. It is still unclear whether CD8$^+$ T-cells play a role in MG and EAMG. Different studies have examined this issue in mouse EAMG, with conflicting results. Mice deficient in $\beta_2$-microglobulin do not express MHC class I molecules and do not have CD8$^+$ T-cells, yet they developed EAMG after immunization with *Torpedo* AChR with higher incidence, earlier onset, and more severe weakness than heterozygous littermates that had CD8$^+$ T-cells *(175)*. These results suggested that CD8$^+$ T-cells in mouse EAMG might have regulatory rather than pathogenic functions. Consistent with these results, another study found that CD8$^+$ T-cell depletion augmented the susceptibility of mice to EAMG *(176)*. In contrast with these conclusions, other studies yielded results that suggested an important pathogenic role of CD8$^+$ T-cells in rodent EAMG. One study found that CD8$^+$ T-cell depletion of Lewis rats decreased the severity of EAMG and the serum concentration of anti-AChR antibodies, compared with control rats *(177)*. Another study found that mice genetically deficient in CD8$^+$ T-cells were resistant to EAMG induction. In short, CD8$^+$ T-cells are probably involved in the pathogenesis of EAMG, although it is still unclear whether they have a pathogenic or a modulatory role, or both.

MG patients do not have detectable cytotoxic CD8$^+$ T-cell responses to the AChR or other components of the NMJ *(7)*: thus, CD8$^+$ T-cells are unlikely to play a significant pathogenic role in MG. However, they might have a modulatory role.

MG patients may have different numbers of blood CD8$^+$ T-cells than normal subjects *(178,179)*. MG patients with modest weakness or in clinical remission had numerous activated CD8$^+$ T-cells in the blood, whereas severely affected patients had very few activated blood CD8$^+$ T-cells; an increase in activated CD8$^+$ T-cells in the blood predicted an improvement in manifestations *(180)*. CD8$^+$ T-cells inhibited the anti-AChR responses of CD4$^+$ T-cells in vitro *(83,84,180)*, and removal of CD8$^+$ T-cells from the BMCs of MG patients caused an increase in antibody-producing B-cells and anti-AChR antibodies *(181,182)*.

CD8$^+$ cells, which recognize proteins expressed by activated anti-AChR CD4$^+$ T-cells, might mediate immunoregulatory circuits in MG patients *(183)*.

Regulatory CD8$^+$ T-cells might recognize epitopes derived from the TCR uniquely expressed by a CD4$^+$ T-cell clone (idiotypic epitopes), or from protein expressed by all activated CD4$^+$ T-cells (ergotypic epitopes). A precarious balance between activated autoimmune CD4$^+$ T-cells and CD8$^+$ T-cells able to modulate autoimmune CD4$^+$ T-cell reactivity might explain the relapsing character of MG and of many other autoimmune diseases.

## THE THYMUS

The thymus plays an important, albeit still obscure, role in the pathogenesis of MG. The thymus of MG patients is usually abnormal, and thymectomy may improve the clinical course of MG *(63)*. Most (70%) of the abnormal MG thymi have lymphoid follicular hyperplasia *(1–4,184,185)*: their perivascular spaces are extended, disrupted, and filled with lymphoid tissue that resembles peripheral immune organs, and active germinal centers are present, similar to the secondary lymph follicles of peripheral lymphoid organs. Hyperplastic MG thymi have abnormally high numbers of mature T-cells (CD4$^+$/CD8$^-$ or CD4$^-$/CD8$^+$), usually present only in peripheral lymphoid organs. Also, they contain anti-AChR T- and B-cells, and transplantation of thymus fragments from MG patients into SCID mice induces the appearance of human anti-AChR antibodies, which bind the mouse NMJ and cause AChR loss *(68)*.

About 10% of MG patients have a thymoma *(1–4,184,185)*. Thymomas are a heterogeneous group of tumors, and their histologic characteristics are not consistent with the presence of an ongoing immune response *(184)*. However, areas of lymphoid follicular hyperplasia frequently surround the thymoma tissue of MG patients.

### *AChR-Like Proteins are Expressed in the Thymus*

The anti-AChR response that occurs in MG thymi with lymphoid follicular hyperplasia may be directed to a protein or proteins similar to muscle AChR, synthesized within the thymus *(1–4,184,185)*. Normal and MG thymi express protein(s) that crossreact with antibodies to the muscle AChR and bind α-bungarotoxin (α-BGT), a specific ligand of muscle AChR *(186–192)*. The thymus AChR might be the original autoantigen that triggers the anti-AChR response in MG *(1,184,185)*.

It is not clear whether the thymus expresses true muscle-type AChR, or AChR-like proteins with different antigenic structure, or if expression of AChR or AChR-like proteins is different in thymi from MG patients than in thymi from normal subjects. Human thymus may express mRNA transcripts for all the muscle AChR subunits. However, although transcripts of the α- and β-subunits have been found consistently *(193–203)*, those of the γ-, δ-, and ε-subunits have not *(90,194,196–199,203,204)*. Some studies found γ-subunit, but not ε-subunit transcript *(90,199)*. In contrast, another study found expression of ε-subunit mRNA, but not of γ-subunit in mRNA, in both normal and MG thymi *(198)*. Some studies found δ-subunit protein or mRNA transcript in thymus tissue and in cultured myoid and epithelial cells *(90,194,199,203)*. Yet other studies found absence, or extreme reduction, or erratic expression of δ-subunit transcripts in human thymi *(196,197,204)*. The results of studies that measure mRNA transcripts rather than the corresponding proteins need to be interpreted with caution, because the amounts of different transcripts in a tissue may not reflect the relative abundance of the encoded proteins. The conclusions of such studies will require verification by measurement of the corresponding AChR proteins.

Expression of even an incomplete set of muscle AChR subunits in the thymus must result in assembly of membrane proteins reminiscent of muscle AChR, because the thymus contains binding sites for α-BGT and for AChR-specific antibodies *(186–192)*. Transfection experiments have shown that an incomplete set of AChR subunits, which included only α-, β-, and γ-subunits, assembled into an AChR-like protein that was inserted in the cell membrane and bound cholinergic ligands: an extra copy of the γ-subunit substituted for the missing δ subunit *(205)*. The inconsistent presence of δ- and ε-subunit transcripts in the thymus led to the suggestion that the thymus expresses "triplet receptors" formed only by α-, β-, and γ-subunits *(197)*. Such receptors, because of their different antigenic structure than muscle AChR, might trigger the autoimmune response in MG. However, thymus tissues from healthy subjects rarely express detectable δ-subunit transcripts, a finding inconsistent with that hypothesis *(196,197,204)*.

In summary, the expression of AChR subunits in human thymus seems to be less tightly regulated than in the muscle; the human thymus may express, at least intermittently, AChR-like proteins that have different subunit composition and antigenic structure than muscle AChR.

The thymus may express other AChR-like proteins. Thymomas of MG patients express an AChR-like protein, which contains a single subunit about three times as large as a true AChR subunit *(184)*. This protein binds anti-AChR antibodies that recognize a linear determinant of the α-subunit, but it does not bind α-BGT or anti-MIR antibodies; it might be involved in the anti-AChR response in MG associated with thymoma. MG patients with thymomas have several unique clinical and immunologic features, which may reflect a different initiation of their immune response *(1–4,184,206)*. Thymomas also contain α-BGT binding proteins, which may be *bona fide* AChRs *(184,206)*.

## Thymus Cells That Express AChR Proteins

Not all the cell types present in the thymus express AChR-like proteins. Also, different types of thymus cells may express different AChRs. Cultured human thymus epithelial cells and myoid cells expressed AChR-like protein; however, epithelial cells expressed the ε-subunit, not the γ-subunit, whereas myoid cells expressed both ε- and γ-subunits *(194,203)*. The different spectrum of AChR subunits expressed in various cell types and the potential heterogeneity in cellular composition of the samples of adult human thymi may contribute to the inconsistent results of the studies on expression of AChR subunits in the thymus.

Several studies examined the expression of AChR subunits in normal and MG thymi; they could not identify any consistent characteristic of MG thymi that related to the anti-AChR response *(184)*. Some studies found an increased synthesis of some AChR subunits in MG thymi, perhaps related to the hyperplastic changes common in MG patients *(193,196)*.

The myoid and epithelial cells have characteristics that make them attractive candidates as the source of AChR antigen, which sensitizes autoimmune CD4[+] T-cells in MG. Myoid cells in both normal and MG thymi express AChR-like proteins, of both embryonic and adult type *(189,192,199,200,203)*. Myoid cells do not express MHC class II molecules. However, hyperplastic MG thymi are close to, and occasionally inside, germinal centers and in intimate contact with HLA-DR-positive reticulum cells *(184,207)*, which might serve as APCs of AChR epitopes.

Epithelial cells in normal and MG thymi contain AChR-like proteins that bind α-BGT *(187)*. Cultured epithelial cells express only AChR proteins that comprise the adult ε-subunit and may not include all the subunits necessary for proper AChR function *(194)*; their AChR-like proteins are nonfunctional, because they do not gate currents upon ACh binding *(208)*. This is in contrast to the functional AChR expressed by cultured myoid cells, which have electrophysiologic characteristics similar to muscle AChR and which include the δ-subunit *(203)*. The inconsistent presence of δ-subunit transcripts in human thymi, especially in samples from MG patients, is consistent with the possibility that the AChR-like proteins of epithelial cells—which are much more numerous than myoid cells—do not include the δ-subunit.

## PATHOGENIC MECHANISMS

The cause or causes of the breakdown of self-tolerance in autoimmune diseases are unknown. Many potentially autoreactive CD4[+] T-cells survive clonal deletion during the immune system development: they include CD4[+]

T-cells specific for self-antigens, which, like muscle AChR, may be targets of autoimmune responses *(1)*. However, in normal subjects their presence does not result in clinically significant autoimmune responses.

Clinical and epidemiologic studies suggest that infections may facilitate the induction and relapses of autoimmune diseases *(209)*. Microbial infections might trigger autoimmune responses by activating potentially self-reactive CD4+ T-cells; this mechanism might apply to MG, because CD4+ T-cells play a crucial role in the synthesis of pathogenic anti-AChR antibodies *(1–4)*. Several models have attempted to explain how this might occur.

One model proposes that molecular mimicry between a microbial epitope recognized by CD4+ T-cells and a similar sequence of a self-antigen activates CD4+ T-cells crossreactive with the self-antigen *(210)*. Many sequence segments of microbial antigens are similar to sequences of human proteins *(211)*; also, amino acid identity may be needed only for a few amino acids within a CD4+ epitope sequence *(212)*. Several sequence regions of human muscle AChR, including sequences forming epitopes recognized by CD4+ T-cells of MG patients, are similar to sequences of common microbes *(84,96)*. This is not surprising, because certain short amino acid sequences—which may correspond to common tridimensional structural motifs—occur in the sequence of proteins much more frequently than expected statistically *(213)*. This may explain why fragments of alien proteins long enough to form CD4+ epitopes frequently share sequence similarities with fragments of self-proteins.

Once tolerance to a self-epitope is broken, T-cells that recognize that epitope and secrete proinflammatory cytokines can migrate into the tissue that contains the antigen and cause an inflammatory response and tissue destruction. This might in turn result in the presentation by APCs able to activate any potential self-reactive CD4+ T-cells of new epitopes derived from the same antigen, and even from other antigens released by the damaged tissue *(81,128)*. Thus, inflammation and intermolecular and intramolecular epitope spreading may become self-maintaining processes *(214)*, which cause chronic tissue destruction and sensitization of CD4+ T-cells to an increasingly large repertoire of epitopes and antigens. This process has been termed *epitope spreading*, and it results in sensitization of CD4+ T-cells to epitopes distinct from, and noncrossreactive with, the inducing epitope *(81)*.

Microbial superantigens may also activate potentially autoimmune T-cells. This mechanism might trigger insulin-dependent diabetes mellitus, rheumatoid arthritis, and perhaps multiple sclerosis *(215–217)*. The action of a superantigen might also explain the relapses common in autoimmune diseases: in mouse strains that develop pathogenic anti-myelin basic protein CD4+ T-cells that use the Vβ8 gene family, the superantigen staphylococcal enterotoxin B, which activates Vβ8+ T-cells, induced EAE relapses in mice that were in clinical remission and triggered paralysis in mice with subclinical disease *(218)*.

The action of a superantigen might trigger MG. In hyperplastic MG thymi, dendritic cells are unusually abundant, and the CD4+ T-cells cluster around them, forming rosette-like structures *(184)*. This might be the place where a superantigen released by virus-infected dendritic cells could activate the anti-AChR CD4+ T-cells and trigger MG. Anti-AChR CD4+ T-cells activated by a superantigen in the thymus could migrate to the periphery and activate anti-AChR B-cells in the lymph nodes. Also, encounter of the anti-AChR CD4+ T-cells with muscle AChR epitopes presented by APCs at the inflamed neuromuscular junctions, damaged by the binding of complement-fixing anti-AChR antibodies, could cause further activation of autoimmune CD4+ T-cells and release of proinflammatory cytokines. This would perpetuate this mechanism by causing further recruitment of professional APCs and epitope spreading of the CD4+ T-cells response.

A third model proposes that a viral infection may activate self-reactive cells and trigger a tissue-specific autoimmune response by *bystander activation*, because of the inflammatory reaction to the virus-infected tissue *(219)*. It has been proposed that the immune system responds to antigens not only according to whether they are perceived as self or non-self, but also whether they are potentially dangerous *(220)*. In this model, self-proteins may elicit an immune response if presented to CD4+ T-cells in situations of danger, that is, by professional APCs in inflamed tissues. The inflammation caused by a viral infection would attract antiviral T-cells that express proinflammatory cytokines and professional APCs able to present epitopes derived from tissue proteins. This would result in the activation of potentially self-reactive CD4+ T-cells recognizing those epitopes. Furthermore, proinflammatory cytokines, like IFN-γ, may stimulate expression of class II MHC molecules in cells that do not express them constitutively, including muscle cells *(131, 132)*; this may facilitate presentation of self-epitopes and expansion of any primed self-reactive CD4+ T-cells.

Thus, an inflammatory response resulting from a viral infection in the thymus could cause professional APCs to present epitopes derived from the thymus AChR proteins. This would activate potentially autoreactive anti-AChR CD4+ T-cells and initiate the autoimmune response in MG. This mechanism is especially attractive to explain the appearance of MG associated with a thymoma. The immune response against the cancer cells expressing AChR-like antigens may trigger an autoimmune response able to involve the muscle AChR and cause MG. This mechanism is similar to that proposed for a variety of paraneoplastic syndromes, including the Lambert-Eaton syndrome *(3)*.

Whatever the mechanism that triggers the anti-AChR response might be, the thymus is an attractive candidate as the tissue where the immune response begins *(1–4,184)*. If so, the anti-AChR CD4⁺ T-cells would become sensitized first to epitopes on the AChR subunits expressed, or best expressed, in the thymus. When the muscle AChR becomes involved in the autoimmune response, the CD4⁺ T-cells repertoire would spread to all muscle AChR subunits, even those that may not be expressed in the thymus. The finding that CD4⁺ T-cells from MG patients responded to the δ-subunit significantly less than to other AChR subunits *(85,87)* is consistent with the possibility that a thymus AChR-like protein lacking the δ-subunit triggered the sensitization of anti-AChR CD4⁺ T-cells. Furthermore, anti-AChR CD4⁺ T-cells of MG patients frequently recognize the γ-subunit *(96)* that is usually expressed in the thymus *(199)* but not in adult muscle *(26)*, consistent with the possibility that the CD4⁺ T-cells had been sensitized to an AChR outside the muscle, and possibly in the thymus.

The beneficial effects of thymectomy in MG *(63)* suggest that the thymus has a role in maintaining MG. The therapeutic effects of thymectomy might be explained by the removal of a source of antigenic stimulation. The improvement usually appears several months after surgery *(63)*, consistent with the long life span of activated antigen-specific T-helper cells *(221)*. Such cells must die out before the effects of thymectomy become evident.

The large number of epitopes recognized by any MG patient *(1)* indicates that when the anti-AChR response has caused obvious myasthenic weakness, the whole AChR is involved in the autoimmune response. However, this does not exclude the possibility that the anti-AChR sensitization was initiated by molecular mimicry between a single viral or bacterial epitope and a small sequence region on the AChR, or by superantigen activation of CD4⁺ T-cells expressing a particular Vβ gene family and recognizing just one, or a limited set, of AChR epitopes: activation of CD4⁺ T-cells against even one epitope may be followed by spreading of the CD4⁺ response to the whole AChR. The thymus, rather than the muscle, would be a likely place for initiation of the anti-AChR CD4⁺ T-cell response because it expresses AChR-like proteins and contains cells that express MHC class II molecules *(184, 207)*. Among these, the reticulum cells have an ideal location for processing and presentation of epitopes derived form the AChR expressed by the myoid cells, as discussed above.

The activated AChR-specific CD4⁺ T-helper cells need to interact with anti-AChR B-cells, in order to produce a pathogenic high-affinity anti-AChR antibody. B-cells secreting antibodies that bind the AChR with low affinity are common: about 10% of the monoclonal IgGs in multiple myeloma patients bind muscle AChR *(222)*. However, myelomas are seldom associated with MG; the low affinity for the AChR of the myeloma antibodies may explain their inability to cause MG. The interaction of activated anti-AChR CD4$^+$ T-helper cells with B-cells that make low-affinity anti-AChR antibodies may trigger the mechanism of somatic mutation of the immunoglobulin genes and lead to the production of high-affinity pathogenic antibodies and myasthenic weakness.

## ACKNOWLEDGMENTS

The studies carried out in the authors' laboratory and included in this review were supported by NINDS grant NS23919 and by research grants from the Muscular Dystrophy Association of America (to B.M.C.-F.).

## REFERENCES

1. Conti-Fine BM, Bellone M, Howard JF Jr, Protti MP. *Myasthenia Gravis: The Immunobiology of an Autoimmune Disease*. Austin, TX, Neuroscience Intelligence Unit, RG Landes, 1997.
2. Engel AG. *The Myasthenic Syndromes*. New York, Oxford University Press, 1999.
3. Richman D. Myasthenia gravis and related diseases. Disorders of the neuromuscular junction. *Ann NY Acad Sci* 1998;841:1–838.
4. Oosterhuis HJGH. *Myasthenia gravis*. Groningen, Neurological Press, 1997.
5. Oldstone MB. Molecular mimicry and immune-mediated diseases. *FASEB J* 1998; 12:1255–1265.
6. Brocke S, Hausmann S, Steinman L, Wucherpfennig KW. Microbial peptides and superantigens in the pathogenesis of autoimmune diseases of the central nervous system. *Semin Immunol* 1998;10:57–67.
7. Mokhtarian F, Pino M, Ofosu-Appiah W, Grob D. Phenotypic and functional characterization of T cells from patients with myasthenia gravis. *J Clin Invest* 1990; 86:2099–2108.
8. Toyka KV, Drachman DB, Griffin DE, et al. Myasthenia gravis. Study of humoral immune mechanisms by passive transfer to mice. *N Engl J Med* 1977;296:125–131.
9. Lindstrom JM, Engel AG, Seybold ME, Lennon VA, Lambert EH. Pathological mechanisms in experimental autoimmune myasthenia gravis. II. Passive transfer of experimental autoimmune myasthenia gravis in rats with anti-acetylcholine receptor antibodies. *J Exp Med* 1976;144:739–753.
10. Oda K, Korenaga S, Ito Y. Myasthenia gravis: passive transfer to mice of antibody to human and mouse acetylcholine receptor. *Neurology* 1981;31:282–287.
11. Lennon VA, Lambert EH. Myasthenia gravis induced by monoclonal antibodies to acetylcholine receptors. *Nature* 1980;285:238–240.
12. Cornelio F, Antozzi C, Confalonieri P, Baggi F, Mantegazza R. Plasma treatment in diseases of the neuromuscular junction. *Ann NY Acad Sci* 1998;841:803–810.
13. Soliven BC, Lange DJ, Penn AS, et al. Seronegative myasthenia gravis. *Neurology* 1998;38:514–517.

14. Wang ZY, Karachunski PI, Howard JF Jr, Conti-Fine BM. Myasthenia in SCID mice grafted with myasthenic patient lymphocytes. Role of CD4$^+$ and CD8$^+$ cells. *Neurology* 1999;52:484–497.

15. Hoch W, McConville J, Helms S, et al. Auto-antibodies to the receptor tyrosine kinase MuSK in patients with myasthenia gravis without acetylcholine receptor antibodies. *Nat Med* 2001;7:365–368.

16. Lindstrom JM. Acetylcholine receptors and myasthenia. *Muscle Nerve* 2000;23: 453–477.

17. Tzartos SJ, Barkas T, Cung MT, et al. The main immunogenic region of the acetylcholine receptor. Structure and role in myasthenia gravis. *Autoimmunity* 1991;8: 259–270.

18. Beroukhim R, Unwin N. Three-dimensional location of the main immunogenic region of the acetylcholine receptor. *Neuron* 1995;15:323–331.

19. Lindstrom J, Einarson B. Antigenic modulation and receptor loss in experimental autoimmune myasthenia gravis. *Muscle Nerve* 1979;2:173–179.

20. Conti-Tronconi BM, Tzartos S, Lindstrom JM. Monoclonal antibodies as a probe of acetylcholine receptor structure. 2. Binding to native receptor. *Biochemistry* 1981; 20:2181–2186.

21. Tzartos SJ, Sophianos D, Efthimiadis A. Role of the main immunogenic region of acetylcholine receptor in myasthenia gravis. An Fab monoclonal antibody protects against antigenic modulation by human sera. *J Immunol* 1985;134:2343–2349.

22. Drachman DB. Myasthenia gravis. *N Engl J Med* 1994;330:1797–1810.

23. Lennon VA, Seybold ME, Lindstrom JM, Cochrane C, Ulevitch R. Role of complement in the pathogenesis of experimental autoimmune myasthenia gravis. *J Exp Med* 1978;147:973–983.

24. Engel AG, Arahata K. The membrane attack complex of complement at the endplate in myasthenia gravis. *Ann NY Acad Sci* 1987;505:326–332.

25. Karachunski PI, Ostlie NS, Monfardini C, Conti-Fine BM. Absence of IFN-γ or IL-12 has different effects on experimental myasthenia gravis in C57BL/6 mice. *J Immunol* 2000;164:5236–5244.

26. Conti-Tronconi BM, McLane KE, Raftery MA, Grando SA, Protti MP. The nicotinic acetylcholine receptor: structure and autoimmune pathology. *Crit Rev Biochem Mol Biol* 1994;29:69–123.

27. Lindstrom JM, Einarson BL, Lennon VA, Seybold ME. Pathological mechanisms in experimental autoimmune myasthenia gravis. I. Immunogenicity of syngeneic muscle acetylcholine receptor and quantitative extraction of receptor and antibody-receptor complexes from muscles of rats with experimental autoimmmune myasthenia gravis. *J Exp Med* 1976;144:726–738.

28. Granato DA, Fulpius BW, Moody JF. Experimental myasthenia in Balb/c mice immunized with rat acetylcholine receptor from rat denervated muscle. *Proc Natl Acad Sci USA* 1976;73:2872–2876.

29. Patrick J, Lindstrom J. Autoimmune response to acetylcholine receptor. *Science* 1973;180:871–872.

30. Tarrab-Hazdai R, Aharonov A, Abramsky O, Silman I, Fuchs S. Proceedings: animal model for myasthenia gravis: acetylcholine receptor-induced myasthenia in rabbits, guinea pigs and monkeys. *Isr J Med Sci* 1975;11:1390.

31. Lennon VA, Lindstrom JM, Seybold ME. Experimental autoimmune myasthenia: a model of myasthenia gravis in rats and guinea pigs. *J Exp Med* 1975;141:1365–1375.

32. Berman PW, Patrick J. Experimental myasthenia gravis. A murine system. *J Exp Med* 1980;151:204–223.

33. Zoda T, Yeh TM, Krolick KA. Clonotypic analysis of anti-acetylcholine receptor antibodies from experimental autoimmune myasthenia gravis-sensitive Lewis rats and experimental autoimmune myasthenia gravis-resistant Wistar Furth rats. *J Immunol* 1991;146:663–670.

34. Biesecker G, Koffler D. Resistance to experimental autoimmune myasthenia gravis in genetically inbred rats. Association with decreased amounts of in situ acetylcholine receptor-antibody complexes. *J Immunol* 1988;140:3406–3410.

35. Christadoss P, Krco CJ, Lennon VA, David CS. Genetic control of experimental autoimmune myasthenia gravis in mice. II. Lymphocyte proliferative response to acetylcholine receptor is dependent on Lyt-1+23- cells. *J Immunol* 1981;126:1646–1647.

36. Fuchs S, Nevo D, Tarrab-Hazdai R, Yaar I. Strain differences in the autoimmune response of mice to acetylcholine receptors. *Nature* 1976;263:329–330.

37. Christadoss P, Lindstrom JM, Melvold RW, Talal N. Mutation at I-A β chain prevents experimental autoimmune myasthenia gravis. *Immunogenetics* 1985;21:33–38.

38. Lindstrom JM, Seybold ME, Lennon VA, Whittingham S, Duane DD. Antibody to acetylcholine receptor in myasthenia gravis. Prevalence, clinical correlates, and diagnostic value. *Neurology* 1976;26:1054–1059.

39. Roses AD, Olanow CW, McAdams MW, Lane RJ. No direct correlation between serum antiacetylcholine receptor antibody levels and clinical state of individual patients with myasthenia gravis. *Neurology* 1981;31:220–224.

40. Bellone M, Ostlie N, Lei SJ, Wu XD, Conti-Tronconi BM. The I-Abm12 mutation, which confers resistance to experimental myasthenia gravis, drastically affects the epitope repertoire of murine CD4+ cells sensitized to nicotinic acetylcholine receptor. *J Immunol* 1991;147:1484–1491.

41. Karachunski PI, Ostlie NS, Okita DK, Conti-Fine BM. Interleukin-4 deficiency facilitates development of experimental myasthenia gravis and precludes its prevention by nasal administration of CD4+ epitope sequences of the acetylcholine receptor. *J Neuroimmunol* 1999;95:73–84.

42. Tzartos S, Hochschwender S, Vasquez P, Lindstrom J. Passive transfer of experimental autoimmune myasthenia gravis by monoclonal antibodies to the main immunogenic region of the acetylcholine receptor. *J Neuroimmunol* 1987;15:185–194.

43. Tzartos SJ, Kokla A, Walgrave SL, Conti-Tronconi BM. Localization of the main immunogenic region of human muscle acetylcholine receptor to residues 67–76 of the α subunit. *Proc Natl Acad Sci USA* 1988;85:2899–2903.

44. Bellone M, Tang F, Milius R, Conti-Tronconi BM. The main immunogenic region of the nicotinic acetylcholine receptor. Identification of amino acid residues interacting with different antibodies. *J Immunol* 1989;143:3568–3579.

45. Barkas T, Gabriel JM, Mauron A, et al. Monoclonal antibodies to the main immunogenic region of the nicotinic acetylcholine receptor bind to residues 61–76 of the α subunit. *J Biol Chem* 1988;263:5916–5920.

46. Manfredi AA, Bellone M, Protti MP, Conti-Tronconi BM. Molecular mimicry among human autoantigens. *Immunol Today* 1991;12:46–47.
47. Gomez CM, Richman DP. Anti-acetylcholine receptor antibodies directed against the α-bungarotoxin binding site induce a unique form of experimental myasthenia. *Proc Natl Acad Sci USA* 1983;80:4089–4093.
48. Conti-Fine BM, Kaminski HJ. Neuroimmunology. *Continuum* 2001;7:56–95.
49. Walker MB. Case showing the effect of prostigmin on myasthenia gravis. *Proc R Soc Med* 1935;28:759–751.
50. Poea S, Guyon T, Bidault J, et al. Modulation of acetylcholine receptor expression in seronegative myasthenia gravis. *Ann Neurol* 2000;48:696–705.
51. Aarli JA, Skeie GO, Mygland A, Gilhus NE. Muscle striation antibodies in myasthenia gravis. Diagnostic and functional significance. *Ann NY Acad Sci* 1998;841: 505–515.
52. Link H, Sun JB, Lu CZ, et al. Myasthenia gravis: T and B cell reactivities to the α-bungarotoxin binding protein presynaptic membrane receptor. *J Neurol Sci* 1992; 109:173–181.
53. Takaya M, Kawahara S, Namba T, Grob D. Antibodies against myofibrillar proteins in myasthenia gravis patients. *J Exp Clin Med* 1992;17:35–39.
54. Mohan S, Barohn RJ, Jackson CE, Krolick KA. Evaluation of myosin-reactive antibodies from a panel of myasthenia gravis patients. *Clin Immunol Immunopathol* 1994;70:266–273.
55. Mohan S, Barohn RJ, Krolick KA. Unexpected cross-reactivity between myosin and a main immunogenic region (MIR) of the acetylcholine receptor by antisera obtained from myasthenia gravis patients. *Clin Immunol Immunopathol* 1992;64: 218–226.
56. Kuks JB, Limburg PC, Horst G, Dijksterhuis J, Oosterhuis HJ. Antibodies to skeletal muscle in myasthenia gravis. Part 1. Diagnostic value for the detection of thymoma. *J Neurol Sci* 1993;119:183–188.
57. Aarli JA. Titin, thymoma, and myasthenia gravis. *Arch Neurol* 2001;58:869–870.
58. Skeie GO. Skeletal muscle titin: physiology and pathophysiology. *Cell Mol Life Sci* 2000;57:1570–1576.
59. Baggi F, Andreetta F, Antozzi C, et al. Anti-titin and antiryanodine receptor antibodies in myasthenia gravis patients with thymoma. *Ann NY Acad Sci* 1998;841: 538–541.
60. Hohlfeld R, Toyka KV, Miner LL, Walgrave SL, Conti-Tronconi BM. Amphipathic segment of the nicotinic receptor alpha subunit contains epitopes recognized by T lymphocytes in myasthenia gravis. *J Clin Invest* 1988;81:657–660.
61. Ahlberg R, Yi Q, Pirskanen R, et al. Treatment of myasthenia gravis with anti-CD4 antibody: improvement correlates to decreased T-cell autoreactivity. *Neurology* 1994;44:1732–1737.
62. Morgutti M, Conti-Tronconi BM, Sghirlanzoni A, Clementi F. Cellular immune response to acetylcholine receptor in myasthenia gravis: II. Thymectomy and corticosteroids. *Neurology* 1979;29:734–738.
63. Gronseth GS, Barohn RJ. Practice parameter: thymectomy for autoimmune myasthenia gravis (an evidence-based review): report of the Quality Standards Subcommittee of the American Academy of Neurology. *Neurology* 2000;55:7–15.

64. Hohlfeld R, Kalies I, Ernst M, Ketelsen UP, Wekerle H. T-lymphocytes in experimental autoimmune myasthenia gravis. Isolation of T-helper cell lines. *J Neurol Sci* 1982;57:265–280.
65. Zhang GX, Xiao BG, Bakhiet M, et al. Both CD4+ and CD8+ T cells are essential to induce experimental autoimmune myasthenia gravis. *J Exp Med* 1996;184:349–356.
66. Kaul R, Shenoy M, Goluszko E, Christadoss P. Major histocompatibility complex class II gene disruption prevents experimental autoimmune myasthenia gravis. *J Immunol* 1994;152:3152–3157.
67. Simpson E, Farrant J, Chandler P. Phenotypic and functional studies of human peripheral blood lymphocytes engrafted in SCID mice. *Immunol Rev* 1991;124:97–111.
68. Schonbeck S, Padberg F, Hohlfeld R, Wekerle H. Transplantation of thymic autoimmune microenvironment to severe combined immunodeficiency mice. A new model of myasthenia gravis. *J Clin Invest* 1992;90:245–250.
69. Martino G, DuPont BL, Wollmann RL, et al. The human-severe combined immunodeficiency myasthenic mouse model: a new approach for the study of myasthenia gravis. *Ann Neurol* 1993;34:48–56.
70. Pette M, Fujita K, Kitze B, et al. Myelin basic protein-specific T lymphocyte lines from MS patients and healthy individuals. *Neurology* 1990;40:1770–1776.
71. Martin R, Jaraquemada D, Flerlage M, et al. Fine specificity and HLA restriction of myelin basic protein-specific cytotoxic T cell lines from multiple sclerosis patients and healthy individuals. *J Immunol* 1990;145:540–548.
72. Sommer N, Harcourt GC, Willcox N, Beeson D, Newsom-Davis J. Acetylcholine receptor-reactive T lymphocytes from healthy subjects and myasthenia gravis patients. *Neurology* 1991;41:1270–1276.
73. Kellermann SA, McCormick DJ, Freeman SL, Morris JC, Conti-Fine BM. TSH receptor sequences recognized by CD4+ T cells in Graves' disease patients and healthy controls. *J Autoimmun* 1995;8:685–698.
74. Marrack P. T cell tolerance. *Harvey Lect* 1993–94;89:147–155.
75. Conti-Fine BM, Navaneetham D, Karachunski PI, et al. T cell recognition of the acetylcholine receptor in myasthenia gravis. *Ann NY Acad Sci* 1998;841:283–308.
76. Diethelm-Okita B, Wells GB, Kuryatov A, et al. Response of CD4+ T cells from myasthenic patients and healthy subjects of biosynthetic and synthetic sequences of the nicotinic acetylcholine receptor. *J Autoimmun* 1998;11:191–203.
77. Fujii Y, Lindstrom J. Specificity of the T cell immune response to acetylcholine receptor in experimental autoimmune myasthenia gravis. Response to subunits and synthetic peptides. *J Immunol* 1988;140:1830–1837.
78. Oshima M, Pachner AR, Atassi MZ. Profile of the regions of acetylcholine receptor α chain recognized by T-lymphocytes and by antibodies in EAMG-susceptible and non-susceptible mouse strains after different periods of immunization with the receptor. *Mol Immunol* 1994;31:833–843.
79. Bellone M, Ostlie N, Lei S, Conti-Tronconi BM. Experimental myasthenia gravis in congenic mice: sequence mapping and H-2 restriction of T helper epitopes on the α-subunits of *Torpedo californica* and murine acetylcholine receptor. *Eur J Immunol* 1991;21:2303–2310.

80. Bellone M, Ostlie N, Karachunski P, Manfredi AA, Conti-Tronconi BM. Cryptic epitopes on the nicotinic acetylcholine receptor are recognized by autoreactive CD4+ cells. *J Immunol* 1993;151:1025–1038.
81. Vanderlugt CL, Begolka WS, Neville KL, et al. The functional significance of epitope spreading and its regulation by co-stimulatory molecules. *Immunol Rev* 1998; 64:63–72.
82. Hohlfeld R, Toyka KV, Tzartos SJ, Carson W, Conti-Tronconi BM. Human T-helper lymphocytes in myasthenia gravis recognize the nicotinic receptor α subunit. *Proc Natl Acad Sci USA* 1987;84:5379–5383.
83. Manfredi AA, Protti MP, Wu XD, Howard JF Jr, Conti-Tronconi BM. CD4$^+$ T-epitope repertoire on the human acetylcholine receptor α subunit in severe myasthenia gravis: a study with synthetic peptides. *Neurology* 1992;42:1092–1100.
84. Manfredi AA, Protti MP, Dalton MW, Howard JF Jr, Conti-Tronconi BM. T helper cell recognition of muscle acetylcholine receptor in myasthenia gravis. Epitopes on the γ and δ-subunits. *J Clin Invest* 1993;92:1055–1067.
85. Wang ZY, Okita DK, Howard J Jr, Conti-Fine BM. T-cell recognition of muscle acetylcholine receptor subunits in generalized and ocular myasthenia gravis. *Neurology* 1998;50:1045–1054.
86. Wang ZY, Okita DK, Howard JF Jr, Conti-Fine BM. CD4+ T cell repertoire on the ε subunit of muscle acetylcholine receptor in myasthenia gravis. *J Neuroimmunol* 1998;91:33–42.
87. Wang ZY, Diethelm-Okita B, Okita DK, et al. T cell recognition of muscle acetylcholine receptor in ocular myasthenia gravis. *J Neuroimmunol* 2000;108:29–39.
88. Horton RM, Manfredi AA, Conti-Tronconi BM. The 'embryonic' γ subunit of the nicotinic acetylcholine receptor is expressed in adult extraocular muscle. *Neurology* 1993;43:983–986.
89. Kaminski HJ, Fenstermaker R, Ruff RL. Adult extraocular and intercostal muscle express the γ subunit of fetal AChR. *Biophys J* 1991;59:444a.
90. Nelson S, Conti-Tronconi BM. Adult thymus expresses an embryonic nicotinic acetylcholine receptor-like protein. *J Neuroimmunol* 1990;29:81–92.
91. Geuder KI, Marx A, Witzemann V, et al. Pathogenetic significance of fetal-type acetylcholine receptors on thymic myoid cells in myasthenia gravis. *Dev Immunol* 1992;2:69–75.
92. Protti MP, Manfredi AA, Straub C, et al. Use of synthetic peptides to establish anti-human acetylcholine receptor CD4+ cell lines from myasthenia gravis patients. *J Immunol* 1990;144:1711–1720.
93. Protti MP, Manfredi AA, Straub C, Howard JF Jr, Conti-Tronconi BM. Immunodominant regions for T helper-cell sensitization on the human nicotinic receptor α subunit in myasthenia gravis. *Proc Natl Acad Sci USA* 1990;87:7792–7796.
94. Protti MP, Manfredi AA, Wu XD, et al. Myasthenia gravis. T epitopes on the δ subunit of human muscle acetylcholine receptor. *J Immunol* 1991;146:2253–2261.
95. Protti MP, Manfredi AA, Howard JF Jr, Conti-Tronconi BM. T cells in myasthenia gravis specific for embryonic acetylcholine receptor. *Neurology* 1991;41:1809–1814.
96. Protti MP, Manfredi AA, Wu XD, et al. Myasthenia gravis. CD4+ T epitopes on the embryonic γ subunit of human muscle acetylcholine receptor. *J Clin Invest* 1992; 90:1558–1567.

97. Moiola L, Karachunski P, Protti MP, Howard JF Jr, Conti-Tronconi BM. Epitopes on the β subunit of human muscle acetylcholine receptor recognized by CD4+ cells of myasthenia gravis patients and healthy subjects. *J Clin Invest* 1994;93: 1020–1028.
98. Collins EJ, Frelinger JA. Altered peptide ligand design: altering immune responses to class I MHC/peptide complexes. *Immunol Rev* 1998;163:151–160.
99. Nicholson LB, Greer JM, Sobel RA, Lees MB, Kuchroo VK. An altered peptide ligand mediates immune deviation and prevents autoimmune encephalomyelitis. *Immunity* 1995;3:397–405.
100. Tsitoura DC, Holter W, Cerwenka A, Gelder CM, Lamb JR. Induction of anergy in human T helper 0 cells by stimulation with altered T cell antigen receptor ligands. *J Immunol* 1996;156:2801–2808.
101. Wang ZY, Okita DK, Howard J Jr, Conti-Fine BM. Th1 epitope repertoire on the α subunit of human muscle acetylcholine receptor in myasthenia gravis. *Neurology* 1997;48:1643–1653.
102. Diethelm-Okita BM, Okita DK, Banaszak L, Conti-Fine BM. Universal epitopes for human CD4+ cells on tetanus and diphtheria toxins. *J Infect Dis* 2000;181: 1001–1009.
103. Sommer N, Melms A, Weller M, Dichgans J. Ocular myasthenia gravis. A critical review of clinical and pathological aspects. *Documenta Ophthalmol* 1993;84: 309–333.
104. Kaminski HJ, Maas E, Spiegel P, Ruff RL. Why are eye muscles frequently involved in myasthenia gravis? *Neurology* 1990;40:1663–1669.
105. Kaminski HJ, Ruff RL. Ocular muscle involvement by myasthenia gravis. *Ann Neurol* 1997;41:419–420.
106. Engel AG, Ohno K, Sine SM. Congenital myasthenic syndromes: experiments of nature. *J Physiol Paris* 1998;92:113–117.
107. Kaminski HJ, Kusner LL, Block CH. Expression of acetylcholine receptor isoforms at extraocular muscle endplates. *Invest Ophthalmol Vis Sci* 1996;37:345–351.
108. Kaminski HJ, Kusner LL, Nash KV, Ruff RL. The γ-subunit of the acetylcholine receptor is not expressed in the levator palpebrae superioris. *Neurology* 1995;45: 516–518.
109. MacLennan C, Beeson D, Buijs AM, Vincent A, Newsom-Davis J. Acetylcholine receptor expression in human extraocular muscles and their susceptibility to myasthenia gravis. *Ann Neurol* 1997;41:423–431.
110. Raju R, Navaneetham D, Protti MP, et al. TCR V β usage by acetylcholine receptor-specific CD4+ T cells in myasthenia gravis. *J Autoimmun* 1997;10:203–217.
111. Melms A, Oksenberg JR, Malcherek G, et al. T-cell receptor gene usage of acetylcholine receptor-specific T-helper cells. *Ann NY Acad Sci* 1993;681:313–314.
112. Garcia KC, Teyton L, Wilson IA. Structural basis of T cell recognition. *Annu Rev Immunol* 1999;17:369–397.
113. Li H, Llera A, Malchiodi EL, Mariuzza RA. The structural basis of T cell activation by superantigens. *Annu Rev Immunol* 1999;17:435–466.
114. Hennecke J, Wiley DC. T cell receptor-MHC interactions up close. *Cell* 2001;104: 1–4.
115. Wei S, Charmley P, Robinson MA, Concannon P. The extent of the human germline T-cell receptor V β gene segment repertoire. *Immunogenetics* 1994;40:27–36.

116. Papageorgiou AC, Acharya KR. Microbial superantigens: from structure to function. *Trends Microbiol* 2000;8:369–375.
117. Rose NR. The role of infection in the pathogenesis of autoimmune disease. *Semin Immunol* 1998;10:5–13.
118. Todd JA, Steinman L. The enviroment strikes back. *Curr Opin Immunol* 1993;5: 863–865.
119. Blackman MA, Woodland DL. Role of the T cell receptor α-chain in superantigen recognition. *Immunol Res* 1996;15:98–113.
120. Tesch H, Hohlfeld R, Toyka KV. Analysis of immunoglobulin and T cell receptor gene rearrangements in the thymus of myasthenia gravis patients. *J Neuroimmunol* 1989;21:169–176.
121. Grunewald J, Ahlberg R, Lefvert AK, et al. Abnormal T-cell expansion and V-gene usage in myasthenia gravis patients. *J Immunol* 1991;34:161–168.
122. Truffault F, Cohen-Kaminsky S, Khalil I, Levasseur P, Berrih-Aknin S. Altered intrathymic T-cell repertoire in human myasthenia gravis. *Ann Neurol* 1997;41:731–741.
123. Xu BY, Giscombe R, Soderlund A, et al. Abnormal T cell receptor V gene usage in myasthenia gravis: prevalence and characterization of expanded T cell populations. *Clin Exp Immunol* 1998;113:456–464.
124. Navaneetham D, Penn AS, Howard JF Jr, Conti-Fine BM. TCR-V β usage in the thymus and blood of myasthenia gravis patients. *J Autoimmun* 1998;11:621–633.
125. Navaneetham D, Diethelm-Okita B, Protti MP, Conti-Fine BM. Manuscript in preparation.
126. Yang XD, Tisch R, McDevitt HO. Selective targets for immunotherapy in autoimmune disease. *Chem Immunol* 1995;60:20–31.
127. Vandenbark AA, Hashim GA, Offner H. T cell receptor peptides in treatment of autoimmune disease: rationale and potential. *J Neurosci Res* 1996;43:391–402.
128. Miller SD, McRae BL, Vanderlugt CL, et al. Evolution of the T-cell repertoire during the course of experimental immune-mediated demyelinating diseases. *Immunol Rev* 1995;144:225–244.
129. Dong C, Flavell RA. Th1 and Th2 cells. *Curr Opin Hematol* 2001;8:47–51.
130. Feldmann M, Brennan FM, Maini R. Cytokines in autoimmune disorders. *Int Rev Immunol* 1998;17:217–228.
131. O'Garra A. Cytokines induce the development of functionally heterogeneous T helper cell subsets. *Immunity* 1998;8:275–283.
132. Abbas AK, Murphy KM, Sher A. Functional diversity of helper T lymphocytes. *Nature* 1996;383:787–793.
133. Yi Q, Ahlberg R, Pirskanen R, Lefvert AK. Acetylcholine receptor-reactive T cells in myasthenia gravis: evidence for the involvement of different subpopulations of T helper cells. *J Neuroimmunol* 1994;50:1771–1786.
134. Yi Q, Lefvert AK. Idiotype- and anti-idiotype-reactive T lymphocytes in myasthenia gravis. Evidence for the involvement of different subpopulations of T helper lymphocytes. *J Immunol* 1994;153:3353–3359.
135. Link J, Fredrikson S, Soderstrom M, et al. Organ-specific autoantigens induce transforming growth factor-β mRNA expression in mononuclear cells in multiple sclerosis and myasthenia gravis. *Ann Neurol* 1994;35:197–203.
136. Moiola L, Protti MP, McCormick D, Howard JF, Conti-Tronconi BM. Myasthenia gravis. Residues of the α and γ subunits of muscle acetylcholine receptor

involved in formation of immunodominant CD4+ epitopes. *J Immunol* 1994;152: 4686–4698.

137. Moiola L, Galbiati F, Martino G, et al. IL-12 is involved in the induction of experimental autoimmune myasthenia gravis, an antibody-mediated disease. *Eur J Immunol* 1998;28:2487–2497.

138. Balasa B, Deng C, Lee J, et al. Interferon γ (IFN-γ) is necessary for the genesis of acetylcholine receptor-induced clinical experimental autoimmune myasthenia gravis in mice. *J Exp Med* 1997;186:385–391.

139. Balasa B, Deng C, Lee J, Christadoss P, Sarvetnick N. The Th2 cytokine IL-4 is not required for the progression of antibody-dependent autoimmune myasthenia gravis. *J Immunol* 1998;161:2856–2862.

140. Zhang GX, Xiao BG, Bai XF, et al. Mice with IFN-γ receptor deficiency are less susceptible to experimental autoimmune myasthenia gravis. *J Immunol* 1999;162: 3775–3781.

141. Ostlie NS, Karachunski PI, Wang W, et al. Transgenic expression of IL-10 in T cells facilitates development of experimental myasthenia gravis. *J Immunol* 2001; 166:4853–4862.

142. Sitaraman S, Metzger DW, Belloto RJ, Infante AJ, Wall KA. Interleukin-12 enhances clinical experimental autoimmune myasthenia gravis in susceptible but not resistant mice. *J Neuroimmunol* 2000;107:73–82.

143. Karachunski PI, Ostlie NS, Okita DK, Conti-Fine BM. Prevention of experimental myasthenia gravis by nasal administration of synthetic acetylcholine receptor T epitope sequences. *J Clin Invest* 1997;100:3027–3035.

144. Baggi F, Andreetta F, Caspani E, et al. Oral administration of an immunodominant T-cell epitope downregulates Th1/Th2 cytokines and prevents experimental myasthenia gravis. *J Clin Invest* 1999;104:1287–1295.

145. Im SH, Barchan D, Fuchs S, Souroujon MC. Mechanism of nasal tolerance induced by a recombinant fragment of acetylcholine receptor for treatment of experimental myasthenia gravis. *J Neuroimmunol* 2000;111:161–168.

146. Wang ZY, Link H, Ljungdahl A, et al. Induction of interferon-γ, interleukin-4, and transforming growth factor-β in rats orally tolerized against experimental autoimmune myasthenia gravis. *Cell Immunol* 1994;157:353–368.

147. Karachunski PI, Ostlie NS, Okita DK, Garman R, Conti-Fine BM. Subcutaneous administration of T-epitope sequences of the acetylcholine receptor prevents experimental myasthenia gravis. *J Neuroimmunol* 1999;93:108–121.

148. Im SH, Barchan D, Fuchs S, Souroujon MC. Suppression of ongoing experimental myasthenia by oral treatment with an acetylcholine receptor recombinant fragment. *J Clin Invest* 1999;104:1723–1730.

149. Monfardini C, Milani M, Ostlie N, et al. Adoptive protection from experimental myasthenia gravis with T cells from mice treated nasally with acetylcholine receptor epitopes. *J Neuroimmunol* 2002;123:123–134.

150. Hagenbaugh A, Sharma S, Dubinett SM, et al. Altered immune responses in interleukin 10 transgenic mice. *J Exp Med* 1997;185:2101–2110.

151. Poussin MA, Goluszko E, Hughes TK, Duchicella SI, Christadoss P. Suppression of experimental autoimmune myasthenia gravis in IL-10 gene-disrupted mice is associated with reduced B cells and serum cytotoxicity on mouse cell line expressing AChR. *J Neuroimmunol* 2000;111:152–160.

152. Ding L, Linsley PS, Huang LY, Germain RN, Shevach EM. IL-10 inhibits macrophage costimulatory activity by selectively inhibiting the up-regulation of B7 expression. *J Immunol* 1993;151:1224–1234.

153. Fiorentino DF, Zlotnik A, Mosmann TR, Howard M, O'Garra A. IL-10 inhibits cytokine production by activated macrophages. *J Immunol* 1991;147:3815–3822.

154. Macatonia SE, Doherty TM, Knight SC, O'Garra A. Differential effect of IL-10 on dendritic cell-induced T cell proliferation and IFN-γ production. *J Immunol* 1993;150:3755–3765.

155. Enk AH, Angeloni VL, Udey MC, Katz SI. Inhibition of Langerhans cell antigen-presenting function by IL-10. A role for IL-10 in induction of tolerance. *J Immunol* 1993;151:2390–2398.

156. Aste-Amezaga M, Ma X, Sartori A, Trinchieri G. Molecular mechanisms of the induction of IL-12 and its inhibition by IL-10. *J Immunol* 1998;160:5936–5944.

157. de Waal Malefyt R, Yssel H, de Vries JE. Direct effects of IL-10 on subsets of human CD4+ T cell clones and resting T cells. Specific inhibition of IL-2 production and proliferation. *J Immunol* 1993;150:4754–4765.

158. Taga K, Mostowski H, Tosato G. Human interleukin-10 can directly inhibit T-cell growth. *Blood* 1993;81:2964–2971.

159. Groux H, Bigler M, de Vries JE, Roncarolo MG. Interleukin-10 induces a long-term antigen-specific anergic state in human CD4+ T cells. *J Exp Med* 1996;184:19–29.

160. Schwartz RH. Models of T cell anergy: is there a common molecular mechanism? *J Exp Med* 1996;184:1–8.

161. Georgescu L, Vakkalanka RK, Elkon KB, Crow MK. Interleukin-10 promotes activation-induced cell death of SLE lymphocytes mediated by Fas ligand. *J Clin Invest* 1997;100:2622–2633.

162. Bromberg JS. IL-10 immunosuppression in transplantation. *Curr Opin Immunol* 1995;7:639–643.

163. Akdis CA, Blaser K. IL-10-induced anergy in peripheral T cell and reactivation by microenvironmental cytokines: two key steps in specific immunotherapy. *FASEB J* 1999;13:603–609.

164. Llorente L, Zou W, Levy Y, et al. Role of interleukin 10 in the B lymphocyte hyperactivity and autoantibody production of human systemic lupus erythematosus. *J Exp Med* 1995;181:839–844.

165. Cross JT, Benton HP. The roles of interleukin-6 and interleukin-10 in B cell hyperactivity in systemic lupus erythematosus. *Inflamm Res* 1999;48:255–261.

166. Huang YM, Kivisakk P, Ozenci V, Pirskanen R, Link H. Increased levels of circulating acetylcholine receptor (AChR)-reactive IL-10-secreting cells are characteristic for myasthenia gravis (MG). *Clin Exp Immunol* 1999;118:304–308.

167. Wogensen L, Lee MS, Sarvetnick N. Production of interleukin 10 by islet cells accelerates immune-mediated destruction of β cells in nonobese diabetic mice. *J Exp Med* 1994;179:1379–1384.

168. Moritani M, Yoshimoto K, Tashiro F, et al. Transgenic expression of IL-10 in pancreatic islet A cells accelerates autoimmune insulitis and diabetes in non-obese diabetic mice. *Int Immunol* 1994;6:1927–1936.

169. Pennline KJ, Roque-Gaffney E, Monahan M. Recombinant human IL-10 prevents the onset of diabetes in the nonobese diabetic mouse. *Clin Immunol Immunopathol* 1994;71:169–175.

170. Moritani M, Yoshimoto K, Ii S, et al. Prevention of adoptively transferred diabetes in nonobese diabetic mice with IL-10-transduced islet-specific Th1 lymphocytes. A gene therapy model for autoimmune diabetes. *J Clin Invest* 1996;98:1851–1859.

171. Kong KM, Waldmann H, Cobbold S, et al. Pathogenic mechanisms in murine autoimmune thyroiditis: short- and long-term effects of in vivo depletion of CD4+ and CD8+ cells. *Clin Exp Immunol* 1989;77:428–433.

172. Pummerer C, Berger P, Fruhwirth M, et al. Cellular infiltrate, major histocompatibility antigen expression and immunopathogenic mechanisms in cardiac myosin-induced myocarditis. *Lab Invest* 1991;65:538–547.

173. Mozes E, Kohn LD, Hakim F, et al. Resistance of MHC class I-deficient mice to experimental systemic lupus erythematosus. *Science* 1993;261:91–93.

174. Rodriguez M, Dunkel AJ, Thiemann RL. Abrogation of resistance to Theiler's virus-induced demyelination in H-2b mice deficient in beta 2-microglobulin. *J Immunol* 1993;151:266–276.

175. Shenoy M, Kaul R, Goluszko E, et al. Effect of MHC class I and CD8 cell deficiency on experimental autoimmune myasthenia gravis. *J Immunol* 1994;153:5330–5335.

176. Shenoy M, Baron S, Wu B, et al. IFN-alpha treatment suppresses the development of experimental autoimmue myasthenia gravis. *J Immunol* 1995;154:6203–6208.

177. Zhang GX, Ma CG, Xiao BG, et al. Depletion of CD8+ T cells suppresses the development of experimental autoimmune myasthenia gravis in Lewis rats. *Eur J Immunol* 1995;25:1191–1198.

178. Miller AE, Hudson J, Tindall RS. Immune regulation in myasthenia gravis: evidence for an increased suppressor T-cell population. *Ann Neurol* 1982;12:341–347.

179. Skolnik PR, Lisak RP, Zweiman B. Monoclonal antibody analysis of blood T-cell subsets in myasthenia gravis. *Ann Neurol* 1982;11:170–176.

180. Protti MP, Manfredi AA, Straub C, Howard JF Jr, Conti-Tronconi BM. CD4+ T cell response to human acetylcholine receptor α subunit correlates with myasthenia gravis severity. A study with synthetic peptides. *J Immunol* 1990;144:1276–1281.

181. Lisak RP, Laramore C, Levinson AI, Zweiman B, Moskovitz AR. Suppressor T cells in myasthenia gravis and antibodies to acetylcholine receptor. *Ann Neurol* 1986;19:87–89.

182. Lisak RP, Laramore C, Levinson AI, et al. In vitro synthesis of antibodies to acetylcholine receptor by peripheral blood cells: role of suppressor T cells in normal subjects. *Neurology* 1984;34:802–805.

183. Yuen MH, Protti MP, Diethelm-Okita B, et al. Immunoregulatory CD8+ cells recognize antigen-activated CD4+ cells in myasthenia gravis patients and in healthy controls. *J Immunol* 1995;154:1508–1520.

184. Hohlfeld R, Wekerle H. The thymus in myasthenia gravis. *Neurol Clin* 1994;12:331–342.

185. Levinson AI, Wheatley LM. The thymus and the pathogenesis of myasthenia gravis. *Clin Immunol Immunopathol* 1996;78:1–5.

186. Aharonov A, Tarrab-Hazdai R, Abramsky O, Fuchs S. Immunological relationship between acetylcholine receptor and thymus: a possible significance in myasthenia gravis. *Proc Natl Acad Sci USA* 1975;72:1456–1459.

187. Engel EK, Trotter JL, McFarlin DE, McIntosh CL. Thymic epithelial cell contains acetylcholine receptor. *Lancet* 1977;1:1310–1311.

188. Ueno S, Wada K, Takahashi M, Tarui S. Acetylcholine receptor in rabbit thymus: antigenic similarity between acetylcholine receptors of muscle and thymus. *Clin Exp Immunol* 1980;42:463–469.

189. Schluep M, Willcox N, Vincent A, Dhoot GK, Newsom-Davis J. Acetylcholine receptors in human thymic myoid cells in situ: an immunohistological study. *Ann Neurol* 1987;22:212–222.

190. Kawanami S, Conti-Tronconi B, Racs J, Raftery MA. Isolation and characterization of nicotinic acetylcholine receptor-like protein from fetal calf thymus. *J Neurol Sci* 1988;87:195–209.

191. Kirchner T, Tzartos S, Hoppe F, et al. Pathogenesis of myasthenia gravis. Acetylcholine receptor-related antigenic determinants in tumor-free thymuses and thymic epithelial tumors. *Am J Pathol* 1988;130:268–280.

192. Kao I, Drachman DB. Thymic muscle cells bear acetylcholine receptors: possible relation to myasthenia gravis. *Science* 1977;195:74–75.

193. Zheng Y, Wheatley LM, Liu T, Levinson AI. Acetylcholine receptor α subunit mRNA expression in human thymus: augmented expression in myasthenia gravis and upregulation by interferon-γ. *Clin Immunol* 1999;91:170–177.

194. Wakkach A, Guyon T, Bruand C, et al. Expression of acetylcholine receptor genes in human thymic epithelial cells: implications for myasthenia gravis. *J Immunol* 1996;157:3752–3760.

195. Andreetta F, Baggi F, Antozzi C, et al. Acetylcholine receptor α-subunit isoforms are differentially expressed in thymuses from myasthenic patients. *Am J Pathol* 1997;150:341–348.

196. Navaneetham D, Penn AS, Howard JF Jr, Conti-Fine BM. Human thymuses express incomplete sets of muscle acetylcholine receptor subunit transcripts that seldom include the δ subunit. *Muscle Nerve* 2001;24:203–210.

197. Marx A, Wilisch A, Gutsche S, et al. Low levels of acetylcholine receptor δ subunit message and protein in human thymuses suggest the occurrence of triplet receptors in thymic myoid cells. In: Christadoss P, ed. *Myasthenia Gravis: Disease Mechanisms and Immunointervention*. New Delhi, Narosa, 2000, pp. 28–34.

198. Kaminski HJ, Fenstermaker RA, Abdul-Karim FW, Clayman J, Ruff RL. Acetylcholine receptor subunit gene expression in thymic tissue. *Muscle Nerve* 1993;16:1332–1337.

199. Geuder KI, Marx A, Witzemann V, et al. Pathogenetic significance of fetal-type acetylcholine receptors on thymic myoid cells in myasthenia gravis. *Dev Immunol* 1992;2:69–75.

200. Wheatley LM, Urso D, Tumas K, et al. Molecular evidence for the expression of nicotinic acetylcholine receptor α-chain in mouse thymus. *J Immunol* 1992;148:3105–3109.

201. Kornstein MJ, Asher O, Fuchs S. Acetylcholine receptor α-subunit and myogenin mRNAs in thymus and thymomas. *Am J Pathol* 1995;146:1320–1324.

202. Hara H, Hayashi K, Ohta K, Itoh N, Ohta M. Nicotinic acetylcholine receptor mRNAs in myasthenic thymuses: association with intrathymic pathogenesis of myasthenia gravis. *Biochem Biophys Res Commun* 1993;194:1269–1275.

203. Wakkach A, Poea S, Chastre E, et al. Establishment of a human thymic myoid cell line. Phenotypic and functional characteristics. *Am J Pathol* 1999;155:1229–1240.

204. Wilisch A, Gutsche S, Hoffacker V, et al. Association of acetylcholine receptor α-subunit gene expression in mixed thymoma with myasthenia gravis. *Neurology* 1999; 52:1460–1466.
205. Sine SM, Claudio T. γ- and δ-subunits regulate the affinity and the cooperativity of ligand binding to the acetylcholine receptor. *J Biol Chem* 1991;266:19,369–19,377.
206. Schonbeck S, Chrestel S, Hohlfeld R. Myasthenia gravis: prototype of the anti-receptor autoimmune diseases. *Int Rev Neurobiol* 1990;32:175–200.
207. Kirchner T, Hoppe F, Schalke B, Muller-Hermelink HK. Microenvironment of thymic myoid cells in myasthenia gravis. *Virchows Arch B Cell Pathol* 1988;54: 295–302.
208. Siara J, Rudel R, Marx A. Absence of acetylcholine-induced current in epithelial cells from thymus glands and thymomas of myasthenia gravis patients. *Neurology* 1991;41:128–131.
209. Rose NR. The role of infection in the pathogenesis of autoimmune disease. *Semin Immunol* 1998;10:5–13.
210. Fujinami RS, Oldstone MB. Amino acid homology between the encephalitogenic site of myelin basic protein and virus: mechanism for autoimmunity. *Science* 1985; 230:1043–1045.
211. Todd JA, Steinman L. The environment strikes back. *Curr Opin Immunol* 1993;5: 863–865.
212. Gautam AM, Lock CB, Smilek DE, et al. Minimum structural requirements for peptide presentation by major histocompatibility complex class II molecules: implications in induction of autoimmunity. *Proc Natl Acad Sci USA* 1994;91:767–771.
213. Ohno S. Many peptide fragments of alien antigens are homologous with host proteins, thus canalizing T-cell responses. *Proc Natl Acad Sci USA* 1991;88:3065–3068.
214. Farris AD, Keech CL, Gordon TP, McCluskey J. Epitope mimics and determinant spreading: pathways to autoimmunity. *Cell Mol Life Sci* 2000;57:569–578.
215. Conrad B, Weidmann E, Trucco G, et al. Evidence for superantigen involvement in insulin-dependent diabetes mellitus aetiology. *Nature* 1994;371:351–355.
216. Paliard X, West SG, Lafferty JA, et al. Evidence for the effects of a superantigen in rheumatoid arthritis. *Science* 1991;253:325–329.
217. Brocke S, Veromaa T, Weissman IL, Gijbels K, Steinman L. Infection and multiple sclerosis: a possible role for superantigens? *Trends Microbiol* 1994;2:250–254.
218. Brocke S, Gaur A, Piercy C, et al. Induction of relapsing paralysis in experimental autoimmune encephalomyelitis by bacterial superantigen. *Nature* 1993;365:642–644.
219. Olson JK, Croxford JL, Miller SD. Virus-induced autoimmunity: potential role of viruses in initiation, perpetuation, and progression of T-cell-mediated autoimmune disease. *Viral Immunol* 2001;14:227–250.
220. Matzinger P. Tolerance, danger, and the extended family. *Annu Rev Immunol* 1994;12:991–1045.
221. Blacklaws BA, Nash AA. Immunological memory to herpes simplex virus type 1 glycoproteins B and D in mice. *J Gen Virol* 1990;71:863–871.
222. Eng H, Lefvert AK, Mellstedt H, Osterborg A. Human monoclonal immunoglobulins that bind the human acetylcholine receptor. *Eur J Immunol* 1987;17:1867–1869.

# 4

# Clinical Presentation and Epidemiology of Myasthenia Gravis

## Jan B.M. Kuks and Hans J.G.H. Oosterhuis

## INTRODUCTION

The signs and symptoms of a postsynaptic neuromuscular junction disorder such as myasthenia gravis (MG) result from fluctuating strength of the voluntary muscles. The degree of weakness is partly dependent on the exertion of a muscle group but also varies spontaneously over longer periods without apparent cause. Remissions occur. All types of voluntary muscle may be involved but usually not to the same extent. In about 15% of the patients with MG, manifestations remain confined to the ocular muscles; among other patients, bulbar symptoms and signs predominate. MG usually begins with a few isolated signs (**Table 1**) and extends to other muscles within a few weeks to a few months, but sometimes even years (see below). Apart from a certain degree of local muscle atrophy, no other neurologic abnormalities are expected.

Most patients with fatiguing weakness suffer from the acquired autoimmune disease myasthenia gravis, but other postsynaptic neuromuscular junction disorders are recognized. Acquired MG, developing at any age after birth, should be distinquished from transient neonatal myasthenia, which occurs in 10–15% of children of myasthenic mothers, and congenital (hereditary) myasthenia, which is usually present at birth but may become apparent in the first years of life, or rarely in adulthood (*see* Chap. 14). The authors find Compston et al.'s (*1*) categorization of patients with acquired MG useful: 1) purely ocular MG (weakness restricted to the palpebral levator and the extraocular muscles); 2) early-onset generalized MG, (clinical onset before age 40 years); 3) late-onset generalized MG (onset after age 40 years); and 4) patients with a thymoma, with onset at any age.

From: *Current Clinical Neurology: Myasthenia Gravis and Related Disorders*
Edited by: H. J. Kaminski © Humana Press Inc., Totowa, NJ

**Table 1**
**Clinical Manifestations of Myasthenia Gravis**[a]

| | Early Onset 1–39 yr | Late Onset 40–85 yr | Thymoma | Total |
|---|---|---|---|---|
| Ocular | | | | |
|   Diplopia | 70 (14) | 84 (36) | 17 (1) | 171 |
|   Ptosis | 55 (16) | 36 (12) | 14 | 105 |
|   Ptosis and diplopia | 64 (10) | 47 (18) | 15 | 126 |
| Bulbar | | | | |
|   Articulation | 43 | 5 | 6 | 54 |
|   Face | 20 | 2 | | 22 |
|   Chewing | 1 | 6 | 3 | 10 |
|   Swallowing | 7 | 4 | 1 | 12 |
|   Neck muscles | 2 | 5 | 4 | 11 |
|   Combined | 23 | 20 | 16 | 59 |
| Oculobulbar | 25 | 17 | 30 | 72 |
| Limbs | | | | |
|   Arms | 15 | 3 | 4 | 22 |
|   Hands or fingers | 12 | 1 | 2 | 15 |
|   Legs | 45 | 6 | 1 | 52 |
|   Combined | 29 | 5 | 5 | 39 |
| Generalized | 4 | 5 | 16 | 25 |
| Respiration | 4 | 2 | 4 | 10 |
| Total | 419 (40) | 248 (66) | 138 (1) | 805 |

[a]Initial manifestations of MG reported by the authors' patients. Data in parentheses are numbers of patients who remained purely ocular during follow-up. This was the case in only one patient with a thymoma, in 9.5% in the early-onset group, and in 26.6% in the late-onset group. The ocular muscles were involved at onset in 59% of all patients, the bulbar muscles in 30%, and the ocular and bulbar muscles combined in 80%. Of the 10 patients with initial respiratory signs, 8 had a prolonged apnea without previous weakness and 2 were children with high fever. The onset with ocular signs was more frequent in the late-onset group than in the early-onset group (74% vs. 51%). Limb muscle weakness was more frequent in the early-onset than in the late-onset group (25% vs. 8%). Patients with thymomas had the highest incidence of bulbar signs at onset (55% vs. 31% in the early-onset and 26% in the late-onset group).

## CLINICAL MANIFESTATIONS

### Ocular

Ocular symptoms are the most frequent manifestations of MG. No consensus is found in the literature about the ocular symptom that most frequently appears first: ptosis or diplopia. Furthermore, any of the extraocular muscles may be involved in isolation or in combination, leading to horizontal, vertical, or diagonal double vision. In many patients, both ptosis and diplopia ultimately are present. The patient is immediately aware of double vision, as it occurs acutely, but a mild ptosis may escape attention. Some patients appreciate fluctuation of the diplopia from onset and are able to analyze the double images themselves. Others only complain of blurred vision, which becomes normal when looking with one eye. Patients with isolated ocular symptoms during the entire period of illness form a distinct group (*see* Chap. 5).

## *Bulbar*

In neurologic jargon, "bulbar muscles" are those innervated by motor neurons originating in the pons and the medulla oblongata (cranial nerves V, VII, IX, X, XI, and XII). Among bulbar symptoms, speech difficulties manifesting as nasality of the voice or a difficulty in articulation are the most common at onset of MG. More than any other symptom, dysarthria is likely to occur initially under the influence of emotions. At first, it is frequently an isolated and fluctuating symptom that disappears after a "silent period" and may be accompanied by difficulties in swallowing and chewing. If the dysarthria is caused by an insufficient function of the palatum, regurgitation of liquids through the nose may occur. A slight insufficiency of the upper pharyngeal muscles results in the sensation that food is sticking in the throat, and this can be documented to be the case by barium swallowing studies. Patients with dysphagia commonly report a preference for cold food. This may relate to improvement in neuromuscular transmission produced by relative cooling of the muscles.

Chewing may be difficult at the end of the meal, or the problem may be first appreciated when chewing bubble gum or eating peanuts. If weakness is severe, the jaw sags open and the patient needs to hold the mouth closed. A characteristic posture is seen in **Fig. 1A**. Most of our patients with chewing problems also have weakness of neck muscles. An important symptom correlating well with the severity of dysphagia is weight loss, and most of our patients with bulbar manifestations lost 5–10 kg of weight in the 3–6 months prior to diagnosis.

Weakness of neck muscles may result in difficulty in balancing the head, which is particularly troublesome if the patient has to perform work in a bent position. Complaints about stiffness, vague pains in the neck and the back of the head, and occasionally paraesthesias are then common and nearly always set the doctor on the wrong track, searching for cervical spine pathology, unless the strength of the neck muscles is formally tested.

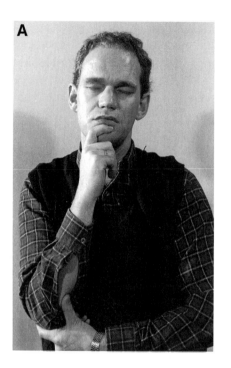
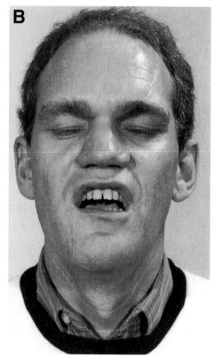

**Fig. 1.** A 36-year-old man with typical facial weakness. (**A**) He needs to support his jaw by holding his mouth closed. (**B**) When he attempts to close his eyelids firmly, his eyelashes remain visible, and the orbicularis oris weakness is evidenced by the straight smile.

Weakness of the facial muscles may occur suddenly—in some patients the initial diagnosis is confused with Bell's palsy—but it more commonly occurs insidiously. The patient's complaint is often stiffness, the sensation known from dental anesthesia, and sometimes paraesthesias or even hypalgesia. Substantial sensory loss, however, is never due to MG. The facial expression may be changed, especially in emotions. Laughing becomes distorted ("we did not know whether she laughed or cried"). Many patients complain of this change of facial expression and avoid social contacts. People ask them why they always look sad or angry. Orbicularis oris weakness is first noticed by the inability to whistle or to kiss, sneeze forcefully, or eat soup with a spoon, or by difficulty in pronouncing certain letters (p, f, s). Some patients complain that their tongues are thick and do not fit in their mouths. The time needed for eating a meal increases, and conversation becomes difficult while eating.

Insufficient strength of the orbicularis oculi may cause problems in keeping the eyes closed while washing the hair. Several of our patients complained that they could not close one eye and keep the other open while taking photographs. If the eyes are not completely closed during sleeping, they may be irritated on awakening. As all these symptoms may be minor and fluctuating, they are often detected retrospectively and do not cause patients to consult a doctor early in the course of the disease.

The most frequent of the bulbar signs among MG patients with more advanced MG is facial weakness. In its most prominent form it is easily recognizable, but it may be subtle and of variable severity, making it easily overlooked at the time of neurologic examination. At rest, facial expression may be unremarkable, but any expression of emotion, and particularly laughing, betrays the loss of normal function. A classical feature is the myasthenic snarl or the *rire verticale* (**Fig. 1B**). Since weakness of the upper part of the face is also present, laughing makes the eyelids droop, even if ptosis is not noticeable at rest. An early and sensitive sign of orbicularis oris weakness is the inability to whistle or to kiss (a neglected part of the neurologic examination). The patient cannot blow out the cheeks without air escaping, if pressure is applied to the cheeks by the examiner's finger. The closed eyes can be opened with one finger by the examiner, or the eyes cannot be closed completely. Facial weakness may be asymmetric, but this is rarely as pronounced as that of the ocular signs. The most sensitive functional test of the muscles of articulation is speaking aloud without interruption. An easy test is counting (101, 102, and so on) or reading aloud. A certain degree of quantitation of examination findings is possible by noting when dysarthria or nasal twang is appreciated compared with the time when the patient becomes unintelligible (**Fig. 2**). In a minority of patients, the voice first becomes weaker in volume, but not dysarthric. Some hoarseness may occur, but aphonia is not a sign of MG. In general, dysarthria and nasality occur while the volume remains normal. Slight palatal weakness may be demonstrated, if peak flow volume measures improve after pinching the nose.

Swallowing difficulties may be caused by weakness of the lips, the tongue, the pharyngeal muscles, or often a combination of these. If observed while eating, some MG patients may be seen to support their jaws, underlips, and floor of the mouth, to counteract gravity and to chew with their hands. Swallowing in some patients improves if they turn their head, probably thus narrowing their (too wide) throat. Regurgitation of fluids through the nose is a sign of palatal weakness. Coughing after swallowing may be a subtle sign of a defective swallowing mechanism. One study demonstrated that elderly patients with bulbar weakness were unable to swallow a 20-mL water bolus

**Dysarthria**

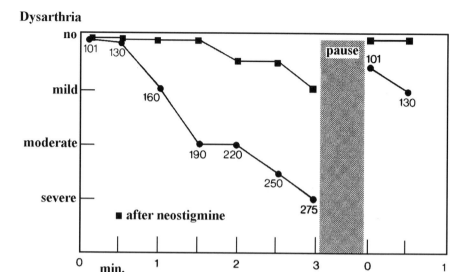

**Fig. 2.** Counting test. Improvement is appreciated by pausing and with neostigmine.

*(2)*. Severe impairment of swallowing manifests with drooling of saliva, choking, and ventilatory insufficiency (*see* Chap. 10).

Weakness of the tongue is apparent by inability of the patient to protrude the tongue and reach the frenulum of the upper lip. If the tongue is pushed against the inner cheek, the degree of weakness can be appreciated directly by the examiner.

Weakness of the masticatory muscles is demonstrated by conventional testing (clenching a tongue depressor). Having the patient repeatedly open and close the mouth vigorously until an audible click is heard is a sign of weakness. This maneuver may be easily performed 100 times in 30 s.

Weakness of the sternocleidomastoids and neck muscles may be appreciated on routine testing. A useful functional test is having the patient lift the head in the recumbent position; the individual should be able to look at the toes for 60 s.

Bulbar weakness is not always easily assessed, and quantification may be difficult. Dysphagia may be evaluated clinically and electrophysiologically. Weijnen et al. *(3–5)* developed several tests and devices that provide quantitative measures of bulbar function among MG patients.

### Limb, Trunk, and Respiratory

Fifteen to 20% of patients complain first of weakness of the arms, hands, or legs. In patients under age 30 years, limb weakness, especially of the legs,

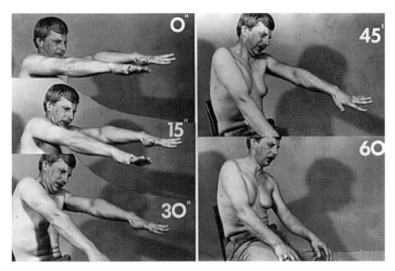

**Fig. 3.** Extended arm test. The patient is asked to lift his arms with hands in pronation. Normally, this position can usually be sustained for at least 3 min. Myasthenic weakness may lead the patient to drop one or both arms. Weakness of one of the extensor digitorum muscles (especially of the fourth finger) may become manifest with this test.

was the first sign in one-third of our patients. This might be explained by younger individuals placing these muscle groups into situations of heavier loading, for example, during sports. Inability to maintain arm position or elevate the upper extremity repetitively, e.g., when hanging laundry, hammering a nail, or washing hair, is a common complaint. Isolated weakness of one or more extensors of the fingers, usually the fourth or fifth, may be difficult for the doctor to interpret and sometimes leads to the misdiagnosis of a peripheral nerve compression.

Leg weakness frequently leads to sudden falls, and several of our patients had MG diagnosed after a fall from stairs. If the first manifestations are weakness of the limbs or trunk muscles, most patients complain of undue fatigability and peculiar feelings of heaviness. If asked about the exact nature of their feelings, they admit that these are different from the normal fatigue after exertion, although some rest is beneficial and restores their normal condition for variable periods. Most patients have arm and leg symptoms, but often one predominates, and the differential fatiguibility may be confirmed by appropriate examination (**Fig. 3**).

Pain in the back and girdle muscles occurs in some patients and is readily explained as an insufficiency of the postural muscles. It usually disappears at rest or after therapy. Chronic pain is not a feature of MG.

Weakness of the respiratory and other trunk muscles is rarely the first, isolated sign of the disease, but it may be the first manifestation that brings a patient to medical care. We have only seen this in rapidly evolving generalized MG in children with coincident infection, or as an effect of curare during narcosis (prolonged apnea). Some patients report short periods of altered awareness with inspiratory stridor, which are often the forerunners of longer lasting and life-threatening attacks. Rarely, short episodes of unconsciousness occur; sudden apneas may not be recognized as the cause. Ventilatory symptoms should always lead to rapid hospitalization. Bilateral vocal fold paralysis was recognized as an initial manifestion of MG in one patient who later developed diplopia, which prompted the evaluation for MG *(6)*.

If a patient is suspected to have MG, it is essential to test muscle strength after exercise. However, we must emphasize that primarily weakness (and not fatigue) is a sign of MG. All tests designed to measure the capacity to do muscle work require the cooperation of the patient. In general this presents no difficulties, but the examiner must discern true weakness from a nonorganic failure to generate maximal muscle force. Frank subterfuge may be a cause of such nonorganic causes of weakness.

The following procedures for assessment of muscle strength and exhaustability are useful. The strength of individual muscle groups is tested after rest. Accuracy is improved by using a hand-held dynamometer and the adoption of fixed postures. After moderate exertion, which does not decrease the strength of normal muscles, the strength of the patient is measured again. Moderate exertion may be standardized as follows *(7)*:

1. The arms, as well as the hands and fingers, are stretched horizontally (**Fig. 3**). This position should be maintained for 3 min without trembling or shaking. The patient may require some encouragement to perform the maneuver. Increasing weakness will produce some shaking or a gradual drooping of arms, hands, or fingers. If weakness is minimal, it may only be detected by measuring the strength again after 3 min of exertion. This test is very sensitive but not specific. Patients with other neuromuscular diseases may not be able to hold arms outstretched for more than 1 min, but strength before and after this effort is the same.
2. Grip strength on repeated contraction may be measured with a hand-held dynamometer. A simple ergometer can be made from a blood pressure manometer.
3. Patients should be able to perform knee bends, or in older people rise, from a standard chair repeatedly without the aid of their arms 20 times.
4. Walking on tiptoes and on the heels at least 30 steps.
5. Straight leg raising to 45° for 1 min in the recumbent position.
6. Vital capacity and peak flow measurements should give normal values five times in a row. A difficulty with these tests may be cased by the weakness of the lips or palate.

In most patients with generalized MG, but without actual or previous dyspnea, a decrease in vital capacity and other respiratory parameters is found; in 40% of pure ocular cases, the vital capacity is even decreased *(8)*. Routine lung function tests show that the vital capacity is decreased to a greater extent than the forced expiratory volume. In most patients, peak flow or vital capacity measurement is a valuable tool in follow-up and is done easily at any time and circumstance. Most of these tests are quantifiable, and the patient can perform some of them at home, to obtain a reliable picture of diurnal and periodic fluctuation. According to the complaints of the individual patient, other tests may be appropriate. A summary of the tests used in our practice is given in **Table 2** *(9)*. The data acquired may show a convincing difference between strength at rest and after exertion. They can also serve as a frame of reference in evaluating the effect of anticholinesterases and other treatments.

## *Muscle Atrophy*

Historically, the observation of focal muscle atrophy has caused much confusion in understanding MG. On the one hand, otherwise typical patients with MG and localized atrophy were included in early series *(10)*, but, on the other hand, muscle atrophy was used as an argument to place such patients in the category of a myasthenic syndrome, with a form of either myopathy, neuropathy, or ophthalmoplegia. Others referred to patients with MG and atrophy as true MG with myopathy, with neuropathy, or with neuromyopathy *(11)*. Osserman *(12)* placed patients with muscular atrophy, comprising 5% of his series, in a separate group and stated that "the histologic changes in the biopsied muscle are indistinguishable from those seen in polymyositis or muscular dystrophy." From a clinical viewpoint, localized muscle atrophy is detectable in about 6–10% of the patients *(11–15)*, and a still higher percentage is reached if patients with permanent ophthalmoplegia are included. Remarkably few details about the distribution of the atrophy are found in the literature *(11,14)*, although atrophy of the tongue is particularly appreciated (**Fig. 4**) *(16)*. In our patients, localized muscle atrophy occurred in 9% of early-onset patients, 8% of late-onset patients, and 12% of thymoma patients *(17)*.

## CLINICAL CLASSIFICATIONS AND QUANTITATIVE TESTS

Several scoring systems of myasthenic signs or the global state of the patient have been proposed *(9)*. The classification of Osserman and Genkins *(18)* is widely used and is in fact a modification of the initial classification of Osserman *(12)* from 1958, altered again by Oosterhuis *(13)* in 1964. In

**Table 2**
**Clinical Investigation of the Patient with Myasthenia Gravis**[a]

Inspection of the head at rest
    Note ptosis of the eyelids (usually asymmetric), ocular deviations, or drooping of the head
    Facial weakness may manifest by disappearance of the nasolabial fold and loss of
        expression
    Weakness of the neck or cheek muscles may be masked by supporting the jaw
    Ptosis may be compensated by lifting the eyebrows
    There may be tilting or rotation of the head to minimalize diplopia
Ocular functions
    Looking straight toward a bright light provokes ptosis
    Looking aside or upward for $60^b$ s provokes ptosis, especially on the side of abduction
    Diplopia may occur after sustained lateral/vertical gaze (maximal $60^b$ s, not further
        than 45° from the midline)
Bulbar Functions
    Test peak expiratory flow or vital lung capacity with and without nose clips to detect
        palatal weakness
    Repeatedly closing the eyes tightly provokes weakness of the ocular orbicular muscle;
        eyelashes may remain visible in spite of firmly closing the eyelids
    Nasal speech may occur after counting from 101 to 199; note the number where dysarthria
        or nasality occurs
    Masseter function may be tested by biting on a spatula before and after 100× closing the
        mouth with click
    Swallowing a glass of water may not be possible without coughing or regurgitation
        through the nose
Neck musculature (tests in horizontal position)
    Keeping the head raised for $120^b$ s ("look at your feet")
    Raising the head repeatedly (20×)
Arm (test in sitting position)
    Arms stretched forward in pronate position (90°) for $240^b$ s
    Note the beginning of trembling or shaking of the arm/hand
    Note drooping of individual fingers
Hand
    Inflation of sphygmomanometer until 300 mmHg
    Fist closing/opening with fingers joined together (no digital abduction allowed; 70×)
    Hand grip with a dynamometer (dominant hand: $45^b$ (men) or $30^b$ (women) kgW;
        nondominant hand: $35^b$ and $25^b$ kgW, respectively)
Leg
    Hip flexion (45° supine in horizontal position) for $100^b$ s
    Deep knee bends (20×)
    Rising from a standard chair without use of the hands
Ventilatory function
    Vital capacity or peak flow in rested condition
    Vital capacity or peak flow may decrease after repeated testing (5–10×)

[a]Test muscle force directly before and after repetitive activity.
[b]Maximal values according to recommendations of the medical scientific advisory board of
the Myasthenia Gravis Foundation of America *(19)*.

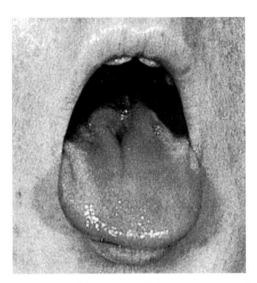

**Fig. 4.** A 60-year-old man with atrophy of the tongue. Note the presence of one medial and two lateral furrows, which define the triple-furrowed tongue. MG existed from early infancy and was diagnosed at age 52.

this classification, juvenile patients and patients with muscle atrophy were excluded as separate entities, and class 1 was confined to ocular myasthenia. It may be used retrospectively to classify patients as a certain type, but it combines localization, severity, and progression and is not well suited to follow individual patients. A Task Force of the Medical Advisory Board of the Myasthenia Gravis Foundation of America proposed an extended modification of this classification scheme in an attempt to provide a standard scheme for use by all investigators *(19)*. Scoring systems exist with categories for ocular, bulbar, limb muscle, and respiratory weakness, based on either description or quantified examinations *(see* Appendix). One system gives a detailed scoring for ocular signs *(20)*.

## COGNITIVE INVOLVEMENT

Clinical experience with MG patients does not raise suspicion of central nervous system involvement. Nonetheless, indications for an organic brain syndrome have been found with abnormalities of visual attention and reaction time. Improvement of memory function during plasma exchange in line with the increase of muscle strength was observed in one study *(21)*, but memory defects were not confirmed in another *(22)*. An auditory vigilance test did not reveal any abnormality *(22)*. Acetylcholine receptor antibodies from MG patients did not bind to the acetylcholine receptors extracted from human brain, which makes it unlikely that central cholinergic receptors are a target of an autoimmune process *(23)*. A review of clinical data regarding cognitive impairment, epilepsy, sleep disturbances, abnormal saccadic eye movements, and psychiatric problems is given elsewhere *(24)*. It is our impression that the data on cognitive and memory dysfunction in MG are currently insufficient and inconclusive (*see* Chap. 16).

## COURSE OF THE DISEASE

The initial manifestations of MG have a highly variable pattern and evolution in the individual patient. When treated and relieved of their symptoms, patients often appreciate that they have suffered from MG longer than they had initially appreciated. Osserman's impression *(12)* was that MG does not have a classical clinical course. There is a tendency toward spread to muscle groups beyond those initially affected, and in only 10% *(25)* to 16% *(26)* of the patients is MG clinically confined to the ocular muscles in the first 3 years; however, after 3 years, generalization occurs in only 3–10% of these purely ocular patients *(12,25,26)* (**Fig. 5**). When the disease is restricted to the ocular muscles for a year, there is a likelihood of 84% that it will remain localized *(27)*. If symptoms are localized, but not to the ocular muscles, then spread of weakness to other muscle groups still occurs over 1–3 years. It is very rare that weakness remains confined to the bulbar muscles or muscles of the extremities.

In most patients the diagnosis is made in the second year after symptom onset, but a much longer delay is not unusual *(12,13)*, especially among early-onset women. One reason for this delay that we found in our study of 100 consecutive patients is the more rapid progression of weakness in men than in women in the first 3 months of disease onset *(28)*. An additional factor appears to be a different diagnostic approach to men and women with early-onset disease. No men underwent psychiatric evaluation compared with 8% of women. Patients with limited or predominant limb muscle weakness had a higher chance of a missed diagnosis. In general, severity of illness increases in the first years of the disease, with a tendency to stabilize, improve, or even resolve after many years. A typical case history is given in **Fig. 6**.

Severe exacerbation of MG leading to myasthenic crisis occurs usually in the first years *(26,29,30)* of the disease and rarely in the first weeks of onset. One exception is for children with MG who have an infection or rapidly progressive bulbar symptoms that lead to choking and a poor cough. In these patients, crises occur more often, with gradually increasing generalized weakness during respiratory infections induced by aspiration. Crisis in MG is life-threatening and demands aggressive treatment with immunomodulating strategies to minimize the duration (*see* Chap. 10).

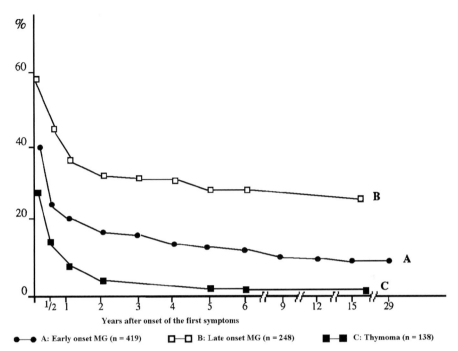

**Fig. 5.** Percentage of patients with ocular signs. Only ocular signs at onset were present in 39% of early-onset, 58% of late-onset, and 27% of thymoma patients. After 3 years, other muscle groups were involved in 84% of early-onset, 68% of late-onset, and 96% of thymoma patients. At the end of the follow-up, 9.6% of early-onset, 26.6% of late-onset, and 1% of thymoma patients remained purely ocular *(17)*.

The mortality of MG has been reduced from 30% to zero in the past decades *(26,28,30–32)*. Spontaneous long-lasting remissions are rare in the first years, but in the long term they are expected in 10–20% of patients *(26,28,30)*. Patients with ocular MG have a higher remission rate than those with the generalized disease *(26,30)*.

## Exacerbating Factors

It is recognized that certain events influence the course of MG unfavorably and may unmask subclinical MG. Of particular importance are infectious diseases with fever, psychological stress (but *see* Chap. 16), hyper- or hypothyroidism, and certain drugs such as antimalaria drugs (quinine, chloroquine), aminoglycosides, β-adrenergic receptor blocking drugs and D-penicillamine *(33)*. Some experts recommend avoidance of vaccinations, but their effects have never been fully investigated. Patients under immunosuppression are advised by some to stop treatment for 2–3 weeks before immunization *(34)*.

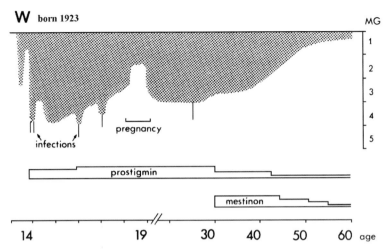

**Fig. 6.** Pictorial representation of a case history of a patient with MG. Onset of MG occurred with dysarthria during a stressful situation with generalization 6 months later; exacerbations during infections and improvement during pregnancy were observed. During a wartime period, oral prostigmin was replaced by subcutaneous injections (0.5 mg 6 times a day) because tablets were scarce. The patient improved very gradually after the age of 30, and after the age of 45 only slight weakness was present. Several major operations in the previous 10 years were performed without development of weakness. She has been reluctant to discontinue medication (Prostigmin® 7.5 mg and Mestinon® 10 mg 3 times a day). The severity of symptoms is expressed using a six-point disability score: 0 = no symptoms; 5 = dependent on artificial ventilation *(35,37)*.

The effect of pregnancy on MG is the subject of conflicting reports: either improvement or deterioration or no influence, each one-third in all the series *(35)*. Most patients improve in the second part of their pregnancy *(35)*. In a prospective investigation of 64 pregnancies, MG worsened in 4 of 23 asymptomatic patients who were not on therapy before conception; in patients under treatment, MG improved in 12 of 31 pregnancies, remained unchanged in 13, and worsened in six. MG worsened after delivery in 15 of 54 pregnancies *(36)*. Minor exacerbations are experienced 3–10 days before menstruation by at least one-third of the women *(13,37)*.

The effect of ambient temperatures has not been studied extensively. Hot weather in particular is reported to increase weakness *(12,38)* and may even induce a crisis *(39)*. In our experience, the individual response varies considerably, and several of our patients are considerably better in warm weather.

## EPIDEMIOLOGY

### *Incidence and Prevalence*

The annual incidence of MG is 3–4/million and the prevalence about 60/ million *(40–46)*; in some surveys, these figures are even higher *(47)*. A striking difference in prevalence was seen between cities and rural areas *(40)*, possibly because of variations in populations and medical facilities. The prevalence seems to be increasing in the last decades, probably influenced by new diagnostic tests and a decrease in mortality rates. In Virginia the incidence and prevalence was found to be higher in the African-American population than in the corresponding Caucasian population. Ocular MG comprised 25% of this group of patients *(42)*, which was higher than observed in previous series.

### *Age, Gender, and Classification*

MG may have its onset at any age. In general, women are affected twice as often as men, in the child-bearing period even three times as frequently, whereas the incidence is about equal before puberty and after the age of 40 *(45,46,48,49)*. The relative incidence is highest in women in the third decade *(18,41,46)*, and in some series a late peak is found in older men *(18,26,46)*. Ocular MG occurs in about 15% of patients and has a higher prevalence in men, especially over the age of 40 *(45,50)*. Age at onset, gender, type, and incidence of thymomas in the author's series of 800 patients are given in **Fig. 7**. A relatively higher onset (22%) in the first decade, or 36% before puberty, is reported from Chinese populations *(51,52)*, and the disease remains restricted to the ocular muscles in more than 50% of patients. However, the incidence of congenital cases is unknown in these series.

### *Acquired Infantile MG*

The prevalence of cases with onset in the first decade in European and American series varies from 1 to 3%, which is lower than the overall prevalence in the population. A relatively greater prevalence was found in Japanese *(50)* and Chinese *(52)* populations, with a peak at the ages of 2–3 years for ocular MG. The relatively higher incidence of ocular MG in prepubertal MG was also found in a European series *(53)*.

The prognosis of MG in infancy is usually favorable, although exacerbations may occur with fevers. In sporadic cases, a fulminating onset with life-threatening respiratory insufficiency may occur *(54)*. The incidence of anti-acetylcholine receptor antibodies is lower than in adults, so this test cannot be used to differentiate between congenital and autoimmune MG. The outcome of infantile (onset at 1–17 years) *(53)* or juvenile MG (onset at 1–20 years) *(55)*

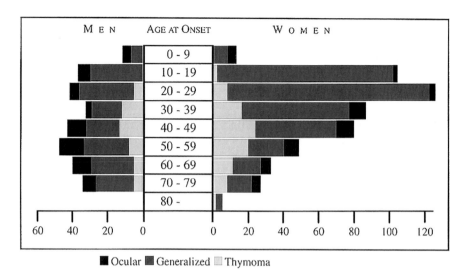

■ Ocular ■ Generalized □ Thymoma

**Fig. 7.** Clinical and demographic data from 805 patients with MG evaluated between 1960 and 1994 *(17)*.

is comparable to that of the adult forms, and the same treatment modalities are used, although it seems justified to be less aggressive with immunomodulation in prepubertal children *(54)*.

*MG in the Elderly*

There are several clinical and epidemiologic reasons to differentiate between patients with late-onset and early-onset MG. [Among series, the defining age of late-onset MG varies between 40, 45, and 50 years *(43,56)*]. Thymoma is more common in late-onset patients, the response to thymectomy is more uncertain than in younger patients, and antibodies to other muscle components than the acetylcholine receptor are more often found among these patients *(2,56,57)*. Although there are no differences between the signs and symptoms in patients with late-onset MG, progression to severe disease may be more common in MG with onset after the age of 50 years. There is a somewhat increased incidence of weakness of bulbar muscles *(32)*, which cannot be attributed to the increased incidence of a thymoma *(2)*. Immunomodulating therapies are effective, but elderly patients may be at increased risk of side effects, particularly for corticosteroids *(2,17,32)*.

*MG and Thymoma*

The incidence for thymoma is about 15% among MG patients *(18,45)*, with late-onset patients being more commonly affected (**Fig. 7**). Generally, the course of MG is more severe, and crises occur more often than in patients without thymomas *(15,25,48)*; however, there are contradictory studies *(58)*. Patients with thymomas more often have onset of MG with bulbar manifestations (**Table 1**). Complications related to the thymoma contribute to a worse outcome, but myasthenic manifestations respond to treatment similarly in thymoma and nonthymoma patients. In our own series *(17)* of 138 patients observed from 1960 and 1994, 16 died from complications of the tumor. In the remaining group, 20 patients (16%) died from MG (all before 1984; only 2 had immunosuppressive therapy), and 55 patients (45%) went into remission with (*n* = 37) or without (*n* = 18) immunosuppression. MG death occurred in 2.8% and full remission in 38% of our 537 nonthymoma patients with generalized disease. Our data also suggest that the natural course of MG with a thymoma is more unfavorable but that the outcome with immunomodulation is the same as in nonthymoma patients with MG.

### Incidence of Autoimmune Diseases

The hypothesis of the autoimmune pathogenesis of MG was partly based on the occurrence of other autoimmune disorders among MG patients *(59)*. Many associations of MG and other autoimmune diseases have been reported in large series of MG patients *(18,25,41,43,46,60)*. The frequencies in these series vary from 2.3 to 24.2%, with a mean of 12.9% compared with that of a United States series of 3.2% *(61)*.

### Genetic Predisposition

Although MG is not considered a hereditary disease with a definite mode of genetic transmission, familial cases are reported in 1–4% of several series *(12,48,62,63)*, with a high of 7.2% *(43)*. In an analysis of 72 familial cases reported up to 1970, 39% belonged to the congenital type (onset before 2 years of age), 22% occurred between 3 and 18 years, and 39% occurred over the age of 18. In 76%, they occurred in one generation, in 24% in two generations, but never in three. In 85% of the families, two members had MG, in 10% three members had MG, and rarely more *(62)*. In twin studies, 6 of 15 monozygotic twins were both affected, but none of 9 dizygotic twins were affected *(64)*.

Recently, four separate families each with two affected members were described out of a total of 800 patients *(65)*. In seven of the eight patients acetylcholine receptor antibodies were found. No association with a single HLA haplotype was found. In another family, 5 of 10 members in one generation (ages 63–77) were described; no genetic abnormalities were found *(66)*. In our own 800 patients *(17)*, 14 had a near family member with acquired

MG (1.7%). Familial autoimmune MG seems to be a rarity, but it can be confused with congenital MG, which is more often familial.

## DIFFERENTIAL DIAGNOSIS

Making the diagnosis of MG in the patient with anti-acetylchloline receptor antibodies is not difficult (*see* Chap. 8 for caveats). If no autoantibodies are found, the history, results of clinical examination, reaction to anticholinesterases, or findings on electrodiagnostic testing may strongly point to the diagnosis. Nevertheless, the diagnosis may remain difficult in a small subgroup of patients. In particular, the diagnosis of ocular MG may be difficult (*see* Chap. 5). Other myasthenic syndromes, especially the Lambert-Eaton syndrome, should always be considered in seronegative patients with fluctuating weakness (some patients with Lambert-Eaton syndrome may have acetylcholine receptor autoantibodies). If the patient has *bulbar symptoms,* one might have reason to include such neuromuscular diseases as amyotrophic lateral sclerosis, oculopharyngeal dystrophy, bulbar spinal atrophy, or myotonic dystrophy in the differential diagnosis. Self-evidently, other (supra) nuclear brainstem pathology may also lead to bulbar manifestations. Some patients with isolated complaints and signs of dysarthria have no organic disease. Isolated dysphagia may be caused by a mechanical impairment or a disturbance in the parasympathetic innervation of the esophagus (achalasia). Focal dyskinesias may also need to be considered in certain patients.

In the seronegative patient with *predominant limb weakness,* the possibility of Lambert-Eaton syndrome surpasses that of MG. Other acquired diseases with more or less fluctuating weakness of limb and trunk muscles may be motor neuron disease, polymyositis, endocrine myopathies, and mitochondrial myopathies. It should be realized that cholinesterase inhibitor treatment might convey a slight benefit in these diseases. Neck extensor weakness may be a prominent or initial manifestation of MG, but it also occurs with motor neuron disease and inflammatory myositis. There is also a benign isolated neck extensor myopathy that develops within 3 months without leading to further weakness *(67)*. Finally, some patients just have complaints of muscle pain or muscle fatigue without objective weakness. These symptoms are not suggestive of MG.

## REFERENCES

1. Compston DAS, Vincent A, Newsom-Davis J, Batchelor JR. Clinical, pathological, HLA-antigen and immunological evidence for disease heterogeneity in myasthenia gravis. *Brain* 1980;103:579–601.
2. Antonini G, Morino S, Gragnani F, Fiorelli M. Myasthenia gravis in the elderly: a hospital based study. *Acta Neurol Scand* 1996;93:260–262.

3. Weijnen FG, van der Bilt A, Wokke J, et al. What's in a smile? Quantification of the vertical smile of patients with myasthenia gravis. *J Neurol Sci* 2000;173:124–128.
4. Weijnen FG, Van der Bilt A, Wokke JHJ, et al. Maximal bite force and surface EMG in patients with myasthenia gravis. *Muscle Nerve* 2000;23:1694–1699.
5. Weijnen FG, Kuks JBM, Van der Bilt, et al. Tongue force in patients with myasthenia gravis. *Acta Neurol Scand* 2000;102:303–308.
6. Osei-Lah A, Reilly V, Capildeo BJ. Bilateral abductor vocal fold paralysis due to myasthenia gravis. *J Laryngol Otol* 1999;113:678–679.
7. Oosterhuis HJGH. *Myasthenia Gravis*. Edinburgh, Churchill Livingstone, 1984, p. 46.
8. Reuther P, Hertel G, Ricker K, Bürkner R. Lungenfunktionsdiagnostik bei myasthenia gravis. *Verh Deutsch Gesell Innere Med* 1978;84:1579–1582.
9. Kuks JBM, Oosterhuis HJGH. Disorders of the neuromuscular junction: outcome measures and clinical scales. In: Guiloff RJ, ed. *Clinical Trials in Neurology*. London, Springer, 2001, pp. 485–499.
10. Oppenheim H. Die *Myasthenische Paralyse (Bulbärparalyse ohne anatomischen Befund)*. Berlin, S Karger, 1901.
11. Oosterhuis HJGH, Bethlem J. Neurogenic muscle involvement in myasthenia gravis. *J Neurol Neurosurg Psychiatry* 1973;36:244–254.
12. Osserman KE. *Myasthenia Gravis*. New York, Grune & Stratton, 1958.
13. Oosterhuis HJGH. Studies in myasthenia gravis. *J Neurol Sci* 1964;1:512–546.
14. Schimrigk K, Samland O. Muskelatrophien bei Myasthenia gravis. *Nervenarzt* 1977;48:65–68.
15. Simpson JA. Evaluation of thymectomy in myasthenia gravis. *Brain* 1958:81:112–145.
16. Kinnier Wilson SA. *Neurology*, vol I. London, Edward Arnolds, 1940, p. 1598.
17. Oosterhuis HJGH. *Myasthenia Gravis*. Groningen, Neurological Press, 1997, pp. 33,34.
18. Osserman KE, Genkins G. Studies in myasthenia gravis: review of a twenty year experience in over 1200 patients. *Mt Sinai J Med* 1971;34:497–537.
19. Task Force of the Medical Scientific Advisory Board of the Myasthenia Gravis Foundation of America. Jartezki A III, Barohn RJ, Ernstoff RM, et al. Myasthenia gravis. Recommendations for clinical research standards. *Neurology* 2000;55:16–23.
20. Schumm F, Wiethoelter H, Fateh-Moghadam A, Dichgans J. Thymectomy in myasthenia gravis with pure ocular symptoms. *J Neurol Neurosurg Psychiatry* 1985; 48:332–337.
21. Tucker DM, Roeltgen DP, Wann PD, Wertheimer RI. Memory dysfunction in myasthenia gravis: evidence for central cholinergic effects. *Neurology* 1988;38:1173–1177.
22. Lewis SW, Ron MA, Newsom-Davis J. Absence of central functional cholinergic deficits in myasthenia gravis. *J Neurol Neurosurg Psychiatry* 1989;52:258–261.
23. Whiting PJ, Cooper J, Lindstrom JM. Antibodies in sera from patients with myasthenia gravis do not bind with nicotinic acetylcholine receptors from human brain. *J Neuroimmunol* 1987;16:205–213.
24. Steiner I, Brenner T, Soffer D, Argov Z. Involvement of sites other than the neuromuscular junction in myasthenia gravis. In: Lisak RP, ed. *Handbook of Myasthenia Gravis and Myasthenic Syndromes*. New York, Marcel Dekker, 1994, pp. 277–294.
25. Oosterhuis HJGH. Myasthenia gravis. A review. *Clin Neurol Neurosurg* 1981;83: 105–135.

26. Grob D, Brunner NG, Namba T. The natural course of myasthenia gravis and the effect of various therapeutic measures. *Ann NY Acad Sci* 1981;377:652–669.
27. Grob D. Natural history of myasthenia gravis. In: Engel AG, ed. *Myasthenia Gravis and Myasthenic Disorders.* New York, Oxford University Press, 1999, pp. 131–145.
28. Beekman R, Kuks JBM, Oosterhuis HJGH. Myasthenia gravis: diagnosis and follow-up of 100 consecutive patients. *J Neurol Sci* 1997;244:112–118.
29. Cohen MS, Younger D. Aspects of the natural history of myasthenia gravis: crisis and death. *Ann NY Acad Sci* 1981;377:670–677.
30. Oosterhuis HJGH. Observations of the natural history of myasthenia gravis and the effect of thymectomy. *Ann NY Acad Sci* 1981:377:678–689.
31. Beghi E, Antozzi C, Batocchi AP, et al. Prognosis of myasthenia gravis: a multicenter follow-up study of 844 patients. *J Neurol Sci* 1991;106:213–220.
32. Donaldson DH, Ansher M, Horan S, Rutherford RB, Ringel SP. The relationship of age to outcome in myasthenia gravis. *Neurology* 1990;40:786–790.
33. Wittbrodt ET. Drugs and myasthenia gravis. An update. *Arch Intern Med* 1997;157: 399–408.
34. Schalke B. Klinische Besonderheiten bei Myasthenia Gravis Patienten. *Akt Neurol* 1998;25:528–529.
35. Plauché WC. Myasthenia gravis in pregnancy: an update. *Am J Obstet Gynecol* 1979; 135:691–697.
36. Batocchi AP, Majolini L, Evoli A, et al. Course and treatment of myasthenia gravis during pregnancy. *Neurology* 1999;52:447–452.
37. Leker RR, Karni A, Abramski O. Exacerbation of myasthenia during the menstrual period. *J Neurol Sci* 1998;156:107–111.
38. Borenstein S, Desmedt JE. Temperature and weather correlates of myasthenia fatigue. Lancet 1974;ii:63–66.
39. Guttman L. Heat-induced myasthenic crises. Arch Neurol 1980;37:671–672.
40. D'Alessandro R, Granieri E, Benassi G, et al. Comparative study on the prevalence of myasthenia gravis in the provinces of Bologna and Ferrara, Italy. *Acta Neurol Scand* 1991;2:83–88.
41. Oosterhuis HJGH. The natural course of myasthenia gravis: a longterm follow-up study. *J Neurol Neurosurg Psychiatry* 1989;52:1121–1127.
42. Phillips LH, Tomer JC, Anderson MS, Cox GM. The epidemiology of myasthenia gravis in central and western Virginia. *Neurology* 1992;42:1888–1893.
43. Pirskanen R. Genetic aspects in myasthenia gravis, a family study of 264 Finnish patients. *Acta Neurol Scand* 1977;56:365–388.
44. Somnier FE, Keiding N, Paulson OB. Epidemiology of myasthenia gravis in Denmark: a longitudinal and comprehensive population survey. *Arch Neurol* 1991;48: 733–739.
45. Sorensen TT, Holm EB. Myasthenia gravis in the county of Viborg, Denmark. *Eur Neurol* 1989;29:177–179.
46. Storm Mathisen A. Epidemiology of myasthenia gravis in Norway. *Acta Neurol Scand* 1984;70:274–284.
47. Robertson NP, Deans J, Compston DAS. Myasthenia gravis: a population based epidemiological study in Cambridgeshire, England. *J Neurol Neurosurg Psychiatry* 1998;65:492–496.
48. Grob D, Arsura EL, Brunner NG, Namba T. The course of myasthenia gravis and therapies affecting outcome. *Ann NY Acad Sci* 1987;505:472–499.

49. Mantegazza R, Beghi E, Pareyson D, et al. A multicentre follow-up study of 1152 patients with myasthenia gravis in Italy. *J Neurol Sci* 1990;237:339–344.
50. Fukuyama Y, Hirayama Y, Osawa M. *Epidemiological and Clinical Features of Childhood Myasthenia Gravis in Japan.* Tokyo, Japan Medical Research Foundation University of Tokyo Press, 1981, p. 19.
51. Hawkins BR, Yu YL, Wong V, et al. Possible evidence of a variant of myasthenia gravis based on HLA and acetylcholine receptor antibody in Chinese patients. *Q J Med* 1989;70:235–241.
52. Wong V, Hawkins BR, Yu YL. Myasthenia gravis in Hong Kong Chinese. *Acta Neurol Scand* 1992;86:68–72.
53. Batocchi AP, Evoli A, Palmisani MT, et al. Early onset myasthenia gravis: clinical characteristics and response to therapy. *Eur J Pediatr* 1990;150:66–68.
54. Oosterhuis HJGH, Kuks JBM, Skallebaek D, et al. Infantile myasthenia gravis. *Muscle Nerve* 2002, in press.
55. Lindner A, Schalke B, Toyka KV. Outcome of juvenile-onset myasthenia gravis: a retrospective study with long term follow-up of 79 patients. *J Neurol* 1997;244: 515–520.
56. Aarli JA. Late-onset myasthenia gravis. *Arch Neurol* 1999;56:25–27.
57. Kuks JBM, Limburg PC, Horst G, Oosterhuis HJGH. Antibodies to skeletal muscle in myasthenia gravis, part 2. Prevalence in non-thymoma patients. *J Neurol Sci* 1993;120:78–81.
58. Bril V, Kojic J, Dhanani A. The long-term clinical outcome of myasthenia gravis in patients with thymoma. *Neurology* 1998;51:1198–1200.
59. Simpson JA. Myasthenia gravis, a new hypothesis. *Scot Med J* 1960;5:419–436.
60. Thorlacius S, Aarli JA, Riise T, Matre R, Johnsen HJ. Associated disorders in myasthenia gravis: autoimmune disease and their relation to thymectomy. *Acta Neurol Scand* 1989;80:290–295.
61. Jacobson DL, Gange SJ, Rose NR, Graham NMH. Epidemiology and estimated population burden of selected autoimmune disease in the United States. *Clin Immunol Immunopathol* 1997;84:223–243.
62. Namba T, Brunner NG, Brown SB, Muguruma M, Grob D. Familial myasthenia gravis. *Arch Neurol* 1971;25:49–60.
63. Szobor A. Myasthenia gravis: familial occurrence, a study of 1100 myasthenia gravis patients. *Acta Med Hung* 1989;4:13–21.
64. Behan P O. Immune disease and HLA association with myasthenia gravis. *J Neurol Neurosurg Psychiatry* 1980;4:611–621.
65. Evoli A, Batocchi AP, Zelano G, et al. Familial autoimmune myasthenia gravis: report of four families. *J Neurol Neurosurg Psychiatry* 1995;58:729–731.
66. Bergoffen J, Zmyewski ChM, Fischbeck KH. Familial autoimmune myasthenia gravis. *Neurology* 1994;44:551–554.
67. Suarez GA, Kelly JJ. The dropped head syndrome. *Neurology* 1992;42:1625–1627.

# 5

# Ocular Myasthenia

## Robert B. Daroff

## INTRODUCTION

Myasthenia gravis (MG) is a generalized disorder that often manifests initially as focal weakness. The most common focal presentation is ocular. Ocular muscle weakness at the onset of MG is present in 85–90% of patients, but the percentage of those without clinical evidence of coexisting bulbar or limb weakness (i.e., pure ocular myasthenia) varies from 15 to 59% in different series *(1)*.

The extraocular muscles (EOMs) and levators are the involved ocular muscles. There may be electrophysiologic evidence of myasthenia in face or limb muscles, but if the weakness is limited to the ocular muscles, it is designated *ocular myasthenia* (OM). Orbicularis oculi weakness is common in OM and is not a sign or predictor of generalization *(2)*.

The marked susceptibility of the EOMs and levators in MG is explained by a variety of factors unique to these muscles *(3–7)*. The very high ocular motor neuron activity (exceeding 600 Hz during saccades) could make EOM fibers particularly susceptible to neuromuscular transmission failure. Singly innervated EOM fibers have less prominent synaptic folds and fewer acetylcholine receptors. The presence of multiply innervated fibers in the EOM differentiate them from other striated muscles and might contribute to their preferential involvement. Expression of the γ-subunit of the acetylcholine receptor in adult EOM is another unique characteristic of these muscles *(8)*, but the levator muscles do not express the γ-subunit *(9)*; thus, ptosis cannot be explained by antibodies specific for the fetal receptor. MG is more likely to be ocular when associated with autoimmune thyroid disease. This may relate to immunologic crossreactivity against shared thyroid and eye muscle antigens *(10)*.

From: *Current Clinical Neurology: Myasthenia Gravis and Related Disorders*
Edited by: H. J. Kaminski © Humana Press Inc., Totowa, NJ

## DIAGNOSIS AND DIFFERENTIAL DIAGNOSIS

The pattern of muscle involvement with OM ranges from weakness of a single EOM or lid to complete external ophthalmoplegia with bilateral ptosis, with any intervening combination. At times, the pattern may mimic a central motility disturbance, such as a gaze palsy or internuclear ophthalmoplegia *(11)*. Although there is a substantial literature on accommodative weakness *(12–14)* and pupillary involvement *(13–17)* in OM, I agree with Glaser and Siatkowski *(11)*, "if pupillary signs are present, another diagnosis must be entertained."

The diagnosis of OM may be strongly suggested by aspects of the history, such as 1) episodes of recurrent unilateral, alternating, or bilateral ptosis; and 2) progressively increasing ptosis or diplopia during the day, with improvement upon awakening in the morning. In addition, the examination may mandate a diagnosis of OM. For example, whereas a third nerve palsy may begin with an isolated ptosis, involvement of EOM soon follows, and the addition of pain and pupillary dilation is frequent. Thus, an isolated painless ptosis is almost certainly diagnostic of OM, with the exception of the extraordinarily rare occurrence of carcinoma metastasizing to the eyelid. Similarly, ophthalmoparesis with rapid saccades within the limited range of eye movements only occurs in MG; all other conditions that restrict ocular amplitude also slow saccadic velocity *(1,18)*. Facial weakness limited to the orbicularis oculi, coexisting with ptosis or EOM weakness, only occurs in MG. Fatigue of EOM and lids during sustained upgaze (**Fig. 1**) suggests OM, although this, as well as Cogan's lid twitch sign,* may also result from midbrain lesions *(19,20)*. Another OM lid sign is enhanced ptosis, in which passive elevation of a ptotic lid causes the opposite lid to droop. The explanation is Hering's law of equal innervation. For instance, if both eyelids are ptotic owing to bilateral levator weakness, and the right is more ptotic than the left, then both sides will receive equivalent increased central innervation to elevate the lids. Because of the asymmetric weakness, the right lid will remain more ptotic than the left. When the right lid is manually elevated, the increased central innervation ceases, and the previously "normal" left lid assumes the ptotic position *(13,21)*.

---

*This sign is commonly present in MG patients with unilateral ptosis. The patient is asked to look down, thereby inhibiting the levator muscles. After about 15 s, the patient looks up to the examiner's nose, or an object at eye level; if the sign is present, the previously ptotic lid overshoots and is transiently higher than the other lid. The retracted lid then slowly drops to its previous ptotic position.

**A**

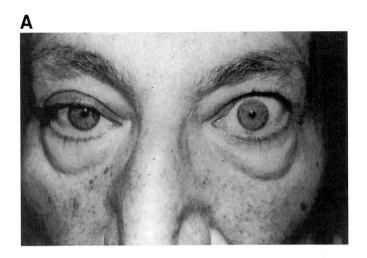

**B**

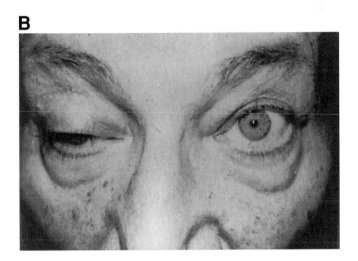

**Fig. 1.** (**A**) The patient is attempting to look up, evidenced by the contraction of the frontalis muscle. Note the slight right ptosis and left lid retraction. (**B**) Lid fatigue that developed during the sustained upward gaze, manifested by marked ptosis on the right, and lessening of the lid retraction on the left. (Photos courtesy of Dr. J. Lawton Smith.)

I must emphasize that no matter how "characteristic" the history and examination is for OM, a dilated pupil or pain negates the diagnosis, unless another disorder coexists with the MG.

## DIAGNOSTIC TESTING

Detection of acetylcholine receptor antibodies is essentially diagnostic of MG. Antibodies are present in approximately 90% of patients with generalized MG; the frequency with OM ranges from 50 to 75% *(16)*. Whereas antibodies to muscle-specific kinase (MuSK) are often present in seronegative patients with generalized MG, anti-MuSK antibodies are not detected in seronegative ocular myasthenics *(22)*.

Approximately 50% of OM patients have a decremental response to repetitive nerve stimulation in limb muscles *(23–25)*. Single-fiber electromyography (SFEMG) in the orbicularis oculi *(26)* and frontalis *(27)* muscles may approach 100% sensitivity in OM.

The mainstay of OM diagnosis in the office is the edrophonium chloride (Tensilon®) test. I regard resolution of eyelid ptosis (**Fig. 2**) or direct observation of the strengthening of at least a single paretic extraocular muscle as the only reliable endpoints. Thus, patients without ptosis or discernible ophthalmoparesis have no valid endpoints *(28)* (**Fig. 3**). Others rely heavily on muscle balance endpoints such as prisms, red glass, Maddox rod, and Lancaster red-green torches *(29)*, but these can yield spuriously positive responses if a nonparetic yolk or antagonist muscle becomes weak after the Tensilon test *(28)*.

A variety of techniques utilize oculography with Tensilon testing *(16,30, 31)*, but, despite being involved in several such published studies in the 1970s, I don't feel their expense or specificity justifies clinical usage, except for research. The same holds for oculographic analysis of saccadic waveforms and optokinetic nystagmus, to quantify EOM weakness or fatigue *(32)*.

Positive Tensilon tests occur occasionally in Lambert-Eaton syndrome, botulism, Guillain-Barré syndrome, and motor neuron disease *(33)*, and in rare patients with brainstem tumors, or compressive cranial neuropathies *(34, 35)*. Indeed, since MG may coexist with an intracranial neoplasm, when in doubt, obtain a magnetic resonance image of the head *(36)*.

Atropine should always be available to counter possible muscarinic side effects of Tensilon, although the amount of Tensilon required to diagnose OM is rarely above 4 mg *(37)*. Some neuroophthalmologists and neurologists seem particularly concerned about the complications of Tensilon. A questionnaire mailed to neuroophthalmologists yielded almost 200 respondents who had performed a combined total of over 23,000 tests in which only 37 (0.16%) were associated with a serious complication, such as bradyarrhythmia and syncope; however, 16% of the respondents preferred an alternative diagnostic procedure, such as the sleep or ice tests *(38)*. Okun et al. *(39)* regard demonstrable fatigue, the ice test, receptor antibodies, EMG, and oral response to anticholin-

**A**

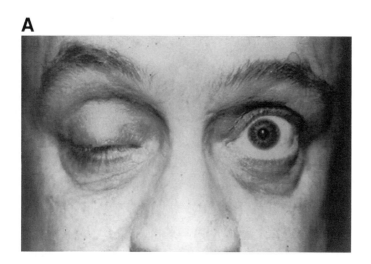

**B**

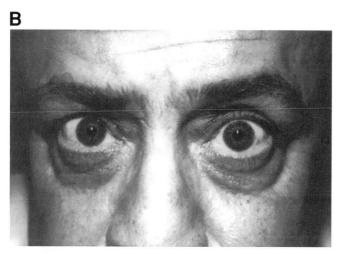

**Fig. 2.** (**A**) An almost complete right ptosis in a patient with ocular myasthenia. The frontalis muscle contraction, elevating the eyebrows, reflects the patient's effort to keep the lids open. (**B**) After administration of intravenous edrophonium chloride (Tensilon), the right ptosis is resolved. (Photos courtesy of Dr. J. Lawton Smith.)

esterase medications as safer and preferable to Tensilon testing. As previously mentioned, fatigue is nonspecific *(19,20)*, and, except for ice, the other tests, although reasonably specific and safe, have the disadvantage of delaying the diagnosis. Never having experienced a complication with Tensilon, absent major contraindications, I prefer this office technique if the patient has appropriate

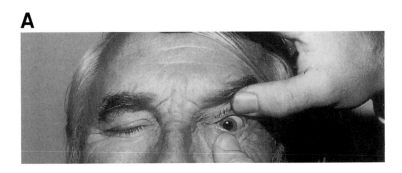

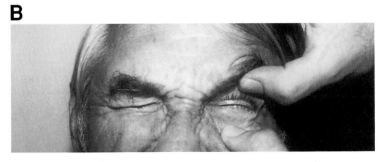

**Fig. 3. (A)** The patient has weakness of eyelid closure, permitting easy opening by the examiner. **(B)** The patient shows much stronger eyelid closure after administration of Tensilon. This patient had myasthenia, demonstrated by EMG and the presence of antibodies. By itself the Tensilon test (which disclosed increased strength of the orbicularis oculi) would not have been conclusive for the diagnosis of MG, since impaired volition could have explained the orbicularis weakness in (A). A Tensilon test with placebo control is unreliable in these circumstances, because iv saline does not cause the same systemic reaction as does Tensilon.

clinical endpoints. Okun et al. *(39)* do provide a good review of Tensilon complications in patients with heart disease and those on drugs such as digoxin and β-blockers.

Odel et al. *(40)* studied the effects of a 30-min rest or sleep in a quiet dark room on ptosis and ophthalmoparesis and found that most patients showed transient improvement immediately upon awakening (positive sleep test), which seems specific for OM.

The ice test is useful in diagnosing myasthenic ptosis, provided it is not complete *(41)*, but it is not particularly helpful for extraocular muscle weakness *(42)*. A surgical glove is filled with ice and placed over a ptotic eyelid for approximately 2 min; correction of the ptosis is a "positive" test. Two studies *(13,43)* found the test to have 100% sensitivity and specificity in OM.

**Table 1**
**Frequency of Generalization of Ocular Myasthenia**

| Series | No. of Patients | Isolated Ocular at Onset (%) | Later Spread of Isolated Ocular (%) |
|---|---|---|---|
| Grob et al. *(2)* | 250 | 46 | 58 |
| Ferguson et al. *(68)* | 75 | 59 | 39 |
| Osserman *(69)* | 325 | 42 | 63 |
| Perlo et al. *(70)* | 470 | 15 | 13 |
| Simpson et al. *(71)* | 295 | 34 | 95 |
| Bever et al. *(48)* | 282 | 51 | 45 |

Jacobson *(44)* suggested that the ice test simply rested the ptotic lid and was really a modified sleep test. Movaghar and Slavin *(45)*, comparing local heat and ice, noted marked improvement with both, the common denominator being inhibition of the levator muscles (i.e., a modified sleep test). Kubis et al. *(46)* compared ice with rest and found that although rest improved ptosis, ice was definitely additive. Since both sleep (or rest) and ice improve myasthenic ptosis, a positive test establishes the diagnosis, despite the uncertain mechanism.

Once the diagnosis of OM is made, the workup is the same as with generalized MG: complete blood count, sedimentation rate, antinuclear antibodies, thyroid function tests, blood glucose, and a computed tomography or magnetic resonance imaging of the chest.

## GENERALIZATION OF OCULAR MYASTHENIA

The major concern in OM is spread to the generalized form. In preparing a chapter for a book that was published in 1980 *(1)*, I constructed a table of various series of OM patients who progressed to generalized disease (*see* **Table 1**, which is updated from the 1980 work). At that time, to my surprise, the range varied from 13 to 95%. Perplexed, I asked MG authority Lewis P. Rowland for his views. He agreed to review his own series and published an abstract *(47)* that I cited in 1980 in a table of my chapter *(1)*. The full report *(48)* of 282 consecutive MG patients indicated that 51% presented as ocular. Over time, 10% of these remitted, and the remaining 90% were basically split between OM and generalized MG. **Table 1** lists the frequency of generalization in the major publications through 1983. In the Bever et al. series *(48)*, there were no predictors of spread, including the presence or absence of antibodies, or decremental EMG response in uninvolved limb muscles. More recent studies indicate that whereas abnormal SFEMG does not predict spread, a normal limb SFEMG provides an 82% likelihood that MG will remain ocular *(49)*.

The largest series from a single institution was that of Grob et al. *(2)*, who found a spread of 66%. In children, reports of the rate of spread varies from 31 to 49% *(50)*. Weizer et al. *(51)* provide a good contemporary review of spread from ocular to generalized MG. These authors found no difference in spread or clinical course in patients who developed OM at age 60 or older. Most OM patients progressed during the first 2 years, but progression may occur up to 24 years after onset *(1)*.

## TREATMENT

The treatment for OM varies among centers *(52–56)*, reflecting the paucity of randomized trials. The spectrum of treatments includes anticholinesterase drugs, usually pyridostigmine bromide (Mestinon®); steroids; immunosuppressants (azathioprine and cyclosporine A); thymectomy; eye patching (for diplopia); or mechanical measures for bilateral ptosis. I will present our treatment approach, followed by those of others.

First we try Mestinon for symptomatic relief. Although it often improves ptosis and diplopia, patients may not be satisfied. For instance, patients with complete unilateral ptosis don't have diplopia; Mestinon may relieve the ptosis and unmask the diplopia. Mestinon usually increases the strength of weak extraocular muscles, but it may not totally correct the weakness, leaving some diplopia. A small amount of diplopia is more disconcerting than a large separation, since it is easier to ignore a diplopic image that is off in the periphery compared with one close to the real image. Thus, eliminating ptosis or substantially reducing diplopia with Mestinon may be more distressing to the patient than their original symptoms.

If we can't correct diplopia with Mestinon, we patch an eye with a clip-on spectacle occluder, frosted lenses, or an occluding contact lens. Ptosis can often be improved with a "crutch" constructed by an optician (**Fig. 4**) or double adhesive tape (Clavin Non-Surgical Eye Lift®; http://www.Clavin.com/).

We use steroids only as a last resort for bilateral total ophthalmoplegia, bilateral ptosis with poor tolerance of crutches, or patient insistence because of overwhelming cosmetic concern *(56)*. The latter refers to a patient who will "kill myself unless you make me look normal again." Besides the usual complications of steroids and the probable necessity of concomitant prophylactic treatment with a biphosphonate to retard osteoporosis *(57,58)*, once started, steroids may be impossible to discontinue without exacerbation of symptoms *(59)*.

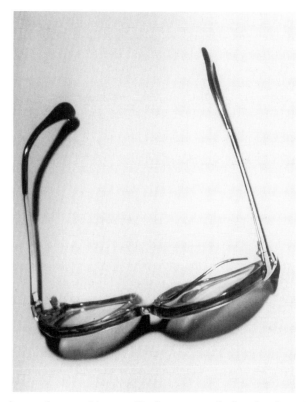

**Fig. 4.** Ptosis crutches are thin metallic frames attached to the rims of eyeglasses. They mechanically elevate the lids but allow blinking. (Photo courtesy of Dr. Robert L. Tomsak.)

I start with prednisone 10 mg qod, increasing by 10 mg every third dose, until the desired clinical effect is achieved. Because the dose increase is slow, patients often reach the desired effect at 40–60 mg qod. The dose is maintained for several months and then decreased by 10 mg a month until 30 mg qod is reached. Any decrease from 30 mg is by increments of 5 mg, and decreases from 20 mg are by increments of 2.5 mg or less. Myasthenics may "crash" with exceedingly small reductions when their qod dose is 20 mg or below. A "crash" in an ocular myasthenic is not particularly problematic, but we never know whether the steroids were masking generalized myasthenia, which might manifest dramatically. I don't use azathioprine, cyclosporine, plasma exchange, or intravenous immunoglobulin (IVIg) in OM, and I do not recommend elective thymectomy.

Kupersmith et al. *(53)* and Agius *(55)* present the arguments for routine steroids in OM. Steroids may not only totally relieve ptosis and diplopia, but, more importantly, they may prevent the patient from developing generalized MG. Our *(56)* counter argument is basically twofold:

1. There is no conclusive evidence that steroids prevent generalization, but they may mask it. If a patient with OM generalizes, we would start steroids.
2. Since 40–60% remain ocular, many patients would be started on a lifetime course of steroids (because of the difficulty in weaning) for no reason other than a cosmetic one, or for symptomatic relief that might otherwise be treated safely with non-pharmacologic measures. The steroid issue will only be resolved by a randomized study.

I start the low-dose, alternate-day prednisone regimen, as does Newsom-Davis *(60)*, because of the recognized early worsening of generalized MG with high-dose steroids. Kupersmith et al. *(53)* found that ocular myasthenics can tolerate a starting dose of 40–80 mg of daily prednisone without worsening. Moreover, they decreased and usually eliminated the drug over 4–6 weeks and felt that subsequent development of generalized MG was reduced.

In addition to steroids, azathioprine *(52,54,61)*, cyclosporine A *(52)*, plasma exchange or IVIg *(55)*, and thymectomy *(52,54,55,62)* have advocates. Evoli et al. *(61)* provide a good recent review of the thymectomy literature in OM.

Rare patients with "fixed" (unchanged for several years) tropias may benefit from corrective strabismus surgery *(63)*. Although lid surgery to improve chronic ptosis is feasible *(64)*, I agree with Sergott *(65)* and do not recommend it. However, blepharoplasty to correct dermatochalasia (redundant, sagging periocular skin) coexisting with MG ptosis may increase the size of the palpebral fissure. Bentley et al. *(63)* used botulinum toxin in a few patients with a fixed tropia to weaken the antagonist of the paretic muscle, thereby straightening the eye. Given the generalized nature of neuromuscular dysfunction in OM, and the distant effect of locally injected botulinum *(66,67)*, the risk seems too great.

## REFERENCES

1. Daroff RB. Ocular myasthenia: diagnosis and therapy. In: Glaser JS, ed. *Neuro-ophthalmology*, vol X. St. Louis, CV Mosby, 1980, pp. 62–71.
2. Grob D, Arsura EL, Brunner NG, Namba T. The course of myasthenia gravis and therapies affecting outcome. *Ann NY Acad Sci* 1987;505:472–499.
3. Porter JD, Baker RS. Muscle of a different 'color': the unusual properties of the extraocular muscles may predispose or protect them in neurogenic and myogenic disease. *Neurology* 1996;46:30–37.
4. Kaminski HJ, Ruff RL. Ocular muscle involvement by myasthenia gravis. *Ann Neurol* 1997;41:419–420.

5. Kaminski HJ. Acetylcholine receptor epitopes in ocular myasthenia. *Ann NY Acad Sci* 1998;841:309–319.
6. Niemann CU, Krag TOB, Khurana TS. Identification of genes that are differentially expressed in extraocular and limb muscle. *J Neurol Sci* 2000;179:76–84.
7. Ubogu EE, Kaminski HJ. The preferential involvement of extraocular muscles by myasthenia gravis. *Neuroophthalmol* 2001;25:219–228.
8. Horton RM, Manfredi AA, Conti-Tronconi BM. The 'embryonic' gamma subunit of the nicotine acetylcholine receptor is expressed in adult extraocular muscle. *Neurology* 1993;43:983–986.
9. Kaminski HJ, Kusner LL, Nash KV, Ruff RL. The gamma subunit of the acetylcholine receptor is not expressed in the levator palpebrae superioris. *Neurology* 1995; 45:516–518.
10. Marino M, Barbesino G, Pinchera A, et al. Increased frequency of euthyroid ophthalmopathy in patients with Graves' disease associated with myasthenia gravis. *Thyroid* 2000;10:799–802.
11. Glaser JS, Siatkowski. Infranuclear disorders of eye movement. In: Glaser JS, ed. *Neuroophthalmology*, 3rd ed. Philadelphia, Lippincott Williams & Wilkins, 1999, pp. 405–459.
12. Cooper J, Kruger P, Panariello G. The pathognomonic pattern of accommodative fatigue in myasthenia gravis. *Binocul Vis Strabismus Q* 1988;3:141–148.
13. Kuncl RW, Hoffman PN. Myopathies and disorders of neuromuscular transmission. In: Miller NR, Newman NJ, eds. *Walsh and Hoyt's Clinical Neuro-Ophthalmology*, 5th ed., vol 1. Baltimore, Williams & Wilkins, 1998, pp. 1351–1431.
14. Loewenfeld IE. *The Pupil: Anatomy, Physiology, and Clinical Applications*. Boston, Butterworth Heinemann, 1999, pp. 1364–1366.
15. Thompson HS, Miller NR. Disorders of pupillary function, accommodation, and lacrimation. In: Miller NR, Newman NJ, eds. *Walsh and Hoyt's Clinical Neuro-opthalmology*, 5th ed., vol 1. Baltimore, Williams & Wilkins, 1998, pp. 961–999.
16. Barton JJS. Ocular aspects of myasthenia gravis. *Semin Neurol* 2000;20:7–20.
17. Valmaggia C, Gottlob I. Cocaine abuse, generalized myasthenia, complete external ophthalmoplegia, and pseudotonic pupil. *Strabismus* 2001;9:9–12.
18. Yee RD, Cogan DG, Zee DS, Baloh RW, Honrubia V. Rapid eye movements in myasthenia gravis. II. Electro-oculographic analysis. *Arch Ophthalmol* 1976;94: 1465–1472.
19. Ragge ML, Hoyt WF. Midbrain myasthenia: fatigable ptosis, 'lid twitch' sign, and ophthalmoparesis from a dorsal midbrain glioma. *Neurology* 1992;42:917–919.
20. Kao Y-F, Lan M-Y, Chou M-S, Chen W-H. Intracranial fatigable ptosis. *J Neuroophthalmol* 1999;19:257–259.
21. Averbuch-Heller L, Poonyathalang A, von Maydell RD, Remler BF. Hering's law for eyelids: still valid. *Neurology* 1996;45:1781–1783.
22. McConville J, Hoch W, Newsom-Davis J, Vincent A. Antibodies to the muscle specific kinase, MuSK, in generalised and ocular myasthenia gravis seronegative for acetylcholine receptor antibodies. *J Neurol Sci* 2001;187(Suppl 1):S122–S123.
23. Oosterhuis HJ. The ocular signs and symptoms of myasthenia gravis. *Doc Ophthalmol* 1982;52:363–378.
24. Sanders, DB. Electrophysiological and pharmacological tests in neuromuscular junction disorders. In: Lisak RP, ed. *Handbook of Myasthenia Gravis and Myasthenic Syndromes*. New York, Marcel Dekker, 1994, pp. 103–148.

25. Binnie CD, Cooper R, Fowler CJ, Mauguière F, Prior PF. EMG, nerve conduction and evoked potentials. In: Osselton JW, ed. *Clinical Neurophysiology.* Boston, Butter-worth Heinemann, 1995, pp. 201–204.

26. Padua L, Stalberg E, LoMonaco M, et al. SFEMG in ocular myasthenia gravis diagnosis. *Clin Neurophysiol* 2000;111:1203–1207.

27. Valls-Canals J, Montero J, Pradas J. Stimulated single fiber EMG of the frontalis muscle in the diagnosis of ocular myasthenia. *Muscle Nerve* 2000;23:779–783.

28. Daroff RB. The office Tensilon test for ocular myasthenia gravis. *Arch Neurol* 1986;43:843–844.

29. Seybold ME. The office Tensilon test for ocular myasthenia gravis. *Arch Neurol* 1986;43:842–843.

30. Barton JJS. Quantitative ocular tests for myasthenia gravis: a comparative review with detection theory analysis. *J Neurol Sci* 1998;155:104–114.

31. Yang Q, Wei M, Sun F, et al. Open-loop and closed-loop optokinetic nystagmus (OKN) in myasthenia gravis and nonmyasthenic subjects. *Exp Neurol* 2000;166: 166–172.

32. Toth L, Toth A, Dioszeghy P, Repassy G. Electronystagmographic analysis of opto-kinetic nystagmus for the evaluation of ocular symptoms in myasthenia gravis. *Acta Otolaryngol* 1999;119:629–632.

33. Oh, SJ, Cho HK. Edrophonium responsiveness not necessarily diagnostic of myas-thenia gravis. *Muscle Nerve* 1990;13:187–191.

34. Dirr LY, Troost BT. A false positive edrophonium test in a patient with a brain stem glioma. *Neurology* 1989;39:865–867.

35. Moorthy G, Behrens MM, Drachman DB, et al. Ocular pseudo-myasthenia or ocu-lar myasthenia "plus": a warning to clinicians. *Neurology* 1989;39:1150–1154.

36. Schmidt D. Signs in ocular myasthenia and pseudomyasthenia. Differential diag-nostic criteria. *Neuroophthalmology* 1995;15:21–58.

37. Kupersmith MJ, Latkany R, Straga J. Ocular myasthenia gravis: steroids, edropho-nium dose, thymoma, and generalization. *Neuroophthalmology* 2001;25:39.

38. Ing EB, Ing SY, Ing T, Ramocki JA. The complication rate of edrophonium testing for suspected myasthenia gravis. *Can J Ophthalmol* 2000;35:141–145.

39. Okun MS, Charriez CM, Bhatti MT, Watson RT, Swift T. Tensilon and the diagno-sis of myasthenia gravis: are we using the Tensilon test too much? *Neurologist* 2001; 7:295–299.

40. Odel JG, Winterkorn JM, Behrens MM. The sleep test for myasthenia gravis. A safe alternative to Tensilon. *J Clin Neuroophthalmol* 1991;11:288–292.

41. Golnick KC, Pena R, Lee AG, Eggenberger ER. An ice test for the diagnosis of myasthenia gravis. *Ophthalmology* 1999;106:1282–1286.

42. Larner AJ, Thomas DJ. Can myasthenia gravis be diagnosed with the 'ice pack test'? A cautionary note. *Postgrad Med J* 2000;76:162–163.

43. Ellis FD, Hoyt CS, Ellis FJ, Jeffery AR, Sondhi N. Extraocular muscle responses to orbital cooling (ice test) for ocular myasthenia gravis diagnosis. *J AAPOS* 2000; 4:271–281.

44. Jacobson DM. The 'ice pack test' for diagnosing myasthenia gravis. *Ophthalmol-ogy* 2000;4:622–623.

45. Movaghar M, Slavin ML. Effect of local heat versus ice on blepharoptosis resulting from ocular myasthenia. *Ophthalmology* 2000;107:2209–2214.

46. Kubis KC, Denesh-Meyer HV, Savino PJ, Sergott RC. The ice test versus the rest test in myasthenia gravis. *Ophthalmology* 2000;107:1995–1998.
47. Bever CT Jr, Aquino AV, Penn AS, Loveless RA, Rowland LP. Prognosis of ocular myasthenia. *Neurology* 1980;30:387.
48. Bever CT, Aquino AV, Penn AS, Lovelace RE, Rowland LP. Prognosis of ocular myasthenia. *Ann Neurol* 1983;14:515–519.
49. Weinberg DH, Rizzo JF, Hayes MT, Kneeland MD, Kelly JJ. Ocular myasthenia gravis: predictive value of single-fiber electromyography. *Muscle Nerve* 1999;22: 1222–1227.
50. Mullaney P, Vajsar J, Smith R, Buncic JR. The natural history and ophthalmic involvement in childhood myasthenia gravis at The Hospital for Sick Children. *Ophthalmology* 2000;107:504–510.
51. Weizer JS, Lee AG, Coats DK. Myasthenia gravis with ocular involvement in older patients. *Can J Ophthalmol* 2001;36:26–33.
52. Drachman DB. Management of ocular myasthenia gravis. In: Tusa RJ, Newman SA, eds. *Neuroophthalmological Disorders, Diagnostic Work-Up and Management.* New York, Marcel Dekker, 1995, pp. 265–275.
53. Kupersmith MJ, Moster M, Bhiyan S, Warren F, Weinberg H. Beneficial effects of corticosteroids on ocular myasthenia gravis. *Arch Neurol* 1996;53:802–804.
54. Sommer N, Sigg B, Melms A, Weller M, et al. Ocular myasthenia gravis: response to long term immunosuppressive treatment. *J Neurol Neurosurg Psychiatry* 1997; 62:156–162.
55. Agius MA. Treatment of ocular myasthenia with corticosteroids. *Arch Neurol* 2000; 57:750–751.
56. Kaminski HJ, Daroff RB. Treatment of ocular myasthenia. *Arch Neurol* 2000;57: 752–753.
57. Lloyd ME, Spector TD, Howard R. Osteoporosis in neurological disorders. *J Neurol Neurosurg Psychiatry* 2000;68:543–549.
58. Smith GDP, Stevens DL, Fuller GN. Myasthenia gravis, corticosteroids and osteoporosis prophylaxis. *J Neurol* 2001;248:151.
59. Beekman R, Kuks JB, Oosterhuis HJ. Myasthenia gravis: diagnosis and follow-up of 100 consecutive patients. *J Neurol* 1997;244:112–118.
60. Newsom-Davis J. Disorders of the neuromuscular junction. In: Scolding N, ed. *Contemporary Treatments in Neurology.* Oxford, Butterworth Heinemann, 2001, pp. 158–169.
61. Evoli A, Batocchi AP, Minisci C, Di Schino C, Tonali P. Therapeutic options in ocular myasthenia gravis. *Neuromuscul Disord* 2001;11:208–216.
62. Sanders DB, Howard JF Jr. Disorders of neuromuscular transmission. In: Bradley WG, Daroff RB, Fenichel GM, Marsden CD, eds. *Neurology in Clinical Practice: The Neurological Disorders*, 3rd ed. Boston, Butterworth Heinemann, 2000, pp. 2167–2185.
63. Bentley CR, Dawson E, Lee JP. Active management in patients with ocular manifestations of myasthenia gravis. *Eye* 2001;15:18–22.
64. Bradley EA, Bartley GB, Chapman KL, Waller RR. Surgical correction of blepharoptosis in patients with myasthenia gravis. *Ophthalmol Plast Reconstr Surg* 2001; 17:103–110.
65. Sergott RC. Ocular myasthenia. In: Lisak RP, ed. *Handbook of Myasthenia Gravis and Myasthenic Syndromes.* New York, Marcel Dekker, 1994, pp. 21–31.

66. Sanders DB, Massey EW, Buckley EG. Botulinum toxin for blepharospasm: single-fiber EMG studies. *Neurology* 1986;36:545–547.
67. Lange DJ, Rubin M, Greene PE, et al. Distant effects of locally injected botulinum toxin: a double-blind study of single fiber EMG changes. *Muscle Nerve* 1991;14: 672–675.
68. Ferguson FR, Hutchinson EC, Liversedge LA. Myasthenia gravis: results of medical management. *Lancet* 1955;2:636–639.
69. Osserman KE. *Myasthenia gravis*. New York, Grune & Stratton, 1955.
70. Perlo VP, Poskanzer DC, Schwab RS, Viets HR, Osserman KE, Genkins G. Myasthenia gravis: evaluation of treatment in 1,355 patients. *Neurology* 1966; 16:431–439.
71. Simpson JF, Westerberg MR, Magee KR. Myasthenia gravis: an analysis of 295 cases. *Acta Neurol Scand* 1966; 42(Suppl):1–27.

# 6

# Thymoma-Associated Myasthenia Gravis

## Alexander Marx and Philipp Stroebel

## INTRODUCTION

Seropositive myasthenia gravis (MG) is an autoimmune disease caused by autoantibodies to the nicotinic acetylcholine receptor (AChR) at the neuromuscular junction *(1,2)*. By contrast, seronegative MG in many patients results from autoantibodies to muscle-specific tyrosine kinases (MuSK) at the endplate *(3)*. Thymoma-associated MG (paraneoplastic MG) is a seropositive MG subtype. Thymoma has an adverse effect on survival among MG patients *(4)*. Thymic pathology occurs in 80–90% of MG patients and is most subtle in seronegative MG *(5,6)*. There are significant associations between different thymic alterations and clinical findings *(7–9)* (**Table 1**). Prior to highlighting the peculiarities of thymoma-associated MG, we begin with a brief review of MG with thymic lymphofollicular hyperplasia (TFH) and thymic atrophy.

## HISTOPATHOLOGY OF THE THYMUS IN MG

### Thymic Lymphofollicular Hyperplasia

TFH occurs in 70% of MG patients *(10)*. It is characterized by lymphoid follicles with or without germinal centers extending perivascular spaces (PVSs). The basal membrane around the PVS is disrupted by lymphoid follicle development *(11)*, resulting in a fusion of the medulla (i.e., a part of the thymus parenchyma) and PVS (thought to belong to the peripheral immune system) *(12,13)*. Myoid cells are noninnervated myoblast- or myotube-like muscle cells that occur in the thymic medulla (outside lymphoid follicles, if present). In the normal thymus and in TFH they are MHC class II-negative *(14)* and probably express both fetal and adult-type AChR *(12,15–17)*. For unknown reasons myoid cells in TFH are frequently located in intimate apposition to dendritic cells *(12)*. Such contacts are rare in normal thymus. The thymic cortex in TFH shows the normal age-dependent morphology.

From: *Current Clinical Neurology: Myasthenia Gravis and Related Disorders*
Edited by: H. J. Kaminski © Humana Press Inc., Totowa, NJ

**Table 1**
**MG Subtypes Related to Thymus Pathology[a]**

| Parameter | Hyperplasia[b] | Thymoma | Atrophy |
|---|---|---|---|
| Age at onset of symptoms (yr) | 10–39 | 15–80 | >40 |
| Sex (male/female) | 1:3 | 1:1 | 2:1 |
| HLA association | B8; DR3 | DR2, A24 | B7; DR2 |
| CTLA-4 polymorphism (allele 104) | Normal | Increased | Normal |
| TNFA*T1/B*2 homozygous | Rare | Very frequent | Frequent |
| TNFA*T2; TNFB1 TNFB*1, C4A *QO, C4B*1, DRB1*03 | Frequent | Rare | Rare |
| Autoantibodies against | | | |
| AChR | 80% | >95% | 90% |
| Striated muscle | 10–20% | >90% | 30–60% |
| Titin | <10% | >90% | 30–40% |
| Ryanodine receptor | <5% | 50–60% | 20% |
| IL-12, IFN-α[b] | Infrequent | 63–88% | Infrequent |

[a]Correlation with clinical, epidemiologic, and genetic findings *(6,9,57–59,70,73,87,114,116, 117,126–130)*. AChR = acetylcholine receptor; IL-12 = interleukin-12; IFN-α = interferon-α.
[b]Early-onset MG.
[c]Cumulative percentage for nonthymoma MG patients was reported to be 12% and that in non-MG thymoma patients 30% *(70)*.

## Thymus Atrophy in MG

Thymic atrophy is encountered in 10–20% of MG patients *(18)*. It is probably not the end stage of TFH, and, except for a slight increase in medullary B-cells and dendritic cells *(19)*, the thymuses in these patients are equivalent to age-matched controls, including a normal number of myoid cells per thymic tissue area *(12,20)*.

## Thymomas in Paraneoplastic MG

Thymoma occurs in about 10% of MG patients. There are rare reports of MG occurring in single cases of a variety of epithelial, mesenchymal, and hematopoietic tumors *(21)*. However, only for MG-associated thymomas is it undisputed that they play a role in the pathogenesis of MG *(7,9,22–27)*.

Thymomas are epithelial tumors of the thymus. Criteria for their histologic diagnosis have recently been defined by the World Health Organization (WHO) *(28,29)*, as follows: types A (medullary), AB (mixed), B1 (organoid), B2 (cortical), B3 (well-differentiated thymic carcinoma), and C. Type C thymomas are carcinomas of the thymus resembling carcinomas in other parts of the body, whereas types A, AB, and B1–3 thymomas are unique to the

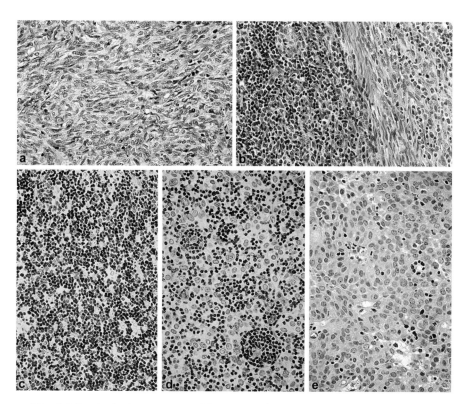

**Fig. 1.** Morphologic spectrum of thymomas that can be associated with paraneo-plastic MG. (**a**) WHO type A (medullary) thymoma with prominent spindle cell features and scarce intermingled lymphocytes, which are mostly of the mature pheno-type. (**b**) WHO type AB (mixed) thymoma with features of both WHO type A and B (cortical) thymomas. In this case, both areas are clearly separated, whereas in other tumors, the type A and B areas may be indistinguishably interwoven. (**c–e**) WHO type B1 (**c**), B2 (**d**), and B3 (**e**) thymoma. High numbers of immature T-cells, lack of cytologic atypia of the thymic epithelium, and presence of numerous Hassal's corpuscles are diagnostic of type B1 thymomas. Type B2 tumors show somewhat reduced numbers of T-cells with marked atypia of the thymic epithelium; occasional Hassal's corpuscles may occur. The picture in type B3 thymomas is clearly dominated by the epithelium, with formation of characteristic perivascular spaces and perivascular palisading. Cytologic atypia is less pronounced in type B3 than in B2 tumors. (Hematoxylin and eosin stain.)

thymus. It is of note that only type A, AB, and B1–3 thymomas exhibit "thymus-like features," i.e., they have the capacity to promote intratumorous T-cell development (see below), and only these thymoma subtypes but not type C thymomas (e.g., squamous cell carcinomas of the thymus) are associated with MG *(21,28)*. Prototypical cases of MG-associated thymoma subtypes are shown in **Fig. 1**. The genetic basis of thymoma oncogenesis is currently being elucidated *(30–32)*.

## PATHOGENIC CONCEPTS IN SEROPOSITIVE MG

### Pathogenesis of MG in Thymic Lymphofollicular Hyperplasia

It is now generally accepted that TFH-associated MG results from an intrathymic pathogenesis, with AChRs on thymic myoid cells being primarily involved as the triggering autoantigen *(33)*. This concept is supported by five findings: 1) a substantial percentage of autoantibodies in TFH/MG patients recognize fetal AChRs *(34)*; 2) fetal AChRs (i.e., AChRs with a γ- instead of an ε-subunit) are expressed only on thymic myoid cells and on a few extraocular muscle fibers *(17,35–37)*; 3) thymus with TFH is the organ where most anti-AChR autoantibodies are produced in absolute terms and on a per plasma cell basis *(38)*, explaining the beneficial effect of thymectomy *(39,40)*; 4) extrathymic immunization with AChR can induce experimental autoimmune MG (EAMG) but does not elicit TFH *(41)*; and 5) by contrast, transplantation of TFH-affected thymus into severe combined immunodeficiency (SCID) mice results in prolonged production of anti-AChR autoantibodies, showing that TFH contains all the constituents of a self-sustaining autoimmune reaction *(42–44)*. Furthermore, clusters of myoid cells and antigen-presenting dendritic cells have been observed in TFH *(12)*. Since myoid cells remain largely negative for MHC class II in MG, they are probably unable to prime AChR-reactive CD4+ T-cells *(45)*. Therefore, dendritic cells may take up AChR from myoid cells and present AChR peptides to potentially AChR-reactive T-cells that occur as nontolerized T-cells in the normal T-cell repertoire *(46–48)* and are increased in TFH *(22,49)*. If activated, such autoreactive T-cells may provide help to B-cells for autoantibody production inside and outside the thymus *(50,51)*. Autoantibodies may react with peripheral muscle and with myoid cells. Whether prominent myoid cell apoptosis in TFH/MG patients *(52)* is caused by autoantibodies, cytotoxic attack, or endogenous instability is not known. However, recent experiments suggest that low-level expression of MHC class II molecules on myoid cells in LFH may stimulate preactivated T-cells *(14)*. Therefore, myoid cell apoptosis in TFH *(52)* might be of pathogenic significance as far as AChR epitope spreading is concerned *(14)*.

TFH occurs frequently in MG *(24)* and commonly in other autoimmune diseases *(18)* but rarely in healthy persons *(53)*. Its actual trigger is not known, but a genetic contribution to the etiology of TFH-associated MG is obvious, as demonstrated for the following polymorphic genes: MHC class I and II

**Table 2**
**Paraneoplastic Diseases Possibly Related to Thymoma**[a]

| | |
|---|---|
| Addison's disease | Neuromyotonia |
| Agranulocytosis | Panhypopituitarism |
| Alopecia areata | Pernicious anemia |
| Aplastic anemia | Polymyositis |
| Autoimmune colitis | Pure red cell aplasia |
| (graft-versus-host-like disease) | Rheumatoid arthritis |
| Cushing's syndrome | Rippling muscle disease |
| Hemolytic anemia | Sarcoidosis |
| Hypogammaglobulinemia | Scleroderma |
| Intestinal pseudo-obstruction | Sensory motor neuropathy |
| Limbic encephalitis | Stiff person syndrome |
| Myasthenia gravis | Systemic lupus erythematosus |
| Myocarditis | Thyroiditis |

[a]In most of these diseases, the immunopathogenesis has not been resolved (reviewed in ref. *21*).

*(54,55)*, interleukin (IL)-1β *(56)* tumor necrosis factor (TNF)-α *(57–59)*, IL-10 *(60)*, and the AChR α-, but not, β-subunit *(61–63)* (**Table 1**). It is unknown whether hyperexpression of bcl-2 in thymic germinal centers *(64)* or of FAS in mature thymic T-cells *(65,66)* is involved in the etiology of thymitis.

## Pathogenesis of Thymoma-Associated MG

### Distinct Autoantigens, Autoantibodies, Genetics, and Associated Autoimmune Paraneoplastic Syndromes in Thymoma Patients

A large body of evidence (**Table 1**) shows that the pathogenesis of thymoma-associated MG differs from that of LFH-associated MG *(5,9,21,67)*. There is a broad spectrum of paraneoplastic autoimmune diseases that occur either in isolation or associated with MG in thymoma (**Table 2**). In some of these paraneoplastic syndromes, the autoantigens and autoantibodies and their pathogenic relevance have been characterized (**Table 3**). Some authors found no increase of nonmuscle autoimmune diseases in MG-positive thymoma patients *(68,69)*. Antibodies to IL-12 and interferon (IFN)-α might be involved in the pathogenesis of paraneoplastic MG and are sensitive markers to detect thymoma recurrences *(70)*. Titers of anti-ryanodine receptor antibodies correlate significantly with clinical MG severity *(71,72)*, whereas anti-titin autoantibodies as markers for disease severity are not unequivocally established *(72,73)*.

**Table 3**
**Autoimmune Diseases with Defined Autoantigens,**
**Pathogenic Relevance of Autoantibodies or Autoreactive T-cells**
**in Thymoma Patients, and Relationship to Histologic Thymoma Subtype[a]**

| Autoimmune Disease | Autoantigen | Pathogenic Relevance of Autoantibodies or Autoreactive T-Cells | Preferred Thymoma Subtype (WHO) |
|---|---|---|---|
| Myasthenia gravis | AChR | Yes | |
| | StrA | Probably no | |
| | IFN-α, IL-12 | Probably yes | WHO type B > AB > A |
| Neuromyotonia | VGKC | Yes | n.k. |
| Peripheral neuropathy | VGKC | Yes | n.k. |
| Stiff person syndrome | GAD | n.k. | n.k. |
| Rippling muscle disease | Neuronal AChR | Probably yes | WHO type AB, B |
| Intestinal pseudo-obstruction | Neuronal AChR | Probably yes | n.k. |
| Limbic encephalitis | Neuronal nuclear antigens | Probably yes | n.k. |
| | Glial antigens | | |
| Red blood cell aplasia, neutropenia, pancytopenia | Unknown | Yes (T-cells) (auto-antibodies?) | WHO type A > B |
| Polymoyositis dermatomyositis | Unknown | Unknown | WHO type B, C |

[a]Data from refs. *21, 27, 115, 131,* and *132.* AChR = acetylcholine receptor; StrA = striational antigens (myosin, titin, ryanodine receptor); VGKC = voltage-gated potassium channel; GAD = glutamic acid decarboxylase; IFN-α = interferon-α; IL-12 = interleukin-12; n.k. = not known.

A major morphologic difference between thymoma and TFH is the presence of AChR-expressing myoid cells in LFH but their absence in thymomas. A striking functional difference is the absence [with few exceptions *(74)*] of autoantibody production inside thymomas *(75).*

*Shared Features Among MG-Associated Thymomas*

Although the pathogenesis of paraneoplastic MG might be heterogeneous, considering the heterogeneous morphologic and functional findings *(21)*, MG-associated thymomas share some common features:

1. All MG-associated thymomas are either type A, AB, or B1–3 thymomas according to the WHO classification, and they share morphologic and functional features with the normal thymus. In particular, they provide signals for the homing of

# MG(+) thymomas      MG(-) thymomas

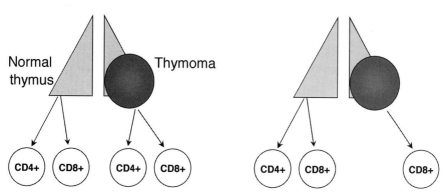

**Fig. 2.** T-cell export from thymus and thymomas to the blood in either MG-positive or MG-negative patients. Statistically significant data on the role of CD4 T-cell export for the pathogenesis of paraneoplastic MG have been obtained in the most frequent WHO type AB and B thymomas but not for the rare type A thymomas *(82, 83)*. Recent data suggest that failure to complete intratumorous CD4 T-cell maturation is the main reason for the different CD4 T-cell export in MG-positive and MG-negative thymomas (Stroebel et al., in press).

immature hematopoietic precursors and promote their differentiation to apparently mature T-cells *(76–78)*. It is not yet clear whether a few type A thymomas might be an exception to this rule since they generate at most very few T-cells. However, thymic carcinomas (type C thymomas), thymic neuroendocrine tumors, and thymic lymphomas do not exhibit intratumorous thymopoiesis and are unassociated with MG *(21)*.

2. MG-associated thymomas are enriched for autoreactive T-cells with specificity for the AChR α- and the ε-subunits *(26,78–81)*. There is strong evidence that some of these are generated by intratumorous, nontolerogenic thymopoiesis *(26,81)*.

3. All MG-associated thymomas export naive mature T-cells *(82)*, and it has been hypothesized that export of autoreactive CD4+ T-cells is of pathogenic relevance. This hypothesis was directly proved by Buckley et al. *(83)* using the quantification of T-cell receptor excision circles (TRECs) in circulating T-cells, showing that both naïve CD4+ and CD8+ T-cells are increased in thymoma patients with MG, whereas there was no clear-cut increase of CD4+ T-cells in thymoma patients without MG (**Fig. 2**). Recently, we found that this difference between MG-positive and MG-negative thymoma patients is associated with the capacity of MG-positive but not MG-negative thymomas to complete intratumorous thymopoiesis, i.e., to generate CD4+/CD45RA+ naive T-cells (in press).

4. Almost all MG-associated thymomas exhibit reduced expression of MHC class II molecules on neoplastic epithelial cells *(84,85)*. In parallel, thymopoiesis in thymomas is quantitatively less efficient *(76,85)*. In addition, reduced MHC class II levels might be one reason why thymopoiesis in thymomas is not tolerogenic, i.e., qualitatively abnormal (see below) *(85,86)*.
5. Concurrent autoimmunity against four apparently unrelated types of autoantigens is highly characteristic of paraneoplastic MG. These autoantigens are
   a. The AChR *(27)*.
   b. Striational muscle antigens, including titin *(87)*.
   c. Neuronal antigens *(88)*.
   d. Cytokines (IL-12, IFN-α) *(70)*.
   Autoimmunity to the ryanodine receptor is also highly characteristic but less frequent *(71,89)*. A common theme shared by MG-associated thymomas is the occurrence of mRNA coding for the autoantigens mentioned *(90–92)*. Except for the cytokines, however, there appears to be an apparent lack of the respective proteins *(89,93–96)*, although the possibility has not been excluded that translation into very small amounts of autoantigenic protein occurs, with potential implications for autoimmunization *(97–100)*.

## Driving Features of MG-Associated Thymomas

Apart from shared features among MG-associated thymomas there are also features that are clearly diverse. One such feature is the abnormal (hyper) expression in neoplastic epithelial cells of proteins that are unrelated to the autoantigens but express AChR-, titin-, or ryanodine receptor-like epitopes *(81,89,93,96)*. These antigens occur in a subset of thymomas only. Although the role of such crossreacting proteins as specific immunogens has been seriously questioned recently *(81,101)*, it appears likely that abnormally expressed proteins might disturb the normal pool of endogenous peptides for presentation by MHC II proteins on thymoma epithelial cells *(86)*. Since quality and quantity of thymic endogenous epithelial cell peptides have a major impact on T-cell selection and tolerance induction *(102–105)*, altered expression of endogenous proteins in thymoma might be an indirect mechanism resulting in nontolerogenic intratumorous T-cell development (see below) *(21)*.

Loss of heterozygosity (LOH) for the MHC locus in neoplastic epithelium mainly of MG-associated thymomas appears to be particularly frequent among MG-positive thymomas, although more cases have to be evaluated. This LOH may result in MHC chimerism between the hemizygous thymoma epithelium (presumed to perform T-cell selection) and the heterozygous intratumorous dendritic cells and the peripheral immune system. MHC chimerism might be one among other mechanisms of nontolerogenic T-cell selection in a subset of thymomas *(21,31)*.

Finally, there is diversity in the occurrence of activated mature T-cells in thymomas. Some type A (medullary) thymomas, which are rarely associated with MG, have been found to harbor increased numbers of activated $CD25^+/CD4^+$ mature T-cells compared with the normal thymus *(77)*. By contrast, almost all type AB, B2, and B3 thymomas (which collectively are frequently MG-associated) are devoid of activated $CD4^+$ T-cells *(25,78,85)*. These findings argue for a different pathogenesis of paraneoplastic MG in type A vs. type AB and B thymomas (see below).

## PATHOGENIC MODEL
## OF PARANEOPLASTIC MYASTHENIA GRAVIS

Taken together, the following findings await explanation through an appropriate pathogenic model:

1. Paraneoplastic MG occurs in thymomas that contain *immature* T-cells and promote their maturation *(21,86)*.
2. Thymomas express reduced levels of MHC class II antigens *(84,106–108)*, and loss of one MHC locus on chromosome 6p21 in many thymomas may result in a qualitatively altered MHC/peptide repertoire on thymoma epithelial cells *(31)*.
3. Thymoma epithelial cells often exhibit hyperexpression of endogenous proteins.
4. MG-associated thymomas are enriched in autoreactive T-cells *(22)*, which are probably generated in the thymoma. They are restricted to the minority HLA isotypes DP14 and DR52a, which are infrequent in MG patients without thymoma *(26)*. Furthermore, intratumorous and blood T-cells exhibit unusual autoantigen specificities *(81)*.
5. Thymomas export CD4 *(83)* and CD8 T-cells *(109)*, and paraneoplastic MG is associated with export of CD4 T-cells *(83,109)*. Lack of CD4 T-cell export from MG-negative thymomas could be explained by a failure of MG-negative thymomas to promote terminal $CD4^+$ T-cell development (Stoebel et al., in press).
6. Intratumorous activation of mature T-cells is restricted to rare type A thymomas *(25)*.
7. Intratumorous autoantibody production is exceptionally rare *(74,75)*.

Furthermore, it has been shown in mice that tolerance induction is influenced by the quantity and quality of MHC/peptide complexes on thymic epithelial cells *(102,103,110,111)*. The MHC level is particularly important when medullary structures (performing negative selection under physiologic conditions) are reduced *(112,113)*. The latter observations might have a bearing for paraneoplastic MG, since a reduction of medullary structures is typical for thymomas *(86)*.

## Thymoma                              Periphery

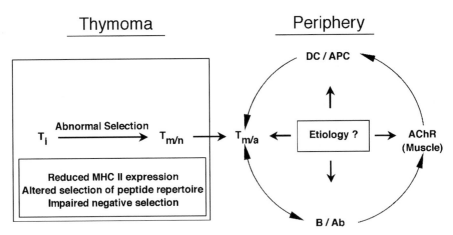

**Fig. 3.** Pathogenic model for paraneoplastic MG in WHO type AB and B thymomas. MG-associated thymomas promote T-cell maturation from immature precursors ($T_i$) to fully mature, naive CD4 T-cells ($T_{m/n}$). Thymocyte maturation might be accompanied by abnormal positive and nontolerogenic negative T-cell selection. After export to the periphery (i.e., residual thymus, lymph nodes, bone marrow, and eventually muscle), naive T-cells are primed by antigen-presenting dendritic cells (DC/APC) to become mature, activated CD4 T-cells ($T_{m/a}$) that provide help to autoantibody-producing B-cells. Whether the acetylcholine receptor (AChR) in skeletal muscle or thymic myoid cells is the primary (triggering) autoantigen or becomes secondarily involved is unknown. Likewise, the events initiating the autoimmune cascade have not been identified. The pathogenesis of MG in WHO type A thymomas, which are virtually nonthymopoietic, has not been resolved.

Taking these data together, we favor the hypothesis that type AB and type B thymomas (90–95% of MG-positive thymoma cases) contribute to autoimmunization by nontolerogenic thymopoiesis and export of naive but potentially autoreactive, mature T-cells to the periphery *(82)* (**Fig. 2**). Export of naive T-cells might gradually replace the normally tolerant, thymus-derived T-cell repertoire by a chimeric autoimmunity-prone T-cell repertoire derived from both the thymoma and the thymus (**Fig. 2**). To become functionally relevant, nonactivated but potentially autoantigen-reactive T-cells have to become activated (by whatever etiologic mechanism; see below) in order to provide help for autoantibody-producing B-cells outside the thymoma *(25)* (**Fig. 3**). At this stage of pathogenesis, a role of a CTLA-4 low phenotype *(114)* and of anti-IL-12 or anti-IFN-α autoantibodies *(70)* can be envisaged facilitating the CD4 T-cell dependent production of anti-AChR autoantibodies.

MG(+)  MG(-)  ps-MG

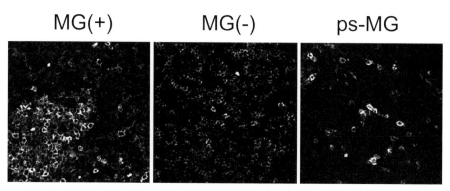

**Fig. 4.** Confocal laser microscope immunofluorescence staining of a thymoma with (MG-positive) and without (MG-negative) associated MG at the time of surgery, and of the thymoma of a patient who developed MG months after surgical removal of the tumor [postsurgery (ps)-MG]. Abundant mature naive CD4 T-cells are found in the MG-positive and ps-MG thymoma. The MG-negative thymoma is virtually depleted of this T-cell subset. Detection of intratumorous mature naive CD4 T-cells in the thymoma of patients without autoimmune phenomena at the time of surgery may indicate an increased risk of developing ps-MG.

## ETIOLOGY OF PARANEOPLASTIC MG

The mechanisms that activate the autoimmunity-prone T-cell repertoire, i.e., the etiologies triggering the MG-provoking autoimmune cascade, have yet to be defined. We have observed paraneoplastic MG following nonspecific infectious or traumatic stimuli, but in most cases no major event can be spotted *(21)*. Whether $CD8^+$ T-cells *(115)* and genetic susceptibility *(116,117)* contribute to the etiologic events has yet to be proved. The periphery (outside the thymoma) where emigrant T-cells become activated can clearly be the residual thymus *(118)*, which we found to be enriched in autoreactive T-cells in many thymoma cases (unpublished data). However, other lymphoid organs and probably the bone marrow also have to play a role in this process *(9)*, given that even complete surgical removal of thymoma plus residual thymus is often *not* followed by a decline of autoantibody titers *(119)*.

## POSTSURGERY MG

MG can occur weeks or even years after thymectomy in a small minority of thymoma patients *(120)*. In accordance with the pathogenic model given in **Fig. 3**, postsurgery MG has been taken as circumstantial evidence for a scenario in which thymomas start to alter the peripheral T-cell repertoire during the nonmyasthenic phase of thymoma growth *(115)*. Furthermore, the model given in **Fig. 3** suggests the testable prediction that postsurgery MG thymomas may generate and export mature naive CD4$^+$ T-cells like MG$^+$ thymomas but unlike true MG-negative thymomas. Recently, this prediction could be verified in a single postsurgery MG thymoma (**Fig. 4**) that harbored fully mature naive CD4$^+$/CD45RA$^+$ T-cells, whereas such cells were virtually absent from all other investigated thymomas that were MG-negative at the time of surgery ($n = 14$). These findings suggest a low risk of developing postsurgery MG for patients who are nonmyasthenic at the time of surgery. However, detection of naive CD4 T-cells in a nonmyasthenic thymoma may indicate that the risk for postsurgery MG is increased. More patients need to be studied to verify this hypothesis.

## MAJOR UNRESOLVED
## QUESTIONS IN PARANEOPLASTIC MG

It has remained enigmatic why nontolerogenic thymopoiesis in type AB and B thymomas results in only a quite narrow spectrum of autoimmune phenomena (**Table 3**) and an even narrower spectrum of autoimmune diseases, with MG outnumbering cytopenias or central nervous system alterations by far *(21,26)*. It is tempting to speculate that the lack of myoid cells in thymomas might play a role in this respect.

Another enigma has been the pathogenesis of paraneoplastic MG in type A thymomas (5% of MG-associated thymomas). In this thymoma subtype the frequency of paraneoplastic MG is the lowest, whereas the frequency of cytopenias, particularly pure red cell aplasia, is the highest among all potentially MG-associated thymoma subtypes (A, AB, B1–3). Type A thymomas usually exhibit minimal or virtually absent intratumorous thymopoiesis (in terms of both immature CD4$^+$/CD8$^+$ and naive CD4$^+$ T-cells) *(77,109)*. Considering the central role of intratumorous thymopoiesis for the pathogenic model given in **Fig. 3** for type AB and B thymomas, we believe that MG in type A thymomas might have another pathogenesis, which may be based on CD8$^+$ T-cells (that appear to be produced by type A thymomas) *(82)* or on CD25$^+$ T-cells that are increased in type A but reduced in all other thymoma subtypes *(25)*.

Finally, it has not been elucidated which autoantigens maintain the prolonged autoantibody response after thymoma surgery; the AChR itself is an obvious candidate. The destruction of skeletal muscle endplates by autoantibodies or cytotoxic T-cells could release AChR and striational antigens, which may be processed and presented to autoreactive T-cells by the intramuscular inflammatory infiltrate *(121)* or by antigen-presenting cells in regional lymph nodes *(9,86)*.

## IS THE PATHOGENESIS OF MG IN THYMIC ATROPHY SIMILAR TO THE PATHOGENESIS OF PARANEOPLASTIC MG?

Pathogenic models based on experimental data have not been suggested for thymic atrophy-associated MG. Heterogeneity of autoantibodies to striational antigens *(6)*, particularly titin *(122,123)*, suggests heterogeneity among MG patients with thymic atrophy. Given that thymoma-associated and MG with thymic atrophy share striational autoantibodies (**Table 1**) and the more protracted effects of thymectomy on MG *(6)*, we speculate that atrophic thymuses might resemble thymomas as to the pathogenesis of MG. Specifically, atrophic thymuses might contribute new, but less efficiently tolerized T-cells to the T-cell repertoire because of age-associated thymic insufficiencies *(20,124,125)*. As in thymomas, the recently exported but autoimmunity-prone T-cells may gradually replace the more tolerant historic T-cell repertoire from the preatrophic era. Individual genetic or environmental susceptibility factors may then determine whether and when tolerance breakdown occurs in the periphery *(29)*. According to this model, activation of autoreactive T-cells should occur outside the atrophic thymus, in agreement with a recent histologic study *(122)*.

## REFERENCES

1. Lindstrom JM, Seybold ME, Lennon VA, Whittingham S, Duane DD. Antibody to acetylcholine receptor in myasthenia gravis: prevalence, clinical correlates, and diagnostic value. 1975 [classical article]. *Neurology* 1998;51:933–939.
2. Tzartos SJ, Barkas T, Cung MT, et al. Anatomy of the antigenic structure of a large membrane autoantigen, the muscle-type nicotinic acetylcholine receptor. *Immunol Rev* 1998;163:89–120.
3. Hoch W, McConville J, Helms S, et al. Autoantibodies to the receptor tyrosine kinase MuSK in patients with myasthenia gravis without acetylcholine receptor antibodies. *Nat Med* 2001;7:365–368.
4. Christensen PB, Jensen TS, Tsiropoulos I, et al. Mortality and survival in myasthenia gravis: a Danish population based study. *J Neurol Neurosurg Psychiatry* 1998;64:78–83.
5. Willcox N, Schluep M, Ritter MA, Newsom-Davis J. The thymus in seronegative myasthenia gravis patients. *J Neurol* 1991;238:256–261.
6. Williams CL, Hay JE, Huiatt TW, Lennon VA. Paraneoplastic IgG striational autoantibodies produced by clonal thymic B cells and in serum of patients with myasthenia gravis and thymoma react with titin. *Lab Invest* 1992;66:331–336.
7. Willcox N. Myasthenia gravis. *Curr Opin Immunol* 1993;5:910–917.
8. Drachman DB. Myasthenia gravis. *N Engl J Med* 1994;330:1797–1810.
9. Marx A, Wilisch A, Schultz A, et al. Pathogenesis of myasthenia gravis. *Virchows Arch* 1997;430:355–364.
10. Muller-Hermelink HK, Marx A. Pathological aspects of malignant and benign thymic disorders. *Ann Med* 1999;31(Suppl 2):5–14.

11. Roxanis I, Micklem K, Willcox N. True epithelial hyperplasia in the thymus of early-onset myasthenia gravis patients: implications for immunopathogenesis. *J Neuroimmunol* 2001;112:163–173.

12. Kirchner T, Schalke B, Melms A, von Kugelgen T, Muller-Hermelink HK. Immunohistological patterns of non-neoplastic changes in the thymus in myasthenia gravis. *Virchows Arch B Cell Pathol Incl Mol Pathol* 1986;52:237–257.

13. Flores KG, Li J, Sempowski GD, Haynes BF, Hale LP. Analysis of the human thymic perivascular space during aging. *J Clin Invest* 1999;104:1031–1039.

14. Curnow J, Corlett L, Willcox N, Vincent A. Presentation by myoblasts of an epitope from endogenous acetylcholine receptor indicates a potential role in the spreading of the immune response. *J Neuroimmunol* 2001;115:127–134.

15. Navaneetham D, Penn AS, Howard JF Jr, Conti-Fine BM. Human thymuses express incomplete sets of muscle acetylcholine receptor subunit transcripts that seldom include the delta subunit. *Muscle Nerve* 2001;24:203–210.

16. Geuder KI, Marx A, Witzemann V, et al. Pathogenetic significance of fetal-type acetylcholine receptors on thymic myoid cells in myasthenia gravis. *Dev Immunol* 1992;2:69–75.

17. Schluep M, Willcox N, Vincent A, Dhoot GK, Newsom-Davis J. Acetylcholine receptors in human thymic myoid cells in situ: an immunohistological study. *Ann Neurol* 1987;22:212–222.

18. Muller-Hermelink HK, Marx A. Thymus. In: Damjanov ILJ, ed. *Anderson's Pathology*. St. Louis, Mosby, 1996, pp. 1218–1243.

19. Kirchner T, Tzartos S, Hoppe F, et al. Pathogenesis of myasthenia gravis. Acetylcholine receptor-related antigenic determinants in tumor-free thymuses and thymic epithelial tumors. *Am J Pathol* 1988;130:268–280.

20. Sempowski GD, Hale LP, Sundy JS, et al. Leukemia inhibitory factor, oncostatin M, IL-6, and stem cell factor mRNA expression in human thymus increases with age and is associated with thymic atrophy. *J Immunol* 2000;164:2180–2187.

21. Muller-Hermelink HK, Marx A. Thymoma. *Curr Opin Oncol* 2000;12:426–433.

22. Sommer N, Willcox N, Harcourt GC, Newsom-Davis J. Myasthenic thymus and thymoma are selectively enriched in acetylcholine receptor-reactive T cells. *Ann Neurol* 1990;28:312–319.

23. Kirchner T, Schalke B, Buchwald J, et al. Well-differentiated thymic carcinoma. An organotypical low-grade carcinoma with relationship to cortical thymoma. *Am J Surg Pathol* 1992;16:1153–1169.

24. Vincent A. Aetiological factors in development of myasthenia gravis. *Adv Neuroimmunol* 1994;4:355–371.

25. Marx A, Schultz A, Wilisch A, et al. Paraneoplastic autoimmunity in thymus tumors. *Dev Immunol* 1998;6:129–140.

26. Nagvekar N, Moody AM, Moss P, et al. A pathogenetic role for the thymoma in myasthenia gravis. Autosensitization of IL-4-producing T cell clones recognizing extracellular acetylcholine receptor epitopes presented by minority class II isotypes. *J Clin Invest* 1998;101:2268–2277.

27. Vincent A. Antibodies to ion channels in paraneoplastic disorders. *Brain Pathol* 1999;9:285–291.

28. Rosai J. Histological typing of tumours of the thymus. In: Sobin L, ed. *WHO International Classification of Tumours*. Berlin, Springer-Verlag, 1999, pp. 1–65.

29. Marx A, Muller-Hermelink HK. From basic immunobiology to the upcoming WHO-classification of tumors of the thymus. The Second Conference on Biological and Clinical Aspects of Thymic Epithelial Tumors and related recent developments [editorial] [In Process Citation]. *Pathol Res Pract* 1999;195:515–533.

30. Parrens M, Labouyrie E, Groppi A, et al. Expression of NGF receptors in normal and pathological human thymus. *J Neuroimmunol* 1998;85:11–21.

31. Zettl A, Ströbel P, Wagner K, et al. Recurrent genetic aberrations in thymoma and thymic carcinoma. *Am J Pathol* 2000;157:257–266.

32. Zhou R, Zettl A, Strobel P, et al. Thymic epithelial tumors can develop along two different pathogenetic pathways. *Am J Pathol* 2001;159:1853–1860.

33. Wekerle H, Ketelsen UP. Intrathymic pathogenesis and dual genetic control of myasthenia gravis. *Lancet* 1977;1:678–680.

34. Weinberg CB, Hall ZW. Antibodies from patients with myasthenia gravis recognize determinants unique to extrajunctional acetylcholine receptors. *Proc Natl Acad Sci USA* 1979;76:504–508.

35. Geuder KI, Marx A, Witzemann V, et al. Genomic organization and lack of transcription of the nicotinic acetylcholine receptor subunit genes in myasthenia gravis-associated thymoma. *Lab Invest* 1992;66:452–458.

36. Kaminski HJ, Kusner LL, Block CH. Expression of acetylcholine receptor isoforms at extraocular muscle endplates [published erratum appears in Invest Ophthalmol Vis Sci 1996;37:6A]. *Invest Ophthalmol Vis Sci* 1996;37:345–351.

37. MacLennan C, Beeson D, Buijs AM, Vincent A, Newsom-Davis J. Acetylcholine receptor expression in human extraocular muscles and their susceptibility to myasthenia gravis [see comments]. *Ann Neurol* 1997;41:423–431.

38. Scadding GK, Vincent A, Newsom-Davis J, Henry K. Acetylcholine receptor antibody synthesis by thymic lymphocytes: correlation with thymic histology. *Neurology* 1981;31:935–943.

39. Nieto IP, Robledo JP, Pajuelo MC, et al. Prognostic factors for myasthenia gravis treated by thymectomy: review of 61 cases [see comments]. *Ann Thorac Surg* 1999;67:1568–1571.

40. Tsuchida M, Yamato Y, Souma T, et al. Efficacy and safety of extended thymectomy for elderly patients with myasthenia gravis [see comments]. *Ann Thorac Surg* 1999;67:1563–1567.

41. Meinl E, Klinkert WE, Wekerle H. The thymus in myasthenia gravis. Changes typical for the human disease are absent in experimental autoimmune myasthenia gravis of the Lewis rat. *Am J Pathol* 1991;139:995–1008.

42. Schonbeck S, Padberg F, Marx A, Hohlfeld R, Wekerle H. Transplantation of myasthenia gravis thymus to SCID mice. *Ann NY Acad Sci* 1993;681:66–73.

43. Spuler S, Marx A, Kirchner T, Hohlfeld R, Wekerle H. Myogenesis in thymic transplants in the severe combined immunodeficient mouse model of myasthenia gravis. Differentiation of thymic myoid cells into striated muscle cells. *Am J Pathol* 1994;145:766–770.

44. Spuler S, Sarropoulos A, Marx A, Hohlfeld R, Wekerle H. Thymoma-associated myasthenia gravis. Transplantation of thymoma and extrathymomal thymic tissue into SCID mice. *Am J Pathol* 1996;148:1359–1365.

45. Baggi F, Nicolle M, Vincent A, et al. Presentation of endogenous acetylcholine receptor epitope by an MHC class II-transfected human muscle cell line to a specific

CD4+ T cell clone from a myasthenia gravis patient. *J Neuroimmunol* 1993;46: 57–65.

46. Melms A, Malcherek G, Gern U, et al. T cells from normal and myasthenic individuals recognize the human acetylcholine receptor: heterogeneity of antigenic sites on the alpha-subunit. *Ann Neurol* 1992;31:311–318.

47. Jermy A, Beeson D, Vincent A. Pathogenic autoimmunity to affinity-purified mouse acetylcholine receptor induced without adjuvant in BALB/c mice. *Eur J Immunol* 1993;23:973–976.

48. Salmon AM, Bruand C, Cardona A, Changeux JP, Berrih-Aknin S. An acetylcholine receptor alpha subunit promoter confers intrathymic expression in transgenic mice. Implications for tolerance of a transgenic self-antigen and for autoreactivity in myasthenia gravis. *J Clin Invest* 1998;101:2340–2350.

49. Melms A, Schalke BC, Kirchner T, et al. Thymus in myasthenia gravis. Isolation of T-lymphocyte lines specific for the nicotinic acetylcholine receptor from thymuses of myasthenic patients. *J Clin Invest* 1988;81:902–908.

50. Hohlfeld R, Wekerle H. The immunopathogenesis of myasthenia gravis. In: Angel AG, ed. *Myasthenia Gravis and Myasthenic Disorders.* Oxford, Oxford University Press, 1999, pp. 87–110.

51. Sims GP, Shiono H, Willcox N, Stott DI. Somatic hypermutation and selection of β cells in thymic germinal centers responding to acetylcholine receptor in myasthenia gravis. *J Immunol* 2001;167:1935–1944.

52. Bornemann A, Kirchner T. An immuno-electron-microscopic study of human thymic B cells. *Cell Tissue Res* 1996;284:481–487.

53. Middleton G, Schoch EM. The prevalence of human thymic lymphoid follicles is lower in suicides. *Virchows Arch* 2000;436:127–130.

54. Compston DA, Vincent A, Newsom-Davis J, Batchelor JR. Clinical, pathological, HLA antigen and immunological evidence for disease heterogeneity in myasthenia gravis. *Brain* 1980;103:579–601.

55. Degli-Esposti MA, Andreas A, Christiansen FT, et al. An approach to the localization of the susceptibility genes for generalized myasthenia gravis by mapping recombinant ancestral haplotypes. *Immunogenetics* 1992;35:355–364.

56. Huang D, Shi FD, Giscombe R, et al. Disruption of the IL-1beta gene diminishes acetylcholine receptor-induced immune responses in a murine model of myasthenia gravis. *Eur J Immunol* 2001;31:225–232.

57. Skeie GO, Pandey JP, Aarli JA, Gilhus NE. TNFA and TNFB polymorphisms in myasthenia gravis. *Arch Neurol* 1999;56:457–461.

58. Huang DR, Pirskanen R, Matell G, Lefvert AK. Tumour necrosis factor-alpha polymorphism and secretion in myasthenia gravis. *J Neuroimmunol* 1999;94:165–171.

59. Franciotta D, Cuccia M, Dondi E, Piccolo G, Cosi V. Polymorphic markers in MHC class II/III region: a study on Italian patients with myasthenia gravis. *J Neurol Sci* 2001;190:11–16.

60. Huang DR, Zhou YH, Xia SQ, et al. Markers in the promoter region of interleukin-10 (IL-10) gene in myasthenia gravis: implications of diverse effects of IL-10 in the pathogenesis of the disease. *J Neuroimmunol* 1999;94:82–87.

61. Garchon HJ, Djabiri F, Viard JP, Gajdos P, Bach JF. Involvement of human muscle acetylcholine receptor alpha-subunit gene (CHRNA) in susceptibility to myasthenia gravis. *Proc Natl Acad Sci USA* 1994;91:4668–4672.

62. Djabiri F, Gajdos P, Eymard B, et al. No evidence for an association of AChR beta-subunit gene (CHRNB1) with myasthenia gravis. *J Neuroimmunol* 1997;78:86–89.
63. Giraud M, Beaurain G, Yamamoto AM, et al. Linkage of HLA to myasthenia gravis and genetic heterogeneity depending on anti-titin antibodies. *Neurology* 2001;57:1555–1560.
64. Onodera J, Nakamura S, Nagano I, et al. Upregulation of Bcl-2 protein in the myasthenic thymus. *Ann Neurol* 1996;39:521–528.
65. Masunaga A, Arai T, Yoshitake T, Itoyama S, Sugawara I. Reduced expression of apoptosis-related antigens in thymuses from patients with myasthenia gravis. *Immunol Lett* 1994;39:169–172.
66. Moulian N, Bidault J, Truffault F, et al. Thymocyte Fas expression is dysregulated in myasthenia gravis patients with anti-acetylcholine receptor antibody. *Blood* 1997;89:3287–3295.
67. Vincent A, Willcox N, Hill M, et al. Determinant spreading and immune responses to acetylcholine receptors in myasthenia gravis. *Immunol Rev* 1998;164:157–168.
68. Aarli JA, Gilhus NE, Matre R. Myasthenia gravis with thymoma is not associated with an increased incidence of non-muscle autoimmune disorders. *Autoimmunity* 1992;11:159–162.
69. Christensen PB, Jensen TS, Tsiropoulos I, et al. Associated autoimmune diseases in myasthenia gravis. A population-based study [see comments]. *Acta Neurol Scand* 1995;91:192–195.
70. Meager A, Vincent A, Newsom-Davis J, Willcox N. Spontaneous neutralising antibodies to interferon-alpha and interleukin-12 in thymoma-associated autoimmune disease [letter]. *Lancet* 1997;350:1596–1597.
71. Mygland A, Aarli JA, Matre R, Gilhus NE. Ryanodine receptor antibodies related to severity of thymoma associated myasthenia gravis. *J Neurol Neurosurg Psychiatry* 1994;57:843–846.
72. Romi F, Skeie GO, Aarli JA, Gilhus NE. The severity of myasthenia gravis correlates with the serum concentration of titin and ryanodine receptor antibodies. *Arch Neurol* 2000;57:1596–1600.
73. Yamamoto AM, Gajdos P, Eymard B, et al. Anti-titin antibodies in myasthenia gravis: tight association with thymoma and heterogeneity of nonthymoma patients. *Arch Neurol* 2001;58:885–890.
74. Fujii Y, Monden Y, Nakahara K, Hashimoto J, Kawashima Y. Antibody to acetylcholine receptor in myasthenia gravis: production by lymphocytes from thymus or thymoma. *Neurology* 1984;34:1182–1186.
75. Newsom-Davis J, Willcox N, Schluep M, et al. Immunological heterogeneity and cellular mechanisms in myasthenia gravis. *Ann NY Acad Sci* 1987;505:12–26.
76. Takeuchi Y, Fujii Y, Okumura M, et al. Accumulation of immature CD3-CD4+CD8-single-positive cells that lack CD69 in epithelial cell tumors of the human thymus. *Cell Immunol* 1995;161:181–187.
77. Nenninger R, Schultz A, Vandekerckhove B, et al. Abnormal T lymphocyte development in myasthenia gravis-associated thymomas. In: Marx A, Müller-Hermelink HK, eds. *Epithelial Tumors of the Thymus. Pathology, Biology, Treatment.* New York, Plenum Press, 1997.
78. Nenninger R, Schultz A, Hoffacker V, et al. Abnormal thymocyte development and generation of autoreactive T cells in mixed and cortical thymomas. *Lab Invest* 1998;78:743–753.

79. Sommer N, Harcourt GC, Willcox N, Beeson D, Newsom-Davis J. Acetylcholine receptor-reactive T lymphocytes from healthy subjects and myasthenia gravis patients. *Neurology* 1991;41:1270–1276.

80. Conti-Fine BM, Navaneetham D, Karachunski PI, et al. T cell recognition of the acetylcholine receptor in myasthenia gravis. *Ann NY Acad Sci* 1998;841:283–308.

81. Schultz A, Hoffacker V, Wilisch A, et al. Neurofilament is an autoantigenic determinant in myasthenia gravis. *Ann Neurol* 1999;46:167–175.

82. Hoffacker V, Schultz A, Tiesinga JJ, et al. Thymomas alter the T-cell subset composition in the blood: a potential mechanism for thymoma-associated autoimmune disease. *Blood* 2000;96:3872–3879.

83. Buckley C, Douek D, Newsom-Davis J, Vincent A, Willcox N. Mature, long-lived CD4+ and CD8+ T cells are generated by the thymoma in myasthenia gravis. *Ann Neurol* 2001;50:64–72.

84. Willcox N, Schluep M, Ritter MA, et al. Myasthenic and nonmyasthenic thymoma. An expansion of a minor cortical epithelial cell subset? *Am J Pathol* 1987;127:447–460.

85. Ströbel P, Hoffacker V, Kalbacher H, Konrad M-HH, Marx A. Evidence for distinct mechanisms in the shaping of the CD4 T-cell repertoire in histologically different myasthenia gravis-associated thymomas. *Dev Immunol* 2001; 8:279–290.

86. Muller-Hermelink HK, Wilisch A, Schultz A, Marx A. Characterization of the human thymic microenvironment: lymphoepithelial interaction in normal thymus and thymoma. *Arch Histol Cytol* 1997;60:9–28.

87. Aarli JA, Skeie GO, Mygland A, Gilhus NE. Muscle striation antibodies in myasthenia gravis. Diagnostic and functional significance. *Ann NY Acad Sci* 1998;841:505–515.

88. Marx A, Kirchner T, Greiner A, et al. Neurofilament epitopes in thymoma and antiaxonal autoantibodies in myasthenia gravis. *Lancet* 1992;339:707–708.

89. Mygland A, Kuwajima G, Mikoshiba K, et al. Thymomas express epitopes shared by the ryanodine receptor. *J Neuroimmunol* 1995;62:79–83.

90. Hara Y, Ueno S, Uemichi T, et al. Neoplastic epithelial cells express alpha-subunit of muscle nicotinic acetylcholine receptor in thymomas from patients with myasthenia gravis. *FEBS Lett* 1991;279:137–140.

91. Skeie GO, Freiburg A, Kolmerer B, et al. Titin transcripts in thymomas. *Ann NY Acad Sci* 1998;841:422–426.

92. Kusner LL, Mygland A, Kaminski HJ. Ryanodine receptor gene expression thymomas. *Muscle Nerve* 1998;21:1299–1303.

93. Marx A, O'Connor R, Geuder KI, et al. Characterization of a protein with an acetylcholine receptor epitope from myasthenia gravis-associated thymomas [see comments]. *Lab Invest* 1990;62:279–286.

94. Siara J, Rudel R, Marx A. Absence of acetylcholine-induced current in epithelial cells from thymus glands and thymomas of myasthenia gravis patients. *Neurology* 1991;41:128–131.

95. Marx A, Osborn M, Tzartos S, et al. A striational muscle antigen and myasthenia gravis-associated thymomas share an acetylcholine-receptor epitope. *Dev Immunol* 1992;2:77–84.

96. Marx A, Wilisch A, Schultz A, et al. Expression of neurofilaments and of a titin epitope in thymic epithelial tumors. Implications for the pathogenesis of myasthenia gravis. *Am J Pathol* 1996;148:1839–1850.

97. Wakkach A, Guyon T, Bruand C, et al. Expression of acetylcholine receptor genes in human thymic epithelial cells: implications for myasthenia gravis. *J Immunol* 1996;157:3752–3760.
98. Wilisch A, Gutsche S, Hoffacker V, et al. Association of acetylcholine receptor alpha-subunit gene expression in mixed thymoma with myasthenia gravis. *Neurology* 1999;52:1460–1466.
99. Klein L, Roettinger B, Kyewski B. Sampling of complementing self-antigen pools by thymic stromal cells maximizes the scope of central T cell tolerance. *Eur J Immunol* 2001;31:2476–2486.
100. Derbinski J, Schulte A, Kyewski B, Klein L. Promiscuous gene expression in medullary thymic epithelial cells mirrors the peripheral self. *Nat Immunol* 2001;2: 1032–1039.
101. Nagvekar N, Jacobson LW, Willcox N, Vincent A. Epitopes expressed in myasthenia gravis (MG) thymomas are not recognized by patients' T cells or autoantibodies. *Clin Exp Immunol* 1998;112:17–20.
102. Fukui Y, Ishimoto T, Utsuyama M, et al. Positive and negative CD4+ thymocyte selection by a single MHC class II/peptide ligand affected by its expression level in the thymus. *Immunity* 1997;6:401–410.
103. Barton GM, Rudensky AY. Requirement for diverse, low-abundance peptides in positive selection of T cells. *Science* 1999;283:67–70.
104. Dongre AR, Kovats S, deRoos P, et al. In vivo MHC class II presentation of cytosolic proteins revealed by rapid automated tandem mass spectrometry and functional analyses. *Eur J Immunol* 2001;31:1485–1494.
105. Wong P, Barton GM, Forbush KA, Rudensky AY. Dynamic tuning of T cell reactivity by self-peptide-major histocompatibility complex ligands. *J Exp Med* 2001; 193:1179–1187.
106. Inoue M, Okumura M, Miyoshi S, et al. Impaired expression of MHC class II molecules in response to interferon-gamma (IFN-gamma) on human thymoma neoplastic epithelial cells. *Clin Exp Immunol* 1999;117:1–7.
107. Kadota Y, Okumura M, Miyoshi S, et al. Altered T cell development in human thymoma is related to impairment of MHC class II transactivator expression induced by interferon-gamma (IFN-gamma). *Clin Exp Immunol* 2000;121:59–68.
108. Ströbel P, Helmreich M, Kalbacher H, Müller-Hermelink HK, Marx A. Evidence for distinct mechanisms in the shaping of the CD4 T cell repertoire in histologically distinct myasthenia gravis-associated thymomas. *Dev Immunol* 2000;8:279–290.
109. Hoffacker V, Schultz A, Tiesinga JJ, et al. Thymomas alter the T-cell subset composition in the blood: a potential mechanism for thymoma-associated autoimmune disease [In Process Citation]. *Blood* 2000;96:3872–3879.
110. Ashton-Rickardt PG, Tonegawa S. A differential-avidity model for T-cell selection. *Immunol Today* 1994;15:362–366.
111. Hogquist KA, Jameson SC, Heath WR, et al. T cell receptor antagonist peptides induce positive selection. *Cell* 1994;76:17–27.
112. Laufer TM, Fan L, Glimcher LH. Self-reactive T cells selected on thymic cortical epithelium are polyclonal and are pathogenic in vivo. *J Immunol* 1999;162:5078–5084.
113. van Meerwijk JP, MacDonald HR. In vivo T-lymphocyte tolerance in the absence of thymic clonal deletion mediated by hematopoietic cells. *Blood* 1999;93:3856–3862.

114. Huang D, Giscombe R, Zhou Y, Pirskanen R, Lefvert AK. Dinucleotide repeat expansion in the CTLA-4 gene leads to T cell hyper-reactivity via the CD28 pathway in myasthenia gravis. *J Neuroimmunol* 2000;105:69–77.
115. Vincent A, Willcox N. The role of T-cells in the initiation of autoantibody responses in thymoma patients. *Pathol Res Pract* 1999;195:535–540.
116. Huang D, Liu L, Noren K, et al. Genetic association of CTLA-4 to myasthenia gravis with thymoma. *J Neuroimmunol* 1998;88:192–198.
117. Machens A, Loliger C, Pichlmeier U, et al. Correlation of thymic pathology with HLA in myasthenia gravis. *Clin Immunol* 1999;91:296–301.
118. Conti-Tronconi BM, McLane KE, Raftery MA, Grando SA, Protti MP. The nicotinic acetylcholine receptor: structure and autoimmune pathology. *Crit Rev Biochem Mol Biol* 1994;29:69–123.
119. Somnier FE. Exacerbation of myasthenia gravis after removal of thymomas [see comments]. *Acta Neurol Scand* 1994;90:56–66.
120. Namba T, Brunner NG, Grob D. Myasthenia gravis in patients with thymoma, with particular reference to onset after thymectomy. *Medicine (Balt)* 1978;57:411–433.
121. Maselli RA, Richman DP, Wollmann RL. Inflammation at the neuromuscular junction in myasthenia gravis. *Neurology* 1991;41:1497–1504.
122. Myking AO, Skeie GO, Varhaug JE, et al. The histomorphology of the thymus in late onset, non-thymoma myasthenia gravis. *Eur J Neurol* 1998;5:401–405.
123. Lubke E, Freiburg A, Skeie GO, et al. Striational autoantibodies in myasthenia gravis patients recognize I-band titin epitopes. *J Neuroimmunol* 1998;81:98–108.
124. Haynes BF, Markert ML, Sempowski GD, Patel DD, Hale LP. The role of the thymus in immune reconstitution in aging, bone marrow transplantation, and HIV-1 infection. *Annu Rev Immunol* 2000;18:529–560.
125. Fagnoni FF, Vescovini R, Passeri G, et al. Shortage of circulating naive CD8(+) T cells provides new insights on immunodeficiency in aging. *Blood* 2000;95:2860–2868.
126. Aarli JA, Stefansson K, Marton LS, Wollmann RL. Patients with myasthenia gravis and thymoma have in their sera IgG autoantibodies against titin. *Clin Exp Immunol* 1990;82:284–288.
127. Romi F, Skeie GO, Aarli JA, Gilhus NE. Muscle autoantibodies in subgroups of myasthenia gravis patients. *J Neurol* 2000;247:369–375.
128. Gautel M, Lakey A, Barlow DP, et al. Titin antibodies in myasthenia gravis: identification of a major immunogenic region of titin. *Neurology* 1993;43:1581–1585.
129. Mygland A, Tysnes OB, Matre R, et al. Ryanodine receptor autoantibodies in myasthenia gravis patients with a thymoma. *Ann Neurol* 1992;32:589–591.
130. Mygland A, Tysnes OB, Aarli JA, Flood PR, Gilhus NE. Myasthenia gravis patients with a thymoma have antibodies against a high molecular weight protein in sarcoplasmic reticulum. *J Neuroimmunol* 1992;37:1–7.
131. Vernino S, Auger RG, Emslie-Smith AM, Harper CM, Lennon VA. Myasthenia, thymoma, presynaptic antibodies, and a continuum of neuromuscular hyperexcitability. *Neurology* 1999;53:1233–1239.
132. Pande R, Leis AA. Myasthenia gravis, thymoma, intestinal pseudo-obstruction, and neuronal nicotinic acetylcholine receptor antibody. *Muscle Nerve* 1999;22:1600–1602.

# 7

# Electrodiagnosis
# of Neuromuscular Junction Disorders

## Bashar Katirji

## INTRODUCTION

The electrodiagnostic (EDX) examination in patients with suspected neuromuscular junction (NMJ) disorders requires a good comprehension of the physiology and pathophysiology of neuromuscular transmission. The EDX studies that are useful in the evaluation of such patients include: 1) motor nerve conduction studies (NCSs); 2) conventional needle electromyography (EMG); 3) repetitive nerve stimulation (RNS); and 4) single-fiber EMG. This chapter reviews, in brief, basic knowledge of neuromuscular transmission as it relates to the EDX studies and discusses in detail the EDX studies and findings in various NMJ disorders.

## BASIC CONCEPTS OF NEUROMUSCULAR TRANSMISSION

Performing EDX studies in NMJ disorders depends on the understanding of a few important concepts inherent to neuromuscular transmission. These physiologic facts dictate the type and frequency of RNS, as well as the type of single-fiber EMG study utilized in the accurate diagnosis of NMJ disorders. The physiology of neuromuscular transmission is discussed in detail in other chapters and is only addressed briefly here (1–4).

### Quantum

A quantum is the amount of acetylcholine (ACh) packaged in a single vesicle, which is approximately 5000–10,000 ACh molecules. Each quantum (vesicle) released results in a 1-mV change in postsynaptic membrane potential. This occurs spontaneously during rest and forms the basis of miniature end plate potential (MEPP).

From: *Current Clinical Neurology: Myasthenia Gravis and Related Disorders*
Edited by: H. J. Kaminski © Humana Press Inc., Totowa, NJ

The number of quanta released after a nerve action potential depends on the number of quanta in the *immediately available (primary) store* and the probability of release, i.e., $m = p \times n$, where $m$ = the number of quanta released during each stimulation, $p$ = the probability of release (effectively proportional to the concentration of calcium and typically about 0.2, or 20%), and $n$ = the number of quanta in the immediately available store. Under normal conditions, a single nerve action potential triggers the release of 50–300 vesicles (quanta), with an average of about 60 quanta (60 vesicles).

## End Plate Potential

The end plate potential (EPP) is the potential generated at the postsynaptic membrane following a nerve action potential and neuromuscular transmission. Since each vesicle (quanta) released causes a 1-mV change in the postsynaptic membrane potential, this release results in about a 60 mV change in the amplitude of the membrane potential.

## Safety Factor

Under normal conditions, the number of quanta (vesicles) released at the NMJ by the presynaptic terminal (about 60 vesicles) far exceeds the postsynaptic membrane potential change required to reach the *threshold* needed to generate a postsynaptic muscle action potential (7–20 mV). In normal NMJ, the safety factor is about 4. The safety factor results in an EPP that always reaches threshold, results in an all-or-none muscle fiber action potential (MFAP), and prevents neuromuscular transmission failure despite repetitive action potentials. In addition to quantal release, several other factors contribute to the safety factor and EPP including ACh receptor conduction properties, ACh receptor density, and ACh-esterase activity, synaptic architecture, and sodium channel density at the NMJ.

## Calcium Influx into the Terminal Axon

Following depolarization of the presynaptic terminal, voltage-gated calcium channels (VGCCs) open, leading to calcium influx. Through a calcium-dependent intracellular cascade, vesicles are docked at active release sites (called active zones) and release ACh molecules. Calcium then diffuses slowly away from the vesicle release site in 100–200 ms. The rate at which motor nerves are repetitively stimulated in the electrodiagnostic laboratory dictates whether calcium accumulation plays a role in enhancing the release of ACh. At a slow rate of RNS (i.e., a stimulus every 200 ms or more, or a stimulation rate of <5 Hz), calcium's role in ACh release is not enhanced, and subsequent nerve action potentials reach the nerve terminal long after calcium has dispersed. In contrast, with rapid RNS (i.e., a stimulus every 100 msec or less, or stimulation rate of >10 Hz), calcium influx is greatly enhanced and the probability of release of ACh quanta increases.

In addition to the immediately available store of ACh-containing synaptic vesicles located beneath the presynaptic nerve terminal membrane, *a secondary (or mobilization) store* starts to replenish the immediately available store after 1–2 s of repetitive nerve action potentials. A large *tertiary (or reserve) store* is also available in the axon and cell body.

## Compound Muscle Action Potential

The *compound muscle action potential (CMAP)* is the summation of all MFAPs generated in a muscle following supramaximal stimulation of all motor axons while recording via surface electrode placed over the belly of a muscle.

## ELECTRODIAGNOSTIC TESTS IN NEUROMUSCULAR JUNCTION DISORDERS

### Routine Motor Nerve Conduction Studies

Motor NCSs are helpful in the evaluation of all disorders affecting the motor unit. In NMJ disorders, CMAP amplitude is the most useful parameter analyzed since motor distal latencies and conduction velocities (as well F-waves, H-reflexes, and sensory NCSs) are always normal. The CMAPs are usually normal in postsynaptic disorders [such as myasthenia gravis (MG)] owing to the presence of the safety factor: after a single supramaximal stimulus, and despite ACh receptor blockade, EPPs achieve thresholds and generate MFAPs in all muscle fibers, resulting in normal CMAP. Occasionally, as in a myasthenic crisis, the CMAPs may be borderline or slightly diminished owing to severe postsynaptic neuromuscular blockade. This situation is usually encountered when recording proximal muscles, but since routine motor NCSs are performed recoding distal limb muscles, CMAP amplitudes usually remain normal even in severe MG. In presynaptic disorders [such as Lambert-Eaton syndrome (LES)], the CMAP amplitudes on routine NCSs are often low since many EPPs do not reach threshold, and many muscle fibers do not fire.

### Conventional Needle Electromyography

The needle EMG is usually normal in NMJ disorders. However, nonspecific changes, more commonly encountered in myopathies or neurogenic disorders, may occasionally be associated with NMJ disorders, particularly when they are chronic and severe.

*Moment-to-Moment Variation of Motor Unit Action Potentials*

In healthy subjects, individual motor unit action potential (MUAP) amplitude, duration, and phases are stable, with little, if any, variation. However, in NMJ disorders such as MG, individual MUAP amplitude and morphology may vary significantly during activation due to intermittent endplate blockade, slowing, or both. During needle EMG recording, moment-to-moment variation should be distinguished from MUAP overlap. This can be achieved by always recording from a single MUAP at a time.

*Short-Duration, Low-Amplitude, and Polyphasic MUAPs*

These MUAPs occur primarily in proximal muscles and are similar in morphology to those seen in myopathies. In NMJ disorders, "myopathic" MUAPs are caused by physiologic blocking and slowing of neuromuscular transmission at endplates during voluntary activation. This leads to exclusion of MFAPs from the MUAP (hence the short duration and low amplitude) and asynchrony of neuromuscular transmission of muscle fibers (hence the polyphasia).

*Fibrillation Potentials*

Fibrillation potentials are rarely encountered in NMJ disorders *(5,6)*. They are usually inconspicuous and present mostly in proximal muscles. The mechanism of fibrillation potentials in NMJ disorders is not clear but may be related to chronic neuromuscular transmission blockade or loss of endplates, resulting in "effective" denervation of individual muscle fibers. Since fibrillation potentials are rare in NMJ disorders, their presence should always raise the suspicion of an alternate diagnosis or associated illness.

### Repetitive Nerve Stimulation

*Techniques*

RNSs often follows routine motor NCSs. Electromyographers and technologists should master the various motor NCS and RNS techniques to avoid false-positive and false-negative results. Certain prerequisites are essential for performing reliable RNSs, as follows:

1. Limb temperature should be maintained at around 33°C since neuromuscular transmission is enhanced in a cool limb, which may mask a CMAP decrement.
2. Patients on ACh-esterase inhibitors (such as pyridostigmine) should be asked to withhold their medication for 12–24 h before RNS, if not contraindicated medically.
3. The limb tested should be immobilized as best as possible. Particular attention should be given to the stimulation and recording sites. Movement at either sites

may result in CMAP amplitude decay or increment, potentially leading to a false diagnosis of a NMJ disorder.

4. Although a supramaximal stimulation (i.e., 10–20% above the intensity level needed for a maximal response) is needed to obtain a CMAP, unnecessary high-intensity or long-duration stimuli should be avoided to prevent movement artifact and excessive pain.
5. The stimulus rate and number of stimuli applied during RNS depend on the clinical problem and the working diagnosis.
   a. Slow RNS is usually done at a rate 2–3 Hz; this rate is low enough to prevent calcium accumulation but high enough to deplete the quanta in the immediately available stores before the secondary (mobilization) stores start to replenish it. A total of three to five stimuli is adequate since the maximal decrease in ACh release occurs after the first four stimuli. There is nothing to be gained in exceeding 9–10 stimuli.
   b. Rapid RNS is done with a frequency of 20–50 Hz to ensure accumulation of calcium in the presynaptic terminal. However, a brief (10-s) period of maximal isometric voluntary exercise has the same effect as rapid RNS at 20–50 Hz. This is much less painful than rapid RNS and hence may be done on multiple motor nerves. Brief exercise can substitute for rapid RNS in cooperative subjects; however, rapid RNS is necessary in patients who cannot exercise (e.g., infants, comatose patients, or patients with severe weakness).
6. The choice of nerve to be stimulated and muscle to be recorded from depends on the patient's manifestations. Useful nerves for RNS are the median and ulnar nerves, recording the abductor pollicis brevis and abductor digiti minimi, respectively. Since the upper limb is easily immobilized, these RNSs are well tolerated and accompanied by minimal movement artifact. However, since distal muscles may be spared in some NMJ disorders (such as MG), recording from a proximal muscle is often necessary. Slow RNS of the spinal accessory nerve is the most common study of a proximal nerve. It is relatively well tolerated, less painful, and subject to less movement artifact compared with RNS of other proximal nerves such as the musculocutaneous or axillary nerves, recording the biceps or deltoid muscles, respectively. Finally, facial slow RNS is indicated in patients with ocular or facial weakness when MG is suspected and other RNSs are normal or equivocal. However, the facial CMAP is low in amplitude and often plagued by large stimulation artifacts. This renders measurement of decrement difficult and subject to error.

## Findings

*Slow RNSs* do not abolish any MFAPs in healthy subjects. Although the second to fifth EPPs fall in amplitude owing to the relative decrease in ACh release, the EPPs remain above threshold (owing to the normal safety factor) and ensure generation of MFAPs with each stimulation (**Fig. 1A**). In addition, the secondary store begins to replace the depleted quanta after the first

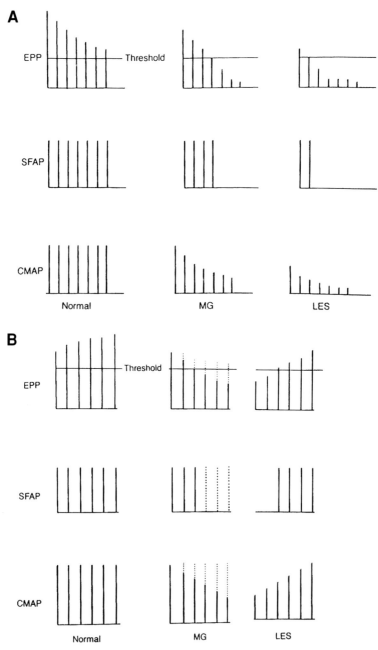

**Fig. 1.** Effects of slow repetitive nerve stimulation (**A**) and rapid repetitive nerve stimulation (**B**) on EPP, single fiber action potential (SFAP), and CMAP in normal subjects, and in patients with MG and LES (marked ELS). (Reproduced with permission from Oh S. *Clinical Electromyography. Neuromuscular Transmission Studies*, Baltimore, Williams & Wilkins, 1988.)

few seconds, with a subsequent rise in the EPP. Thus, with slow RNS, all muscle fibers generate MFAPs, and the CMAP does not change. In postsynaptic NMJ disorders (such as MG), the safety factor is reduced since there are fewer ACh receptors available for binding to ACh. Hence, the baseline EPP is reduced but is usually still above threshold. Slow RNS results in some EPPs falling below threshold at many endplates, and MFAPs will not be generated. The decline in the number of MFAPs is reflected by a decrement of the CMAP amplitude *(7,8)*. In presynaptic disorders (such as LES), the baseline EPP is low, with many endplates often not reaching threshold, and many muscle fibers do not fire. This results in low baseline CMAP. Slow RNS causes a CMAP decrement, owing to further decline of ACh release with the subsequent stimuli, resulting in further loss of many MFAPs *(9,10)*.

*Rapid RNS* in healthy subjects increases EPP amplitude but has no ultimate effect on MFAPs since all EPPs are and remain above threshold (**Fig. 1B**). In patients with a presynaptic disorder (such as LES), the baseline CMAP is low in amplitude since many muscle fibers do not reach threshold owing to inadequate release of quanta after a single stimulus. However, calcium influx is greatly enhanced with rapid RNS, resulting in larger releases of quanta and larger EPPs. This leads to increasingly more muscle fibers reaching the threshold required for the generation of MFAPs. Thus, more MFAPs are generated and hence the increment of the CMAP *(9–11)*. In patients with a post-synaptic disorder, the depleted stores are compensated for by the calcium influx induced by rapid RNS, usually resulting in no change of CMAP. In severe postsynaptic defect (such as during myasthenic crisis), the increased quantal release cannot compensate for the marked NMJ blockade, resulting in a drop in EPP amplitude. Hence, fewer MFAPs are generated, resulting in CMAP decrement.

## Measurements

After establishing a supramaximal CMAP, slow RNS is usually performed by applying three to five stimuli to a mixed or motor nerve at a rate of 2–3 Hz. Calculation of the decrement with slow RNS is accomplished by comparing the baseline (first) CMAP amplitude with the lowest CMAP amplitude (usually the third or fourth). In NMJ disorders, the CMAP decrement generally plateaus or begins to improve by the fifth or sixth response, owing to the mobilization store resupplying the immediately available store (**Fig. 2**). The CMAP decrement is expressed as a percentage and is calculated as follows:

$$\% \; decrement = \frac{amplitude \; (1st \; response) - amplitude \; (3rd/4th \; response)}{amplitude \; (1st \; response)} \times 100$$

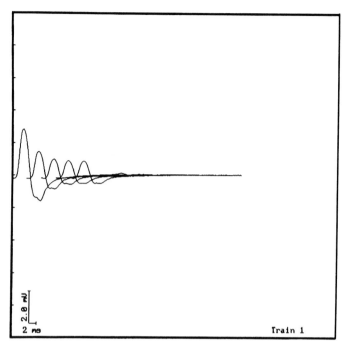

**Fig. 2.** Slow repetitive nerve stimulation (3 Hz) of the median nerve (recording thenar muscles) in a patient with myasthenic crisis. The largest decrement is between the first and the second CMAPs (45%), and the maximal decrement is between the first and third CMAP (65%). Note that the CMAP amplitude plateaus after the third response and that the baseline (first) CMAP amplitude is slightly diminished during myasthenic crisis (see text).

Stimulation at rest should be repeated after an interval of 1–2 min to confirm a normal or abnormal response. A decrement of more than 10% is considered abnormal and eliminates false positives. A decrement less than 10% is equivocal and not diagnostic. If there is a reproducible decrement at rest (≥10%), slow RNS should be repeated after the patient exercises for 10 s to demonstrate repair of the decrement (*postexercise facilitation*). If there is no or equivocal decrement (≥10%) with slow RNS at rest, the patient should perform maximal voluntary exercise for 1 min (exercise for 30 s, rest for 5 s, and exercise for another 30 s). Immediately after exercise, slow RNS is repeated at 1, 2, 3, 4, and 5 min later. Since the amount of ACh released with each stimulus is at its minimum 2–5 min after exercise, slow RNS after exercise provides a high chance of detecting a defect in NMJ by demonstrating a worsening CMAP decrement (*postexercise exhaustion*).

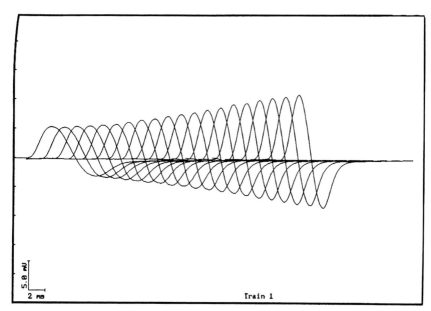

**Fig. 3.** Rapid repetitive nerve stimulation (30 Hz) of the median nerve (recording thenar muscles) in an infant with botulism. There is a 110% increment of CMAP amplitude between the baseline (first) and last (20th) responses.

Rapid RNS is most useful in patients with suspected presynaptic NMJ disorders such as LES or botulism. The optimal frequency is 20–50 Hz for 2–10 s (**Fig. 3**). A typical rapid RNS applies 200 stimuli at a rate of 50 Hz (i.e., 50 Hz for 4 s). Calculation of CMAP increment after rapid RNS is as follows:

$$\% \; increment = \frac{amplitude \; (highest \; response) - amplitude \; (1st \; response)}{amplitude \; (1st \; response)} \times 100$$

A CMAP increment of more than 50–100% is considered abnormal. A modest increment of 25–40% may occur in normal individuals, probably caused by increased synchrony of MFAPs following tetanic stimulation (*physiologic posttetanic facilitation or pseudofacilitation*) *(3,4)*. Brief (10-s) periods of maximal voluntary isometric exercise have the same effect as rapid RNS, are much less painful, and are a good substitute in cooperative subjects *(11)*: a single supramaximal stimulus is applied to generate a baseline CMAP, and then the patient performs a 10-s maximal isometric voluntary contraction, which is followed by another stimulus that produces a postexercise CMAP. Calculation of CMAP increment after a brief (10 s) voluntary contraction is similar to the calculation of the increment following rapid RNS, as follows:

$$\% \text{ increment} = \frac{\text{amplitude of postexercise response} - \text{amplitude of preexercise response}}{\text{amplitude of preexercise response}} \times 100$$

## Single-Fiber EMG

Single-fiber EMG (SFEMG) is the selective recording of a small number (usually two or three) of MFAPs innervated by a single motor unit. SFEMG recording requires special expertise and understanding of the microenvironment of motor unit physiology. Although the examination may be applied to many neuromuscular disorders, SFEMG jitter study is most useful in the diagnosis of NMJ disorders, particularly MG *(12–14)*.

### Techniques

SFEMG jitter study has specific requirements, which are essential for the completion and accurate interpretation of data *(3,12)*:

1. SFEMG is performed by inserting a single-fiber concentric needle into a muscle. This electrode has a small recording surface (25 µm), which restricts the number of recordable MFAPs and results in an effective recording area of 300 µm$^3$, compared with a concentric needle electrode that records from approximately 1 cm$^3$ (**Fig. 4**).
2. A 500-Hz low-frequency filter attenuates signals from distant fibers (>500 µm from the electrode). Filter settings should be set at 500 Hz for the high-pass filter and 10–20 kHz for the low-pass filter.
3. Selected single MFAPs should have a rise time of 300 µs and a preferable peak-to-peak amplitude of 200 µV or more.
4. An amplitude threshold trigger and delay line are needed to allow recording from a single MFAP by triggering on it on a screen with a delay line capability.
5. Computerized equipment assists in calculating individual and mean interpotential intervals (IPIs) and jitters (see below).

*Voluntary (recruitment) SFEMG* is a common method for recording MFAPs in which the patient activates and maintains the firing rate of the motor unit. This technique is not possible if the patient cannot cooperate (e.g., a child or individual with dementia or encephalopathy, or in coma, or with severe weakness) and is difficult if the patient is unable to maintain a constant firing rate (e.g., individuals with tremor, dystonia, or spasticity). The small recording area of an SFEMG needle only registers signals from muscle fibers in its immediate vicinity, usually 5–7 fibers at any time. Given the normal mosaic distribution of muscle fibers within motor units, these fibers may be innervated by up to 5–7 different motor units. By using an amplitude threshold to trigger the oscilloscope trace on the closest MFAP (the action potential with

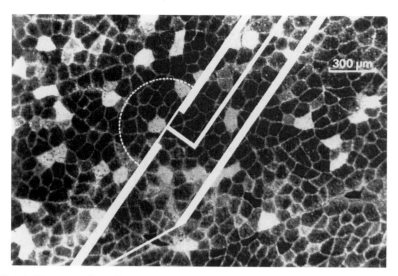

**Fig. 4.** Cross-section of a muscle stained for glycogen after stimulating an isolated motor axon to show the muscle fiber distribution of one motor unit. (The fibers of the motor unit become depleted of glycogen and therefore appear pale.) A single-fiber EMG electrode is superimposed to show the uptake area. The strategy of recording jitter is to position the electrode (as shown) in order to record from two muscle fibers belonging to the same motor unit. (Reproduced with permission from Stålberg E, Trontelj JV. *Single Fiber Electromyography. Studies in Healthy and Diseased Muscle*, 2nd ed. New York, Raven Press, 1994.)

the sharpest rise time and the greatest amplitude), MFAPs from other motor units are excluded from the oscilloscope screen. With minimal voluntary activation, the needle is positioned until two muscle potentials (a pair) from a single motor unit are recognized (**Fig. 4**). When a muscle fiber pair is identified, one fiber triggers the oscilloscope (triggering potential) and the second precedes or follows the first (slave potential). By recording multiple consecutive firings of these two muscle fiber pairs (usually about 50–100 consecutive discharges), one may determine the consecutive IPIs and calculate the difference between consecutive IPIs (**Fig. 5**). Comparison of consecutive IPIs illustrates the slight variation in transmission at the NMJ, termed the *neuromuscular jitter*. Jitter is most accurately determined by calculating a mean consecutive difference (MCD; see Measurements, below). Although jitter analysis may be obtained from any skeletal muscle, the most common muscles examined by voluntary SFEMG are the extensor digitorum communis, frontalis, and orbicularis oculi. These muscles are ideal because of their frequent involvement

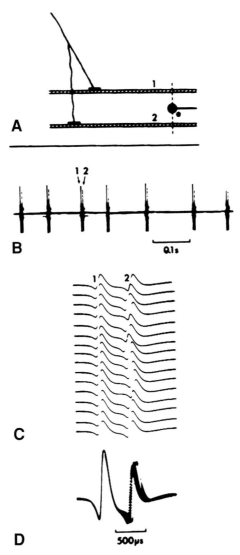

**Fig. 5.** Principle of voluntary single fiber jitter recording. (**A**) The single-fiber EMG electrode is positioned by the electromyographer until it is possible to record from muscle fiber pair (1 and 2) innervated by the same motor axon (see also **Fig. 4**). (**B**) Muscle fiber action potentials firing at a low degree of voluntary activation. (**C**) As in B, but with a faster sweep speed, a sweep triggered by the first potential (the triggering potential), and showing successive discharges of the pair in a raster mode. (**D**) As in C, but shown in a superimposed mode illustrating the variability in the inter-potential intervals (IPIs), which reflect the neuromuscular jitter. (Reproduced with permission from Stålberg E, Trontelj JV. *Single Fiber Electromyography. Studies in Healthy and Diseased Muscle*, 2nd ed. New York, Raven Press, 1994.)

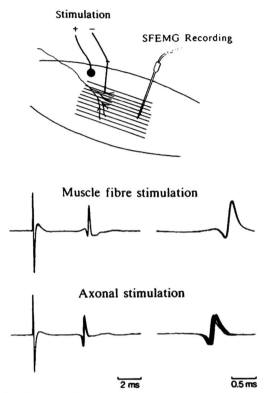

**Fig. 6.** Principle of stimulation single-fiber jitter recording. A monopolar needle stimulating cathode is inserted into the muscle near the motor point; the anode is a surface electrode. The lower tracing discloses normal jitter with axonal stimulation, and the upper tracing discloses a very low jitter (<4 μs) resulting from direct muscle stimulation. (Reproduced with permission from Stålberg E, Trontelj JV. *Single Fiber Electromyography. Studies in Healthy and Diseased Muscle*, 2nd ed. New York, Raven Press, 1994.)

in NMJ disorders and the ability of most patients to control and sustain their voluntary activity to a minimum as required for the test.

*Stimulation SFEMG* is an alternative method of motor unit activation. It has the advantage of not requiring patient participation and may thus be performed on children or uncooperative or comatose patients. It is performed by inserting another monopolar needle electrode near the intramuscular nerve twigs and stimulating at a low current and constant rate. Then the SFEMG is moved slightly until one or more MFAPs are recorded (**Fig. 6**). This technique is slightly more demanding for the electromyographer, who has to manipulate two electrodes, a stimulating and a recording electrode. The IPI is calculated between a stimulus artifact and a single potential generated by stimulating a motor unit near the endplate zone. In contrast to voluntary SFEMG, in which jitter is calculated as the variation in IPIs between two MFAPs (since one potential is time-locked by the trigger, all the variation of both endplates is expressed by the jitter of the slave potential), the IPI in stimulated SFEMG is measured as the latency between the stimulation and the single MFAP (i.e., only one endplate is involved). Hence, stimulation SFEMG jitter values are smaller than their voluntary counterparts. Another advantage of the stimulation technique is that the rate of stimulation can be adjusted from a slow rate (2–3 Hz) to a rapid rate (20–50 Hz). This is helpful in differentiating presynaptic from postsynaptic disorders since the jitter improves significantly with RNS in LES, whereas it does not change or worsens in MG (see below) *(15,16)*.

*Findings*

*Neuromuscular jitter* is defined as the random variability of the time interval between two MFAPs innervated by the same motor unit. In normal subjects, there is a slight variability in the amount of ACh released at the synaptic junction from one moment to another. Although a nerve action potential results in a muscle action potential at all times, the rise of endplate potential is variable, resulting in a small variation of the muscle pair's IPI. *Neuromuscular blocking* is defined as the failure of transmission of one of the potentials. Blocking represents the most extreme abnormality of the jitter.

Jitter analysis is highly sensitive but not specific. It is frequently abnormal in MG and other NMJ disorders, but it may also be abnormal in a variety of neuromuscular disorders including neuropathies, myopathies, and anterior horn cell disorder. Thus a diagnosis of MG by jitter analysis has to be considered in the context of the patient's clinical manifestations, nerve conduction studies, and needle EMG findings.

*Measurements*

The jitter is the MCD of all IPIs recorded of the muscle pair *(12,17)*. It is calculated as follows:

$$MCD = \frac{(IPI1 - IPI2) + (IPI2 - IPI3) + \ldots + (IPIN1 - IPIN)}{N - 1}$$

Where IPI1 is the interpotential interval of the first discharge, IPI 2 of the second discharge, and so on, and *N* is the number of discharges recorded. After analyzing 10–20 muscle fiber pairs, a mean jitter (MCD) is reported.

Normal values for jitter differ between muscles and tend to increase with age (**Table 1**) *(18,19)*. As jitter values obtained by stimulation SFEMG are calculated on the basis of one endplate, the normal values are lower than

**Table 1**
**Reference Values for Jitter Measurements During Voluntary Muscle Activation[a]**

| Muscle | Age (yr) | | | | | | | | |
|---|---|---|---|---|---|---|---|---|---|
| | 10 | 20 | 30 | 40 | 50 | 60 | 70 | 80 | 90 |
| Frontalis | 33.6/49.7 | 33.9/50.1 | 34.4/51.3 | 35.5/53.5 | 37.3/57.5 | 40.0/63.9 | 43.8/74.1 | | |
| Orbicularis oculi | 39.8/54.6 | 39.8/54.7 | 40.0/54.7 | 40.4/54.8 | 40.9/55.0 | 41.8/55.3 | 43.0/55.8 | | |
| Orbicularis oris | 34.7/52.5 | 34.7/52.7 | 34.9/53.2 | 35.3/54.1 | 36.0/55.7 | 37.0/58.2 | 38.3/61.8 | 40.2/67.0 | 42.5/74.2 |
| Tongue | 32.8/48.6 | 33.0/49.0 | 33.6/50.2 | 34.8/52.5 | 36.8/56.3 | 39.8/62.0 | 44.0/70.0 | | |
| Sternocleidomastoid | 29.1/45.4 | 29.3/45.8 | 29.8/46.8 | 30.8/48.8 | 32.5/52.4 | 34.9/58.2 | 38.4/62.3 | | |
| Deltoid | 32.9/44.4 | 32.9/44.5 | 32.9/44.5 | 32.9/44.6 | 33.0/44.8 | 33.0/45.1 | 33.1/45.6 | 33.2/46.1 | 33.3/46.9 |
| Biceps | 29.5/45.2 | 29.6/45.2 | 29.6/45.4 | 29.8/45.7 | 30.1/46.2 | 30.5/46.9 | 31.0/48.0 | | |
| Extensor digitorum communis | 34.9/50.0 | 34.9/50.1 | 35.1/50.5 | 35.4/51.3 | 35.9/52.5 | 36.6/54.4 | 37.7/57.2 | 39.1/61.1 | 40.9/66.5 |
| Abductor digiti minimi | 44.4/63.5 | 44.7/64.0 | 45.2/65.5 | 46.4/68.6 | 48.2/73.9 | 51.0/82.7 | 54.8/96.6 | | |
| Quadriceps | 35.9/47.9 | 36.0/48.0 | 36.5/48.2 | 37.5/48.5 | 39.0/49.1 | 41.3/50.0 | 44.6/51.2 | | |
| Tibialis anterior | 49.4/80.0 | 49.3/79.8 | 49.2/79.3 | 48.9/78.3 | 48.5/76.8 | 47.9/74.5 | 47.0/71.4 | 45.8/67.5 | 44.3/62.9 |

[a]Data are in µs: 95% confidence limits for upper limit of mean jitter/95% confidence limits for jitter values of individual fiber pairs (Adapted from ref. *18*.)

163

those obtained by voluntary activation. To calculate the normal stimulation jitter value, it is recommended that the reference data for voluntary activation be multiplied by 0.80. Blocking is measured as the percentage of discharges of a motor unit in which a single fiber potential does not fire. For example, in 100 discharges of the pair, if a single potential is missing 30 times, the blocking is 30%. In general, blocking occurs when the jitter values are significantly abnormal.

The results of SFEMG jitter study are expressed by 1) the mean jitter of all potential pairs; 2) the percentage of pairs with blocking; and 3) the percentage of pairs with normal jitter *(3,12,13)*. The jitter is considered abnormal when one or more of the following criteria are met (for individuals above than 60 year of age, the first criteria is not used):

1. Mean jitter value exceeds the normal limit.
2. More than 10% of pairs have jitter greater than the upper limit of normal.
3. Blocking is frequently seen in most fiber pairs in a muscle.

## FINDINGS IN NEUROMUSCULAR JUNCTION DISORDERS

### Myasthenia Gravis

Slow RNS is an essential part of the EDX study of patients with suspected MG. This study is particularly useful in patients with seronegative MG or in patients with negative or equivocal edrophonium (Tensilon®) test or neurologic findings. The EDX study of patients with suspected MG should be tailored to the patient's symptomatology.

#### Baseline Compound Muscle Action Potentials

Routine motor NCSs, including CMAP amplitudes, are normal in MG. A single supramaximal stimulus to a motor nerve results in ACh release and a postsynaptic EPP, which reaches threshold despite ACh receptor blockade. Hence, MFAPs are generated in all fibers, resulting in a normal CMAP. Occasionally, as in the midst of a myasthenic crisis, the CMAPs may be borderline or sightly diminished owing to severe postsynaptic neuromuscular blockade (**Fig. 2**). Also, in patients taking large quantities of cholinesterase inhibitors, such as pyridostigmine, there may be a tendency to record multiple CMAPs after a single stimulus applied to the nerve.

#### Slow Repetitive Nerve Stimulation

Slow RNS results in a decrease in quantal release owing to the depletion of the immediate ACh stores. This causes progressive loss of MFAPs since many EPPs do not reach threshold. The end result is a decremental CMAP on slow RNS. The greatest decrease in CMAP amplitude occurs between the first and the second responses, but the decrement continues to the third or fourth responses *(2–4,7,8)*. Often, after the fifth or sixth stimulus, the secondary stores are mobilized, and no further loss of MFAP occurs (**Fig. 2**). This results in stabilization, or sometimes slight improvement of the CMAP after the fifth or sixth stimulus, giving the characteristic U-shaped decrement. A CMAP decrement of >10% is abnormal and eliminates false positives. This should be reproducible and show the typical decrement described above (maximal at 3–5 CMAP, with plateau after 5–6 CMAPs).

The diagnostic yield of slow RNS in MG is increased by:

1. Recording from clinically weakened muscles. This often means recording from a proximal muscle (such as the trapezius) in generalized MG, or from a facial muscle (such as orbicularis oris or nasalis) in ocular MG (**Fig. 7**). This strategy increases the diagnostic sensitivity of slow RNS in the diagnosis of MG *(20)*.
2. Obtaining slow RNS after exercise, looking for postexercise exhaustion. After performing slow RNS at rest, patients are asked to exercise the tested muscle for 1 min. Then slow RNS is repeated every 30–60 s for 4–5 min. Postexercise exhaustion usually lasts for 4–6 min and is particularly useful in patients with suspected MG and equivocal (<10%) CMAP decrement at rest.
3. Warming the extremity studied (hand skin temperature should be >32°C) decreases false-negative results since cooling improves neuromuscular transmission and can mask the decrement.

## Rapid Repetitive Nerve Stimulation

Rapid RNS is not useful in the diagnosis of MG. It should be considered when a presynaptic NMJ disorder (such as LES or botulism) is suspected and needs to be excluded. However, CMAP evaluation after brief (10-s) exercise is often sufficient in these situations and eliminates the severe pain induced by rapid RNS. With rapid RNS (or following brief exercise), the depleted vesicle stores that result in the decremental response observed in MG are usually compensated by the accumulation of calcium, resulting in no change in CMAP amplitude. In severe myasthenics, rapid RNS may cause a decrement when the increased ACh release cannot compensate for the marked postsynaptic neuromuscular blockade. This is in contrast to the CMAP increment seen in patients with a presynaptic NMJ disorder such as LES or botulism (see below).

## Single-Fiber EMG

Evaluation of neuromuscular transmission in patients with suspected MG is the most common indication for performing SFEMG. Commonly tested muscles in patients with suspected MG are the extensor digitorum communis and orbicularis oculi and frontalis. The latter two are particularly helpful in evaluation of ocular myasthenia.

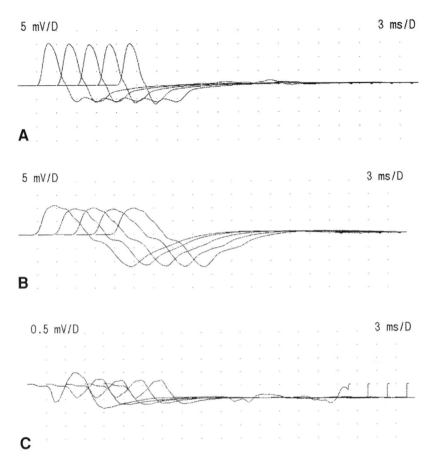

**Fig. 7.** Slow repetitive stimulation in a 35-year-old man with binocular diplopia
and a history of ptosis, revealing (**A**) no decrement in simulating the median nerve
(recording thenar muscles), (**B**) mild and equivocal decrement (10%) in stimulating
the spinal accessory nerve (recording upper trapezius muscle), and (**C**) significant
decrement (40%) in simulating the facial nerve (recording orbicularis oculi muscle).

In patients with MG, abnormal jitter values are common (**Fig. 8**), frequently accompanied by neuromuscular blocking. This reflects the failure
of one of the muscle fibers to transmit an action potential owing to the failure of EPP to reach threshold. SFEMG is extremely sensitive in detecting
MG; a normal SFEMG jitter study in a weak muscle virtually excludes the
diagnosis of MG. The published diagnostic sensitivity ranges from 90 to
99% (**Fig. 9**) *(12–14,19,21)*. This makes SFEMG the most sensitive diagnostic study in MG *(20)*. In contrast, abnormal jitter is nonspecific, since this

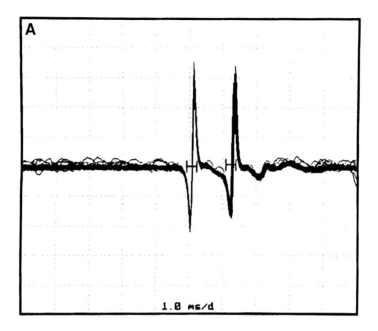

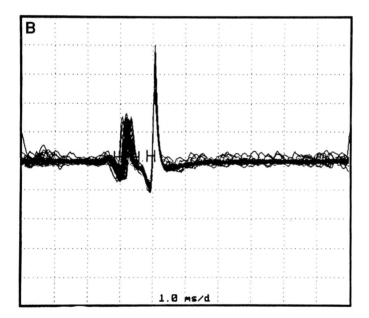

**Fig. 8.** Neuromuscular jitter recordings in the frontalis muscle with voluntary activation in a 22-year-old patient with ptosis (shown in a superimposed mode; also see **Fig. 5**). (**A**) Normal jitter [mean consecutive discharge (MCD) = 18.5 µs]. (**B**) Abnormal jitter (MCD = 65 µs).

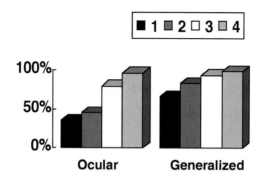

1 = *Slow RNS recording distal (hand) muscle*

2 = *Slow RNS recording proximal (shoulder) muscle*

3 = *Single Fiber EMG of forearm muscle (extensor digitorum communis)*

4 = *Single Fiber EMG of facial muscle (frontalis)*

**Fig. 9.** The diagnostic sensitivity of slow repetitive nerve stimulation and single-fiber EMG in the diagnosis of myasthenia gravis. (Data compiled from OH SJ, Kim DE, Kuruoglu R, Bradley RJ, Dwyer D. Diagnostic sensitivity of the laboratory tests in myasthenia gravis. *Muscle Nerve* 1992;15:720–724 and from Howard JF, Sanders DB, Massey JM. The electrodiagnosis of myasthenia gravis and the Lambert-Eaton syndrome. *Neurol Clin* 1994;12:305–330.)

often occurs in a variety of neuromuscular disorders. Hence, SFEMG jitter findings should be correlated with the history, examination, and conventional needle EMG.

*Conventional Needle EMG*

The needle EMG examination in evaluation of MG serves two purposes. The first is to confirm the diagnosis of MG. Although needle EMG in MG is often normal, the presence of certain findings solidifies the diagnosis. These include moment-to-moment variation of MUAP configuration and short-duration, low-amplitude, and polyphasic MUAPs. These findings usually occur in patients with moderate or severe MG and are most evident in proximal muscles. Fibrillation potentials are rarely seen in MG and represent chronic blockade or loss of endplates (5). Fasciculations may be encountered in patients being treated with large doses of cholinesterase inhibitors, such as pyridostigmine. All these findings are, however, not specific and are more likely to be seen in denervating or myopathic illnesses. The second goal of needle EMG is to exclude other neuromuscular causes of weakness such as motor neuron disease, neuropathies, or myopathies.

## Lambert-Eaton Syndrome

The EDX abnormalities encountered in LES constitute the mainstay of diagnosis as described originally by Lambert and Eaton *(9,10,22,23)*.

### Baseline Compound Muscle Action Potential

In LES, the CMAPs, obtained during routine motor NCSs, are low in amplitude since many endplates do not reach threshold owing to inadequate release of synaptic vesicles after a single stimulus. Thus, low numbers of MFAPs are generated, leading to low-amplitude CMAP. This finding occurs in all muscles, resulting in diffusely low CMAP amplitudes, and may be the first clue that a patient with weakness may have LES. In fact, the electromyographer may be the first to diagnose LES in the EMG laboratory by evaluating post-exercise CMAP in patients with universally low CMAP amplitude referred for a variety of reasons *(24)*.

### Rapid Repetitive Nerve Stimulation

Rapid RNS (usually 20–50 Hz) or post-brief exercise CMAP evaluation enhance calcium influx into the presynaptic terminal, which results in larger releases of quanta and larger EPPs. Although many EPPs do not reach threshold after the first stimulus, many muscle fibers achieve the threshold required for generation of MFAPs with the subsequent stimuli. Hence, rapid RNS results in a CMAP amplitude increment (**Fig. 10**). This posttetanic facilitation should exceed 50% and preferably 100% to be diagnostic, but it is often more than 200% in patients with LEMS *(9–11,22,23,25,26)*.

### Slow Repetitive Nerve Stimulation

Slow RNS (usually 2–3 Hz) is not useful in LES diagnosis since it results in decrement of the CMAP, similar to postsynaptic disorders. With slow RNS, ACh release is reduced further because of the depletion of the immediately available stores, and calcium does not accumulate in the presynaptic terminal. The end result is further loss of many MFAPs and a decrement of CMAP amplitude.

### Single-Fiber EMG

SFEMG jitter is abnormal in LES, similar to the findings in MG *(3,12,13, 15,27)*. However, a stimulation SFEMG technique may help to distinguish these two disorders: the jitter improves significantly with rapid rate stimulation (20–50 Hz) in LES, whereas it does not change or worsens in MG.

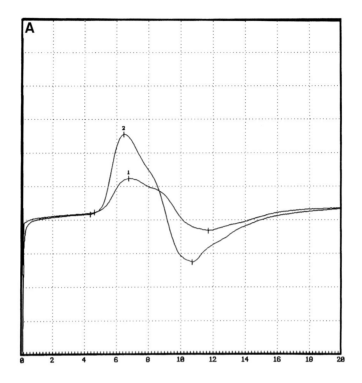

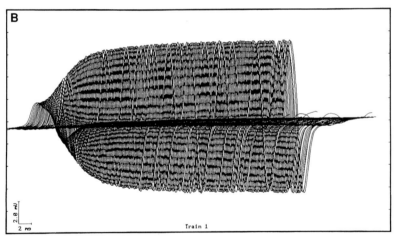

**Fig. 10.** Posttetanic compound muscle action potential (CMAP) evaluation in a patient with LES by stimulating the ulnar nerve (recording hypothenar muscles). (**A**) Baseline low-amplitude CMAP at 2.0 mV (waveform 1). Following 10 s of voluntary maximal isometric exercise, there is a significant CMAP increment (waveform 2) to 4.8 mV (increment = 140%); sensitivity 2 mV/division. (**B**) Rapid (50-Hz) stimulation revealing marked increment of CMAP amplitude (250%).

### Conventional Needle EMG

The findings on needle EMG in LES are very similar to those in MG, although the changes are often more conspicuous but only present in severe cases.

## Botulism

EDX studies are a rapid and readily available method of diagnosing for patients with suspected botulism but who have pending or negative bioassays for botulinum toxin, or negative stool cultures for *Clostridium botulinum*. The EDX findings are compatible with a presynaptic defect of neuromuscular transmission and are somewhat similar to the findings in LES *(6,21,28–30)*. However, the results of EDX studies are variable and depend on the amount of toxic exposure and the timing of the study. During the early course of the disease, it is common for the EDX results to change significantly from day to day.

### Baseline CMAP

Low CMAP amplitudes are the most consistent finding and are present in 85% of patients, particularly when one is recording from weak muscles (usually proximal) *(6,21)*.

### Rapid Repetitive Nerve Stimulation

Rapid RNS, or CMAP following 10 s of isometric exercise, results in CMAP increment between 30 and 100% (**Fig. 3**). This is modest compared with the increment in LES, which often surpasses 200% (**Table 2**) *(6,21,30)*. The increment may be absent, especially in severe cases such as those caused by type A toxin, presumably owing to the degree of presynaptic blockade.

### Slow Repetitive Nerve Stimulation

Slow RNS may cause a decrement of CMAP amplitude. However, this is infrequent and mild not exceeding 8–10% of baseline.

### Single-Fiber EMG

Increased jitter with blocking may be observed by single-fiber EMG *(28, 29)*. Stimulation jitter usually improves during rapid stimulation.

### Conventional Needle EMG

The needle EMG in botulism is variable and depends on the amount of toxic exposure. Often, needle EMG reveals an increase in the number of short-duration, low-amplitude, and polyphasic MUAPs, occasional fibrillation potentials, and variations in MUAP configurations. In severe cases, rapid recruitment of only a few MUAP may be apparent.

**Table 2**
**Baseline CMAP and Repetitive Stimulation**
**Findings in Neuromuscular Junction Disorders**[a]

| NMJ Disorder | NMJ defect | CMAP amplitude | Slow RNS | Rapid RNS[b] |
|---|---|---|---|---|
| Myasthenia gravis | Postsynaptic | Normal | Decrement | Normal or decrement |
| Lambert-Eaton syndrome | Presynaptic | Low in all muscles | Decrement | Marked (>200%) increment in all muscles |
| Botulism | Presynaptic | Low in proximal and weak muscles | Decrement | Modest increment in weak muscles (50–100%) |

[a]NMJ = neuromuscular junction; CMAP = compound muscle action potential; RNS = repetitive nerve stimulation.
[b]Or postexercise CMAP amplitude.

## Congenital Myasthenic Syndromes

Congenital myasthenias are caused by genetic defects of the presynaptic or postsynaptic apparatus. Many congenital myasthenic syndromes, regardless of primary etiology, demonstrate a degeneration of the postsynaptic region and simplification of junctional folds, often with a concomitant reduction of ACh Receptors *(31)*.

Given the similar anatomic pathology of all the congenital myasthenic syndromes, slow RNS often produces a decremental response, which may be absent during rest and only elicited after several minutes of exercise. In cholinesterase deficiency and slow-channel syndrome (the best characterized of the congenital myasthenic syndromes), a single electrical stimulation leads to repetitive CMAPs, similar to the findings in organophosphate poisoning and in patients taking large doses of cholinesterase inhibitors.

## ELECTRODIAGNOSTIC STRATEGY FOR A SUSPECTED NEUROMUSCULAR JUNCTION DEFECT

The EDX study of a patient with suspected NMJ disorder should start with a detailed history and comprehensive neurologic examination. Sensory and motor NCSs in two limbs (preferably an upper and a lower extremity) should be the initial studies. The clinical situation and baseline CMAP amplitudes dictate the next steps *(2,24)*:

1. If the CMAP amplitudes are low, a presynaptic defect should be suspected and ruled out (**Fig. 11**).
2. If the diagnosis of LES is clinically suspected, baseline and postexercise CMAPs of at least two distal motor nerves is a sufficient screening test. In LES, CMAP

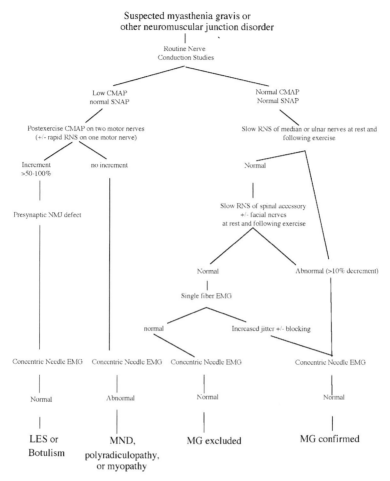

**Fig. 11.** Electrodiagnostic strategy in patients with suspected neuromuscular junction disorder. CMAP = compound muscle action potential; EMG = electromyography; LES = Lambert-Eaton syndrome; MG = myasthenia gravis; MND = motor neuron disease; RNS = repetitive nerve stimulation; SNAP = synaptic vesicle-associated protein.

increment often surpasses 200%. A rapid RNS of one distal nerve, which is extremely painful, is usually sufficient for confirmation if there are CMAP increments after exercise.

3. If the diagnosis of botulism is considered, the choice of muscle should include clinically weak muscles. In botulism, the CMAP increment is usually 30–100%. Also, the study may be repeated in 1–2 days, particularly if the initial evaluation was done during the early phase of the illness.

4. If the diagnosis of MG is clinically suspected, slow RNS at rest and for 4–5 min following a 1-min exercise should be performed on at least two motor nerves. The

selection of nerves and muscles is dependent on the clinical manifestations, with the goal of recording from clinically weak muscles. One should start by performing slow RNS on a distal hand muscle (such as the abductor digiti minimi or abductor pollicis brevis) and then move on to a proximal muscle such as the upper trapezius. Facial RNS should be reserved for patients with oculobulbar manifestations and normal slow RNS recording from distal and proximal muscles (**Fig. 11**). SFEMG of one or two muscles (such as the frontalis, orbicularis oculi, or extensor digitorum communis) should be considered if the diagnosis of MG is still considered despite normal RNS studies and absent serum AChR antibodies.

5. If the CMAPs obtained on motor NCSs in a patient with suspected MG are low or borderline, postexercise CMAP screening should always be done to exclude LES. A misdiagnosis of MG is often made if postexercise CMAP evaluation is not done and a slow RNS shows a CMAP decrement.

6. Postexercise CMAP screening is recommended for patients with weakness associated with a malignancy (particularly a small cell lung cancer), or if the clinical situation does not clearly differentiate between LEMS and MG.

## REFERENCES

1. Boonyapisit K, Kaminski HJ, Ruff RL. The molecular basis of neuromuscular transmission disorders. *Am J Med* 1999;6:97–113.
2. Katirji B. *Electromyography in Clinical Practice. A Case Study Approach.* St. Louis, Mosby, 1998, pp. 171–191, 233–244, and 265–287.
3. Oh SJ. *Electromyography: Neuromuscular Transmission Studies.* Baltimore, Williams & Wilkins, 1988, pp. 87–110, 243–253.
4. Preston DC, Shapiro BE. *Electromyography and Neuromuscular Disorders.* Boston, Butterworth-Heinemann, 1998, pp. 63–73, 503–504.
5. Barberi S, Weiss GM, Daube JR. Fibrillation potentials in myasthenia gravis. *Muscle Nerve* 1982;5:S50.
6. Cherrington M. Botulism. In: Katirji B, Kaminski HJ, Preston DC, Ruff RL, Shapiro EB, eds. *Neuromuscular Disorders in Clinical Practice.* Boston, Butterworth-Heinemann, 2002, pp. 942–952.
7. Desmedt JE, Borenstein S. Diagnosis of myasthenia gravis by nerve stimulation. *Ann NY Acad Sci* 1976;74:174–188.
8. Ozdemir C, Young RR. The results to be expected from electrical testing in the diagnosis of myasthenia gravis. *Ann NY Acad Sci* 1976;74:203–222.
9. Eaton LM, Lambert EH. Electromyography and electric stimulation of nerves in diseases of motor unit: observations on myasthenic syndrome associated with malignant tumors. *JAMA* 1957;163:1117–1124.
10. Lambert EH, Eaton LM, Rooke ED. Defect of neuromuscular conduction associated with malignant neoplasms. *Am J Physiol* 1956;187:612–613.
11. Tim RW, Sanders DB. Repetitive nerve stimulation studies in the Lambert-Eaton myasthenic syndrome. *Muscle Nerve* 1994;17:995–1001.
12. Stålberg E, Trontelj JV. *Single Fiber Electromyography. Studies in Healthy and Diseased Muscle,* 2nd ed. New York, Raven, 1994, pp. 45–83.

13. Sanders DB, Stålberg EV. Single fiber electromyography. *Muscle Nerve* 1996;19: 1069–1083.
14. Sanders DB, Howard JF. Single fiber EMG in myasthenia gravis. *Muscle Nerve* 1986;9:809–819.
15. Trontelj JV, Stålberg E. Single motor endplates in myasthenia gravis and Lambert Eaton myasthenic syndrome at different firing rates. *Muscle Nerve* 1990;14:226–232.
16. Sanders DB. The effect of firing rate on neuromuscular jitter in Lambert-Eaton myasthenic syndrome. *Muscle Nerve* 1992;15:256–258.
17. Ekstedt J, Nilsson G, Stålberg E. Calculation of the electromyographic jitter. *J Neurol Neurosurg Psychiatry* 1974;37:526–539.
18. Gilchrist JM. Ad hoc committee of the AAEM special interest group on SFEMG. Single fiber EMG reference values: a collaborative effort. *Muscle Nerve* 1992;15: 151–161.
19. Gilchrist JM. Single fiber EMG. In: Katirji B, Kaminski HJ, Preston DC, Ruff RL, Shapiro EB, eds. *Neuromuscular Disorders in Clinical Practice*. Boston, Butterworth-Heinemann, 2002, pp. 141–150.
20. Oh SH, Kim DE, Kuruoglu R, Bradley RJ, Dwyer D. Diagnostic sensitivity of the laboratory tests in myasthenia gravis. *Muscle Nerve* 1992;5:720–724.
21. Cherrington M. Electrophysiologic methods as an aid in diagnosis of botulism: a review. *Muscle Nerve* 1982;5:528–529.
22. Lambert EH, Rooke ED, Eaton LM, et al. Myasthenic syndrome occasionally associated with bronchial neoplasm: neurophysiologic studies. In: Viets HR, ed. *Myasthenia Gravis: The Second International Symposium Proceedings 1959*. Springfield, IL, CC Thomas, 1961, pp. 362–410.
23. O'Neil JH, Murray NMF, Newsom-Davis J. The Lambert-Eaton myasthenic syndrome: a review of 50 cases. *Brain* 1988;111:577–596.
24. Katirji B, Kaminski HJ. An electrodiagnostic approach to the patient with neuromuscular junction disorder. *Neuro Clin* 2002;20:557–586.
25. Maddison P, Newsom-Davis J, Mills KR. Distribution of electrophysiological abnormality in Lambert-Eaton myasthenic syndrome. *J Neurol Neurosurg Psychiatry* 1998; 5:213–217.
26. Maddison P, Newsom-Davis J. The Lambert-Eaton myasthenic syndrome. In: Katirji B, Kaminski HJ, Preston DC, Ruff RL, Shapiro EB, eds. *Neuromuscular Disorders in Clinical Practice*. Boston, Butterworth-Heinemann, 2002, pp. 931–941.
27. Oh SJ, Hurwitz EL, Lee KW, Chang CW, Cho HK. The single-fiber EMG in the Lambert-Eaton myasthenic syndrome. *Muscle Nerve* 1989;12:159–161.
28. Schiller HH, Stålberg E. Human botulism studied with single-fiber electromyography. *Arch Neurol* 1978;35:346–349.
29. Padua L, Aprile I, Monaco ML, Fenicia L, Anniballi F, Pauri F, Tonali P. Neurophysiological assessment in the diagnosis of botulism: usefulness of single-fiber EMG. *Muscle Nerve* 1999;22:1388–1392.
30. Cornblath DR, Sladky JT, Sumner AJ. Clinical electrophysiology of infantile botulism. *Muscle Nerve* 1983;6:448–652.
31. Engel AG. Congenital myasthenic syndromes. In: Katirji B, Kaminski HJ, Preston DC, Ruff RL, Shapiro EB, eds. *Neuromuscular Disorders in Clinical Practice*. Boston, Butterworth-Heinemann, 2002, pp. 953–963.

# 8

# Specific Antibodies in the Diagnosis and Management of Autoimmune Disorders of Neuromuscular Transmission and Related Diseases

## Mark A. Agius, David P. Richman, and Angela Vincent

### INTRODUCTION

The term *neuromuscular junction* (NMJ), which denotes the synapse between the motor nerve and the muscle fiber, includes the motor nerve terminal and the endplate region of the postsynaptic muscle fiber. A number of molecules, which include ion channels and other proteins at the NMJ, may be targeted by the immune system, resulting in disordered neuromuscular transmission. In this context antibodies to acetycholine receptors (AChRs), resulting in the clinical picture of acquired myasthenia gravis (MG), were the first to be demonstrated to be pathogenic. More recently, additional targets in both the nerve terminal and muscle cell have been identified, including calcium and potassium ion channels in the motor nerve terminal and components of the AChR clustering mechanisms at the NMJ, as well as proteins located within the muscle fiber. In most cases, the antibodies that bind to these proteins appear to be pathogenic; their identification allows for specific treatments and in certain situations may suggest modifications to current treatment.

Thus one of the most satisfying aspects of our current understanding of the role of antibodies in MG and other diseases of the NMJ is the ability to measure these antibodies effectively in the laboratory. This is largely owing to the use of certain neurotoxins that bind specifically and with high affinity to the ion channels that are the targets for these antibodies. Alternative approaches are needed for autoantibody detection against other proteins, for example, the muscle-specific kinase (MuSK), and various intracellular proteins. Here we start by discussing some general principles and then go on to describe

From: *Current Clinical Neurology: Myasthenia Gravis and Related Disorders*
Edited by: H. J. Kaminski © Humana Press Inc., Totowa, NJ

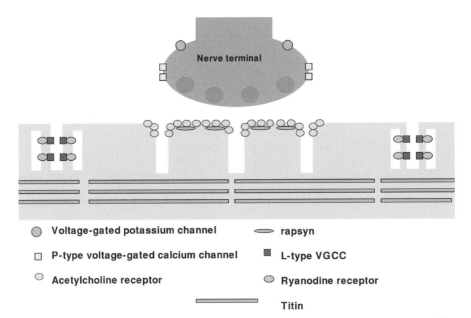

**Fig. 1.** Diagram of the neuromuscular junction with proteins that are targeted for autoimmune attack. VGCC = voltage-gated calcium channel.

the clinical syndromes and the methods that can be used to investigate the pathogenic role of autoantibodies.

## SPECTRUM OF ANTIBODIES TO TARGETS AT THE NMJ AND ASSOCIATED MOLECULES

Most of the proteins targeted in autoimmune myasthenic disorders and related conditions are located in the cell membrane of the motor nerve or muscle endplate with an extracellular domain that is accessible to circulating substances. A functional blood-nerve barrier, composed of endothelial cells and gap junctions, is not present at the NMJ, exposing it to the circulation. In some instances, however, the autoimmune targets appear to be intracellular. Whereas a pathogenic role for autoimmunity against NMJ proteins with an extracellular domain is well characterized, it is also suspected that an immune attack against intracellular components is significant in the pathophysiology of these conditions.

The molecules identified to be targets in the NMJ are illustrated in **Fig. 1**. These include calcium and potassium channels in the motor nerve terminal, AChRs and MuSK postsynaptically, and rapsyn, titin, and ryanodine receptor intracellularly in the muscle cell.

## IDENTIFYING A PATHOGENIC ROLE
## FOR ANTIBODIES IN ANTIBODY-MEDIATED DISORDERS

The classic studies demonstrating a role for autoantibodies in the disorders discussed in this volume are described elsewhere. Here we shall just draw attention to the important principles underlying these observations. In MG, four observations were crucial in leading to the identification of the autoimmune basis of the condition. First, active immunization of animals with purified AChR led to the development of experimental autoimmune myasthenia gravis (EAMG) *(1)*. Second, there was a reduction in AChRs at the motor endplates of patients *(2)*. Third, patients with MG had antibodies to AChR *(3)*, and fourth, it was possible to transfer the signs of the disease by injecting IgG of MG patients into mice *(4)*. These observations made the case that MG was an autoimmune disease so compelling that it was justifiable to attempt plasma exchange as an experimental treatment *(5)*.

In Lambert-Eaton syndrome (LES) and neuromyotonia (NMT), by contrast, active immunization has still not been carried out satisfactorily. However, the combination of clinical response to plasma exchange and passive transfer of immunoglobulins to mice *(6–8)*, or occasionally other species, has shown that these conditions are caused by autoantibodies, and the identification of the target antigens (or some of them) has followed.

## DISEASE PHENOTYPES
## IN AUTOIMMUNE MYASTHENIC DISORDERS

In immune-mediated diseases, the clinical syndrome generated is related to the target antigen and its role in the function of the NMJ and the muscle fiber. At the same time, overlapping phenotypes occur as a consequence of immune attacks directed at distinct molecular targets. For instance, both AChR and MuSK antibodies can be associated with MG but are likely to disturb neuromuscular transmission by different mechanisms. Identification of these mechanisms may allow for improved diagnosis and treatment.

Patients with acquired MG with AChR antibodies fall into three distinct groups, early-onset MG patients without thymoma, patients with thymoma, and patients with late-onset MG without thymoma (**Table 1**) *(9)*. The late-onset group may include at least two further subpopulations of patients.

## HETEROGENEITY AND PATHOPHYSIOLOGIC
## EFFECTS OF AChR ANTIBODIES

Serum AChR antibodies provide a specific marker for MG. When present in humans, they invariably mediate AChR loss, simplification of the postsynaptic membrane, dysfunction of NMJ transmission, and clinical disease. In

**Table 1**
**Autoantigens in Myasthenia Gravis (MG) Subtypes**[a]

| Type of MG | AChR | Titin | MuSK | Thymic Pathology | Age of Onset (yr) |
|---|---|---|---|---|---|
| Early-onset | +++[a] | – | – | Germinal centers | <50 |
| Thymoma | + | + | – | Thymoma | Any |
| Late-onset[b] | + | – | – | | >40 |
| Late-onset with titin antibodies | + | + | – | Atrophy | >50 |
| Seronegative | – | – | + | – | |

[a] +++ = high serum antibody concentration: + = low serum antibody concentration. AChR = acetylcholine receptor; MuSK = muscle-specific kinase.
[b] Late-onset MG is classified into titin-positive and -negative patients.

patients with MG, plasma exchange-induced reduction in serum anti-AChR levels is generally associated with a clinical improvement *(10)* that is often marked *(11)*. The duration of benefit, as in other antibody-mediated diseases in general, may last from 1 to 3 months. In individual patients there is often a rough correlation between severity of disease and the concentration of serum AChR antibodies *(12)*.

In order to understand the effects of antibodies on NMJ function, it is necessary to refer to the animal model, EAMG, that results from active immunization against purified AChR. The majority of anti-AChR antibodies in EAMG bind to a conformational determinant, known as the main immunogenic region (MIR), on the extracellular aspect of the AChR. This region includes the α-subunit 67–76-amino acid sequence *(13)*. Complement activation, leading to the deposition of membrane attack complex, by these antibodies is pivotal to the development of AChR loss in EAMG. C4-deficient guinea pigs do not develop EAMG, and prevention of complement activation prevents EAMG *(14)*. The antibodies crosslink the AChRs in the membrane, and their Fc regions mediate C1q binding and macrophage activation. However, since efficient complement activation requires binding of C1q by crosslinked adjacent immunoglobulin molecules, this may be reduced or prevented by decreased AChR density or distortion of the postsynaptic membrane. In fact, the macrophage infiltration induced by injection of AChR monoclonal antibodies correlates with AChR density *(15)*.

Human MG is characterized by postsynaptic membrane simplification and reduced AChR content. This pathology is induced and maintained by anti-AChR antibodies and is also mediated by complement activation *(16)*. In addition, macrophages invade the postsynaptic membrane in human MG, albeit in relatively few numbers *(17)*. Anti-AChR antibodies may have additional effects on the target molecules by blocking ion channel function *(18)*. A further mechanism is the increased internalization, or antigenic modulation, of the AChR molecules by specific antibody *(19)*. Passive transfer of these modulating antibodies does not cause overt EAMG when complement activation is prevented *(20)*.

The lack of a precise correlation between serum AChR antibody concentrations and clinical weakness in patients with MG, therefore, is likely to be dependent on several confounding factors. These include variables related to the structure and function of the antibodies themselves, including the nature of the variable region forming the binding site and (consequently) determining the AChR site to which it binds. Effector functions of the constant regions also probably influence clinical expression. These are a function of the class and subclass of the antibodies and their interactions with components of the innate immune system, particularly complement and macrophages. Most AChR antibodies in human MG belong to the IgG1 and IgG3 subclasses and are strong activators of complement. Nevertheless, the polyclonal B-cell response means that changes in subpopulations of pathogenic antibodies may result in changes in the clinical manifestations, independent of the total level of the antibody. The relationship between the serum antibody concentration and pathology also involves equilibration between serum and tissue concentrations. The density and organization of the target epitopes is an additional factor, as is the presence of co-occurring antibodies directed at additional targets.

## Binding Antibodies Measured by Immunoprecipitation

This is the assay that tends to be most useful in clinical practice. It uses extracted human skeletal muscle AChR labeled with radioiodinated α-bungarotoxin (α-BGT) (**Table 2**). It detects AChR antibodies in 85% of patients with generalized MG *(21,22)* and 75% of patients with purely ocular MG *(22)*. The patients with early-onset MG with generalized weakness tend to have the highest concentrations of serum AChR antibody levels compared with other patients with MG (**Table 1**). The AChR antibody-positive, or seropositive, patients with ocular MG tend to have serum AChR concentrations that are lower than those of seropositive patients with generalized disease. This finding suggests that the clinical manifestations may, at least in part, be a function of the absolute AChR antibody concentration. A particular susceptibility of ocular muscle NMJs for clinical manifestations of NMJ dysfunction is also suggested by the occurrence of ocular muscle involvement early in the course of disease in many patients with botulism *(23)* or with other neurotoxins. It is also possible that the antigenic targets in the NMJs

**Table 2**
**Neurotoxins Used to Quantitative**
**Assays for Ion Channel Autoantibodies**[a]

| Antigen | Source | Neurotoxin | Source | Use |
|---|---|---|---|---|
| AChR | Muscle or muscle cell lines (TE671 cells) | α-Bungarotoxin | *Bungarus multicinctus* | Diagnosis of MG |
| VGCC | Human or rabbit cerebellum or neuronal or small cell lung cancer lines | ω-Conotoxin$_{MVIIC}$ | *Conus magus* | Diagnosis of LES and investigation of some CNS disorders |
| VGKC | Human or rabbit cortex | Dendrotoxins | *Dendroaspis* species | Diagnosis of NMT and investigation of some CNS disorders |

[a] AChR = acetylcholine receptor; LES = Lambert-Eaton syndrome; MG = myasthenia gravis; NMT = neuromyotonia; VGCC = voltage-gated calcium channel; VGKC = voltage-gated potassium channel.

of extraocular muscles and levator palpebrae provide distinct epitopes for the autoimmune process *(24)*. The patients with generalized MG, who are consistently negative for AChR antibodies, appear to manifest a different disease mechanism despite similar clinical features and course (see below).

### Blocking Antibodies

Blocking antibodies that inhibit the binding of radiolabeled α-BGT to the AChR probably compete for binding to the ACh binding site *(25)*, although in theory they may be noncompetitive and result in allosteric inhibition. AChR blocking antibodies may be detected in many patients with MG. They appear to represent a minority of the AChR antibodies and usually occur in association with AChR binding antibodies. They are suggested to be important pathogenically in an acute severe exacerbation of MG, but blocking antibodies do not necessarily interfere with AChR function. Antibodies that do inhibit function can be detected by measuring ion flux through the AChR or ACh-induced currents *(26,27)*.

### Assays to Detect Modulating Antibodies

The application of serum from patients with MG to muscle cell lines can interfere not only with function but also with AChR expression *(19)*. This is because the antibodies crosslink the AChR in the membrane and increase their rate of degradation. The AChR are measured by binding of radiolabeled-α-BGT after exposure to the serum for 16 h. It is a relatively nonspecific test, and the results should be compared with suitable control sera. The detection of these antibodies is most useful when the AChR binding test yields a negative result *(25)*. It is possible that in some instances, however, the decrease in AChR concentration occurs as a consequence of antibodies directed to postsynaptic targets adjacent to the AChR, rather than to the AChR itself. In general, modulating antibodies directed at the AChR also tend to be positive in immunoprecipitation assays.

## *Other Autoantibodies*

Apart from antibodies to molecular targets located at the NMJ, patients with MG may possess other autoimmune antibodies. These include antibodies directed against thyroglobulin, thyroid microsomes, parietal cells and intrinsic factor, and nuclear antigens. Other autoantibodies are less common *(25)*. The association between these autoantibodies (or other autoimmune diseases) and generalized or ocular MG appears to lie in thymic hyperplasia. Thymic hyperplasia with intramedullary germinal centers is invariably present in patients with early-onset MG. It has also been described in patients with thyroid autoimmune disease and other autoimmune conditions including Addison's disease and pemphigus. Thyrotropin appears to be expressed in the thymus, and the association between thymic hyperplasia and thyroid disease may also be related to loss of tolerance in the thymus *(28)*.

## AUTOIMMUNE MG IN ASSOCIATION WITH THYMOMA

One hundred percent of patients with thymoma and MG have detectable serum AChR antibodies *(29)*. In addition, patients with thymoma without clinically detectable MG frequently, but not invariably, have AChR antibodies, suggesting the presence of subclinical disease. The antibodies and their epitopes may differ in their fine specificities from those in patients with early-onset autoimmune MG without thymoma *(30)*. The serum concentrations of AChR antibodies in thymoma cases tend to be lower than in those with generalized disease.

Complement-activating, striated muscle antibodies were initially described in 1960 by immunofluorescence in patients with MG *(31)*. Most of the striational antibodies are directed against the large structural protein, titin *(32)*. Ryanodine receptor (RyR), and possibly other proteins, constitute additional autoimmune targets *(33)*. Ninety-five percent of patients with thymoma and MG also have titin antibodies, whereas 75% of patients with thymoma and MG possess anti-RyR antibodies *(34)*. Patients with detectable RyR antibodies invariably also possess titin antibodies. The clinical pattern of weakness and fatigability of patients with MG and thymoma is usually indistinguishable from those with MG without thymoma. However, some differences between patients in these two groups may represent the effects of distinct antibodies. Thus, some patients with thymoma, titin, and RyR antibodies may have a myocarditis or a focal myositis *(29)*. The involvement of skeletal and heart muscle is suspected to be a consequence of the striated muscle antibodies providing additional disease-producing potential. In addition, the MG patients with titin antibodies appear to have a more severe course despite lower AChR antibody concentrations compared with those without detectable titin antibodies *(34)*. A more severe course tends to occur in patients with titin antibodies, in the presence or absence of thymoma.

Patients with thymoma require thymectomy to prevent complications stemming from local extension of the tumor (including the superior vena cava syndrome). Thymectomy in these patients, however, may not be followed by clinical improvement. Furthermore, the course of MG may be more severe after thymectomy, and on occasion MG may be precipitated in the postoperative period. It is suggested that the more severe clinical course of MG often characterizing patients with thymoma may be related to pathogenic effects of titin and RyR antibodies *(34–36)*. Patients with thymoma occasionally have been reported to possess antibodies to other autoimmune targets. These include potassium channels *(37)* and calcium channels, as well as rapsyn *(38,39)* and other proteins including glutamic acid decarboxylase *(40)*. Titin and RyR antibodies are also present in a high proportion of the subgroup of patients with late-onset MG who do not have a thymoma *(34,41)* (see below).

## Striated Muscle Antibody Assays

Titin and RyR antibodies may be detected by enzyme-linked immunosorbent assay (ELISA) or immunoblot. An epitope for titin, MGT30, reacting with 90% of titin antibodies is employed for the titin assays, and a commercial assay is available. Striated muscle antibody assays detected by immunofluorescence are also commercially available and may be used in lieu of specific titin and RyR antibody assays. The detection of striated antibodies may be useful diagnostically in patients when AChR antibodies are negative. However, this situation is uncommon. A more important diagnostic role for striated muscle antibodies is to suggest the presence of a thymoma when present in patients under the age of 60 years *(41)*. The sensitivity and specificity of RyR antibodies for thymoma is 70% *(34)*.

## LATE-ONSET MG NOT ASSOCIATED
## WITH A DETECTABLE THYMOMA

The mean AChR antibody concentration in these patients tends to be significantly lower than the early-onset MG group without thymoma *(34)*. The use of antibody profiles utilizing AChR, titin, and RyR antibodies has characterized two subpopulations of patients in this group. Patients who do not have detectable antistriated muscle antibodies may resemble the early-onset MG group and usually present before 60 years of age *(41)*, whereas the patients with titin antibodies present later. Like the patients with thymoma, patients with late-onset MG with titin or RyR antibodies tend to have a poorer response to thymectomy than those with late-onset MG without detectable titin or RyR antibodies *(36)*.

## ROLE OF ANTIBODIES IN DIAGNOSIS
## AND TREATMENT IN PATIENTS WITH MG

Patients with AChR serum antibodies almost invariably have MG. These antibodies provide a valuable diagnostic tool and indicate a mechanism of disease pathogenesis that is more precise than can be obtained by electrophysiologic studies. At this time, the usefulness of following serum concentrations of AChR antibodies to monitor treatment in individual patients is questioned. Identification of subsets of pathogenically important antibodies (including antibodies to additional targets) and measuring their concentration could prove to be important.

The presence of antibodies to targets, other than the AChR, may also influence treatment decisions. Since titin antibodies appear to correlate with disease severity, their presence in patients with thymoma may suggest a role for more aggressive management early in the course of the disease, prior to thymectomy. Similarly, the presence of titin antibodies in patients without thymoma and with onset of disease above the age of 50 may suggest a more aggressive immunosuppression regimen early in the course of the disease and the avoidance of thymectomy.

## SERONEGATIVE MG

The observations indicating that seronegative MG, defined as autoimmune MG without detectable AChR antibodies, was a distinct antibody-mediated condition are summarized below.

### *Plasma Exchange and Passive Transfer*

In seronegative MG, as in LES and NMT, the clinical and experimental evidence for antibody-mediated disease preceded the identification of a target antigen. Several authors showed that the patients responded well to plasma exchange and that passive transfer to mice produced some electrophysiologic evidence of MG *(42,43)*.

## Functional and Binding Studies

The identification of the target antigen(s), however, has been difficult. The possibilities are several. There could be low-affinity antibodies to AChRs that are not detected by radioimmunoassay (RIA) but that nevertheless bind effectively in vivo. This is probably not the case, as shown by binding of seronegative MG IgG to cell lines expressing human AChR. Antibodies from seropositive MG patients bound, but those from AChR antibody-negative patients did not *(44)*. Moreover, when seronegative MG plasma was injected into mice, the AChRs extracted from the mouse muscles were not complexed with IgG *(42)*.

Another explanation is the presence of antibodies binding to another muscle surface antigen. This is supported by the evidence that both AChR antibody-positive and -negative sera bound to TE671 cells, which are derived from a rhabodmyosarcoma and express muscle antigens in addition to AChR *(44)*. This finding suggests that, if not binding to the AChR itself, the serum antibodies must be binding to other muscle proteins.

This hypothesis was confirmed by showing that application of plasma or serum from seronegative MG patients to TE6712 cells leads to a rapid reduction in AChR function, as demonstrated by ion flux studies or by patch clamp *(45,46)*. In order to affect AChR function, without binding directly to it, the antibodies would need to be altering the function of some other membrane protein, perhaps one that stimulated an intracellular pathway. There are various intracellular pathways in muscle that could affect AChR function. In particular, the membrane receptors that stimulate protein kinase A or protein kinase C, such as calcitonin gene-related peptide and ATP receptors, are thought to be present at the neuromuscular junction and could be targets for seronegative MG antibodies. However, these pathways do not appear to be involved in seronegative MG, because inhibitors of either protein kinase A or C do not prevent the effects of the antibodies on AChR function *(46)*.

## Antibodies to a Candidate Antigen

These functional studies suggested that the antibodies might be binding to another type of receptor. An attractive candidate was MuSK. The protein is known to be present at the NMJ and to be a receptor tyrosine kinase that causes autophosphorylation followed by phosphorylation of rapsyn and AChR. Therefore, it is clearly closely associated with AChR at the mature as well as the developing neuromuscular junction. Moreover, seronegative MG IgG

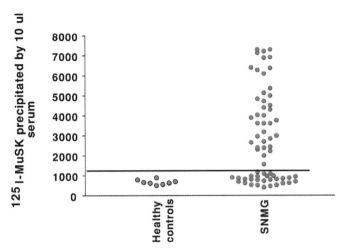

**Fig. 2.** Immunoprecipitation of [$^{125}$I]muscle-specific kinase (MuSK) by sera from patients with seronegative MG. The recombinant extracellular domain of rat MuSK was provided by Dr. Werner Hoch (University of Bristol). The seronegativeMG sera tested were provided by Professor John Newsom-Davis (University of Oxford) and Dr. Amelia Evoli (Catholic University of Rome).

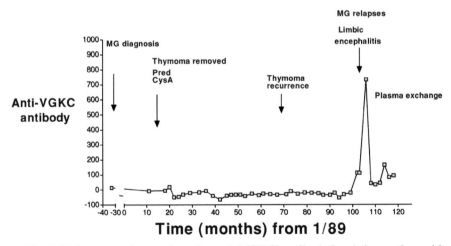

**Fig. 3.** Voltage-gated potassium channel (VGKC) antibody levels in a patient with a 13-year history of thymoma-associated myasthenia gravis (MG). She developed a single episode of limbic signs (memory loss, confusion, disorientation, agitation), associated with a peak of antibodies to VGKC. The antibody levels fell following plasma exchange, and her clinical state improved. Pred = prednisone; CysA = cyclosporine A. [From Buckley et al. *(71)*.] (*See* discussion on pp. 190–191.)

binds strongly to COS cells expressing MuSK *(47)*. To provide a screening assay for MuSK antibodies, Hoch et al. *(47)* used the soluble extracellular domain of recombinant MuSK. Antibodies from seronegative MG patients bound specifically to MuSK, and positive results were initially found in about 70% of patients with well-established disease using a 1:20 dilution of serum.

ELISA is not very easy to use if the concentration of human serum required is relatively high. Nonspecific binding to the plates or to other antigens contaminating the purified recombinant protein can make analysis of the results difficult. Immunoprecipiation of directly labeled rat MuSK is not difficult, and the results correlate strongly with the ELISA data (**Fig. 2**). Cloning and similar expression of human MuSK should provide a suitable antigen for commercial use in the future.

MG in the absence of detectable AChR antibodies, in turn, does not appear to represent a homogenous disease entity. It is likely that patients with seronegative MG, who do not possess detectable antibodies to MuSK, may possess antibodies directed at other proteins at the NMJ. These targets include other proteins involved in the clustering of AChRs at the endplate including intracellular proteins such as rapsyn *(39)*. Furthermore, some MG patients, who are seronegative for AChR antibodies at initial presentation, develop detectable serum anti-AChR antibodies over time. It is possible that at presentation these patients have serum concentrations of AChR antibodies that are below the assay sensitivity.

## LAMBERT-EATON SYNDROME AND CEREBELLAR ATAXIA

### Plasma Exchange and Passive Transfer

Early studies showed that LES was associated with certain autoantibodies and other autoimmune diseases *(48)* and that plasma exchange was an effective treatment *(49)*. Particularly important was the demonstration that injection of patient IgG into mice resulted in a reduction in the quantal release of ACh and an altered number and distribution of active zone particles. The results mirrored the findings in patients *(50,51)*.

### Functional and Binding Studies

To begin to define the nature of the antigen, functional studies on cell lines were used. These started by looking for a candidate antigen, voltage-gated calcium channel (VGCC), on small cell lung cancer cells and by showing that the LES IgGs, when applied for several days in culture, were able to downregulate the VGCC numbers *(52)*. A number of small cell lung cancer cells have been used subsequently, and in all cases VGCCs have been demonstrated and the effects of LES antibodies confirmed *(53,54)*. The main target of the LES antibodies appears to be the P/Q-type VGCCs, which contain an α1a-subunit. These VGCCs are expressed at the motor nerve terminal *(55)* and also on the Purkinje cells in the cerebellum *(56)*.

### Radioimmunoprecipitation Assays

The radioimmunoprecipitation assay for VGCC antibodies was made possible by the discovery in the late 1980s of the cone snail toxins (**Table 2**) *(57)*. The various species of cone snails live on the seabed and produce a rich variety of neurotoxins that are specific for both pre- and postsynaptic ion channels. The first snail toxin to be used to identify VGCCs in LES sera was from *Conus geographus*. This neurotoxin binds to the N-type VGCCs, which are expressed widely in the nervous and neuroendocrine systems. Using VGCCs extracted from human cerebellum or cortex labeled by $[^{125}I]$ω-conotoxin GVIA, about 40% of LES patients are positive *(58)*. However, using the P/Q-type selective ω-conotoxin MVIIC under very similar conditions, up to 90% of LES patients are positive *(59,60)*. These results emphasize the exquisite specificity of these toxins. By contrast, the source of tissue is probably not as important. Similar results are found with rabbit or human cerebellum, indicating that the VGCCs are highly conserved in evolution and antigenically similar between species *(61)*.

RIA has been used extensively as a diagnostic test, and some studies report serial estimations during treatment. For instance, VGCC antibodies are found to fall by 30% on average in patients treated with intravenous immunoglobulin *(62)*. The fall does not start until 2 weeks after the treatment, suggesting that it is not a direct result of "blocking" antibodies. The VGCC levels return to pretreatment levels by about 8 weeks, roughly correlating with clinical manifestations.

Although the VGCC antibody assay is principally used as a diagnostic test for LES, it has other applications. It has been established that a proportion of patients with small cell lung cancer have LES and that VGCC antibodies are present in such patients even without clear clinical evidence of LES *(63, 64)*. Moreover, some patients with cerebellar ataxia with and without clinical evidence of LES have VGCC antibodies. Thus serum from patients who are at risk of small cell lung cancer and who present with a cerebellar or myasthenic syndrome should be tested for VGCC antibodies.

## ACQUIRED NEUROMYOTONIA

### Plasma Exchange and Passive Transfer

Acquired NMT, like LES, was not thought to be autoimmune until clinical studies showed a response of some patients to plasma exchange or intravenous immunoglobulin therapies. In the few reports of passive transfer, enhancement of neuromuscular transmission with resistance to the action of curare was induced in mouse nerve muscle preparations after passive transfer of NMT IgG *(65)*.

## Functional and Binding Assays

A functional effect of NMT IgG on neuronal cell lines was successfully demonstrated by using dorsal root ganglion cells, which developed repetitive action potentials, very similar to those found in the presence of 4-diamino-pyridine, a potassium channel blocker *(7)*. In the PC-12 and NB-1 neuroblastoma cell lines, incubating the cells overnight in NMT IgGs led to a reduction in the voltage-gated potassium channel (VGKC) currents without any observable change in the current/voltage density. These alterations, which were not seen with briefer incubation times, suggest that the antibodies are not blocking channel function directly but rather reducing the number of VGKCs *(66–68)*.

Using cell lines expressing VGKC, it is possible to detect binding of some antibodies from NMT patients, but the sensitivity is not sufficient for routine analysis (unpublished data). Ideally, one would use cell lines expressing different VGKC isotypes, so as to test involvement of different targets in the disease process. Immunohistochemistry on *Xenopus* oocytes expressing some VGKC subtypes demonstrated antibody binding *(69)*, but this approach is time-consuming and has not been evaluated further.

## Radioimmunoprecipitation Assays

There are numerous subtypes of VGKC, particularly of the shaker type. Present nomenclature identifies these as Kv1.1–1.9. To date, it has only been possible to identify autoantibody binding to Kv1.1, 1.2, and 1.6 (and perhaps 1.3) using the *Dendroaspis* neurotoxins that bind specifically to these subtypes (**Table 2**) *(69)*.

The sensitivity of the assay depends on using high specific activity dendrotoxin to label VGKC extracted from human or rabbit cortex, but with this product it is not possible to saturate binding sites. About 40% of NMT patients are positive by this approach *(7,70)*. The antibodies do not appear to inhibit binding of dendrotoxin to the VGKC. Few serial studies of VGKC antibodies have thus far been performed. Perhaps the most striking report is that of a woman with MG and thymoma who following a thymoma recurrence developed an episode of "limbic encephalitis" *(71)*. This responded strikingly to plasma exchange, strongly implying an antibody-mediated basis for the central disease. In a retrospective analysis of VGKC antibodies in over 80 sera collected from this patient over 13 years, a single peak of VGKC antibodies was found, corresponding closely to the time of appearance of her limbic manifestations (**Fig. 3**, *see* p. 187) *(71)*. VGKC antibodies and a clinical response to plasma exchange were found in a patient with classical Morvan's syndrome *(72)*, which includes neuromyotonia with sleep disorder, limbic manifestations, and autonomic dysfunction.

## STIFF PERSON SYNDROME

Autoimmune disorders involving components of central nervous system synapses have been identified with similarity to the peripheral disorders discussed above. Stiff person syndrome (SPS), a condition characterized by muscle rigidity and spasms, was suspected to have an autoimmune basis because of its association with autoantibodies and other autoimmune conditions. Furthermore, patients with SPS respond to immune treatments including plasma exchange *(73)*. The molecular autoimmune targets have been identified to be components of CNS synapses at which γ-aminobutyric acid (GABA) is a neurotransmitter. GABA is the major inhibitory neurotransmitter in the CNS. Ninety percent of patients with SPS possess antibodies directed at glutamic acid decarboxylase (GAD), the rate-limiting enzyme involved in the synthesis of GABA. High serum GAD antibodies are specific for SPS, and cerebrospinal fluid GAD-specific antibodies also occur in SPS *(74)*. Diabetes mellitus is often present, and GAD antibodies are also present in patients with insulin-dependent diabetes mellitus in the absence of SPS. Patients with diabetes mellitus without SPS may have lower serum concentrations than those with SPS and tend to have antibodies to the 65-kDa isoform, whereas patients with SPS may have antibodies to both the 65- and the 67-kDa isoforms *(75)*. Some patients with SPS in association with cancer are reported to not have detectable GAD antibodies but to have serum antibodies to synapse-related proteins including amphiphysin *(76)* and, in one case, gephyrin, a protein that anchors GABA receptors *(77)*. Thus, autoimmune SPS may represent a disease phenotype or syndrome that may result as a consequence of distinct immunopathogenesis and etiology.

## CONCLUSIONS

Acquired MG may be considered the prototypic autoimmune disorder. Observations pertaining to MG are also pertinent to other autoimmune disorders of the NMJ and related disorders. Thus, in MG, phenotypic variations are at least in part a function of different mechanisms of disease. The antibody target, the concentration of antibodies, and the fraction of antibodies that are complement activating are all factors likely to influence the clinical presentation and the course. Serologic testing is of value in the diagnosis as well as the treatment of individual patients. AChR is the main autoantigen in most patients with acquired MG. However, it is not the only potential target. We are developing a clearer picture of a broader spectrum of antigenic targets and how antibodies to these targets may influence the disease course and treatment. Although in most instances the diseases do not overlap, e.g., MG and LES or MG and seronegative MG, in other instances the antibody syndromes occur together, as often occurs in MG in association with thymoma. Patients with AChR antibody-positive MG with early-onset appear to have disease mechanisms that are distinct from those with thymoma and MG. Seronegative MG represents a separate autoimmune condition. Further identification of additional targets of the autoimmune disease is likely to lead to better understanding of the etiology of these disorders.

## REFERENCES

1. Patrick J, Lindstrom J. Autoimmune response to acetylcholine receptor. *Science* 1973;180:871–872.
2. Fambrough DM, Drachman DB, Satyamurti S. Neuromuscular junction in myasthenia gravis: decreased acetylcholine receptors. *Science* 1973;182:293–295.
3. Lindstrom JM, Seybold ME, Lennon VA, Whittingham S, Duane DD. Antibody to acetylcholine receptor in myasthenia gravis: prevalence, clinical correlates, and diagnostic value. *Neurology* 1976;26:1054–1059.
4. Toyka, KV, Drachman, DB, Griffin DE, et al. Myasthenia gravis: study of humoral immune mechanisms by passive transfer to mice. *N Engl J Med* 1977;296:125–131.
5. Pinching AJ, Peters DK, Newsom-Davis JN. Remission of myasthenia gravis following plasma exchange. *Lancet* 1976;2:1373–1376.
6. Lang B, Newsom-Davis J, Prior C, Wray D. Antibodies to motor nerve terminals: an electrophysiological study of a human myasthenic syndrome transferred to a mouse. *J Physiol (Lond)* 1983;344:335–345.
7. Shillito P, Molenaar PC, Vincent A, et al. Acquired neuromyotonia: evidence for autoantibodies directed against $K^+$ channels of peripheral nerves. *Ann Neurol* 1995; 38:714–722.
8. Mossman S, Vincent A, Newsom-Davis J. Passive transfer of myasthenia gravis by immunoglobulins: lack of correlation between antibody bound, acetylcholine receptor loss and transmission defect. *J Neurol Sci* 1988;84:15–28.
9. Compston DA, Vincent A, Newsom-Davis J, Batchelor JR. Clinical, pathological, HLA antigen and immunological evidence for disease heterogeneity in myasthenia gravis. *Brain* 1980;103:579–601.
10. Newsom-Davis J, Pinching AJ, Vincent A, Wilson SG. Function of circulating antibody to acetycholine receptor in myasthenia gravis: investigated by plasma exchange. *Neurology* 1978;28:266–272.
11. Dau PC. Plasmpheresis therapy in mysthenia gravis. *Muscle Nerve* 1980;3:468–482.
12. Oosterhuis HJGH, Limburg PC, Hummel-Tappel E. Anti-acetylcholine receptor antibodies in myasthenia gravis. Part 2. Clinical and serological follow-up of individual patients. *J Neurol Sci* 1983;58:371–385.

13. Tzartos SJ, Loutrari HV, Tang F, et al. Main immunogenic region of *Torpedo* electroplax and human muscle acetylcholine receptor: localization and microhetero-geneity revealed by the use of synthetic peptides. *J Neurochem* 1990;54:51–61.

14. Lennon VA, Seybold ME, Lindstrom JM, Cochrane C, Ulevitch R. Role of complement in the pathogenesis of experimental autoimmune myasthenia gravis. *J Exp Med* 1978;147:973–983.

15. Corey AL, Richman DP, Agius MA, Wollmann RL. Refractoriness to a second episode of experimental myasthenia gravis: correlation with AChR concentration and morphologic appearance of the postsynaptic membrane. *J Immunol* 1987;138: 3269–3275.

16. Gomez CM, Richman DP. Chronic experimental autoimmune myasthenia gravis induced by monoclonal antibody to acetycholine receptor: biochemical and electro-physiological criteria. *J Immunol* 1987;139:73–76.

17. Maselli RA, Richman DP, Wollmann RL. Inflammation at the neuromuscular junction in myasthenia gravis. *Neurology* 1991;41:1497–1504.

18. Gomez CM, Richman DP. Anti-acetylcholine receptor antibodies directed against the alpha bungarotoxin binding site induce a unique form of experimental myasthenia. *Proc Natl Acad Sci USA* 1983;80:4089–4093.

19. Drachman DB, Adams RN, Josifek LF, Self SG. Functional activities of autoantibodies to acetylcholine receptors and the clinical severity of myasthenia gravis. *N Engl J Med* 1982;307:769–775.

20. Dupont BL, Twaddle GM, Richman DP. Suppression of passive transfer acute experimental myasthenia by F(Ab')2 fragments. *J Neuroimmunol* 1987;16:47.

21. Howard FM, Lennon VA, Finley J, Matsumoto J, Elveback LR. Clinical correlations of antibodies that bind, block or modulate human acetylcholine receptors in myasthenia gravis. *Ann NY Acad Sci* 1987;505:526–538.

22. Vincent A, Newsom-Davis J. Anti-acetycholine receptor antibodies. *J Neurol Neurosurg Psychiatry* 1980;43:590–600.

23. Maselli RA, Ellis W, Mandler RN, et al. Cluster of wound botulism in California: clinical, electrophysiologic, and pathologic study. *Muscle Nerve* 1997;20:1284–1295.

24. Kaminski, HJ. Acetylcholine receptor epitopes in ocular myasthenia. *Ann NY Acad Sci* 1998;841:309–319.

25. Lennon VA. Serological diagnosis of myasthenia gravis and the Lambert Eaton myasthenic syndrome. In: Lisak RP, ed. *Handbook of Myasthenia Gravis and Myasthenic Syndromes*. New York, Marcel Dekker, 1994, pp. 149–164.

26. Lang B, Richardson G, Rees J, Vincent A, Newsom-Davis J. Plasma from myasthenia gravis patients reduces acetylcholine receptor agonist-induced Na+ flux into TE671 cell line. *J Neuroimmunol* 1988;19:141–148.

27. Bufler J, Pitz R, Czep M, Wick M, Franke C. Purified IgG from seropositive and seronegative patients with myasthenia gravis reversibly blocks currents through nicotinic acetylcholine receptor channels. *Ann Neurol* 1998;43:458–464.

28. Murakami M, Hosoi Y, Araki O, et al. Expression of thyrotropin receptors in rat thymus. *Life Sci* 2001;68:2781–2787.

29. Aarli J. Myasthenia gravis and thymoma. In: Lisak RP, ed. *Handbook of Myasthenia Gravis and Myasthenic Syndromes*. New York, Marcel Dekker, 1994, pp. 207–224.

30. Lefvert AK, Bergstrom K, Mattel G, Osterman PO, Pirksanen R. Determination of acetycholine receptor antibody in myasthenia gravis: clinical usefulness and pathogenetic implications. *J Neurol Neurosurg Psychiatry* 1978;41:394–403.

31. Strauss AJ, Seegal BC, Hsu JC, et al. Immunofluorescence demonstration of a muscle binding, complement fixing serum globulin fraction in myasthenia gravis. *Proc Soc Exp Biol (NY)* 1960;195:184–191.
32. Aarli JA, Stefansson K, Marton LSG, Wollmann RL. Patients with myasthenia gravis and thymoma have in their sera IgG autoantibodies against titin. *Clin Exp Immunol* 1990;82:284–288.
33. Skeie GO, Lunde PK, Sejersted OM, et al. Autoimmunity against the ryanodine receptor in myasthenia gravis. *Acta Physiol Scand* 2001;171:379–384.
34. Romi F, Skeie GO, Aarli JA, Gilhus NE. Muscle autoantibodies in subgroups of myasthenia gravis patients. *J Neurol* 2000;247:369–375.
35. Romi F, Skeie GO, Aarli JA, Gilhus NE.The severity of myasthenia gravis correlates with the serum concentration of titin and ryanodine receptor antibodies. *Arch Neurol* 2000;57:1596–1600.
36. Romi F. Muscle autoantibodies in myasthenia gravis (MG): clinical, immunological and therapeutic implications. Thesis, University of Bergen, 2001.
37. Mygland A,Vincent A, Newsom-Davis J, et al. Autoantibodies in thymoma-associated myasthenia gravis with myositis or neuromyotonia. *Arch Neurol* 2000;57: 527–531.
38. Lee E-K, Maselli RA, Ellis WG, Agius MA. Morvan's fibrillary chorea: a paraneoplastic manifestation of thymoma. *J Neurol Neurosurg Psychiatry* 1998;65:857–862.
39. Agius MA, Zhu S, Kirvan CA, et al. Rapsyn antibodies in myasthenia gravis. *Ann NY Acad Sci* 1998;841:516–524.
40. Hagiwara H, Enomoto-Nakatani S, Sakai K, et al. Stiff-person syndrome associated with invasive thymoma: a case report. *Neurol Sci* 2001;193:59–62.
41. Buckley C, Newsom-Davis J, Willcox N, Vincent A. Do titin and cytokine antibodies in MG patients predict thymoma or thymoma recurrence? *Neurology* 2001; 57:1579–1582.
42. Mossman S, Vincent A, Newsom-Davis J. Myasthenia gravis without acetylcholine-receptor antibody: a distinct disease entity. *Lancet* 1986;1:116–119.
43. Evoli A, Batocchi AP, Lo Monaco M, et al. Clinical heterogeneity of seronegative myasthenia gravis. *Neuromuscul Disord* 1996;6:155–161.
44. Blaes F, Beeson D, Plested P, Lang B, Vincent A. IgG from "seronegative" myasthenia gravis patients binds to a muscle cell line, TE671, but not to human acetylcholine receptor. *Ann Neurol* 2000;47:504–510.
45. Yamamoto T, Vincent, A. Ciulla TA, et al. Seronegative myasthenia gravis: a plasma factor inhibiting agonist-induced acetylcholine receptor function copurifies with IgM. *Ann Neurol* 1991;30:550–557.
46. Plested CP, Newsom-Davis J, Vincent A. Seronegative myasthenia plasmas and non-IgG fractions transiently inhibit nAChR function. *Ann NY Acad Sci* 1998;841: 501–504.
47. Hoch W, McConville J, Helms S, et al. Autoantibodies to the receptor tyrosine kinase MuSK in patients with myasthenia gravis without acetylcholine receptor antibodies. *Nat Med* 2001;7:365–368.
48. Lennon VA, Lambert EH, Whittingham S, Fairbanks V. Autoimmunity in the Lambert-Eaton myasthenic syndrome. *Muscle Nerve* 1982;5:S21–S25.

49. Newsom-Davis J, Murray NM. Plasma exchange and immunosuppressive drug treatment in the Lambert-Eaton myasthenic syndrome. *Neurology* 1984;34:480–485.
50. Fukunaga H, Engel AG, Osame M, Lambert EH. Paucity and disorganization of presynaptic membrane active zones in the Lambert-Eaton myasthenic syndrome. *Muscle Nerve* 1982;5:686–697.
51. Fukuoka T, Engel AG, Lang B, et al. Lambert-Eaton myasthenic syndrome: I. Early morphological effects of IgG on the presynaptic membrane active zones. *Ann Neurol* 1987;22:139–199.
52. Roberts A, Perera S, Lang B, Vincent A, Newsom-Davis J. Paraneoplastic myasthenic syndrome IgG inhibits $^{45}Ca^{2+}$ flux in a human small cell carcinoma line. *Nature* 1985;317:737–739.
53. Johnston I, Lang B, Leys K, Newsom-Davis J. Heterogeneity of calcium channel autoantibodies detected using a small cell lung cancer line derived from a Lambert-Eaton syndrome patient. *Neurology* 1994;44:334–338.
54. Viglione MP, O'Shaughnessy TJ, Kim Y. Inhibition of calcium currents and exocytosis by Lambert-Eaton myasthenic syndrome antibodies in human lung cancer cells. *J Physiol Lond* 1995;488:303–317.
55. Protti DA, Reisen R, MacKinley TA, Uchitel OD. Calcium channel blockers and transmitter release at the normal human neuromuscular junction. *Neurology* 1996;46:1391–1396.
56. Pinto A, Gillard S, Moss F, et al. Human autoantibodies specific for $\alpha_{1A}$ calcium channel subunit reduce both P-type and Q-type calcium currents in cerebellar neurones. *Proc Natl Acad Sci USA* 1998;95:8328–8333.
57. Espiritu DJ, Watkins M, Dia-Monje V, et al. Venomous cone snails: molecular phylogeny and the generation of toxin diversity. *Toxicon* 2001;39:1899–1916.
58. Sher E, Comola M, Nemni R, Canal N, Clementi F. Calcium channel autoantibody and non-small-cell lung cancer in patients with Lambert-Eaton syndrome. *Lancet* 1990;335:413.
59. Motomura M, Johnston I, Lang B, Vincent A, Newsom-Davis J. An improved diagnostic assay for Lambert-Eaton myasthenic syndrome. *J Neurol Neurosurg Psychiatry* 1995;58:85–87.
60. Lennon VA, Kryzer TJ, Greismann GE, et al. Calcium channel antibodies in the Lambert-Eaton myasthenic syndrome and other paraneoplastic syndromes. *N Engl J Med* 1995;332:1467–1474.
61. Motomura M, Lang B, Johnston I, Palace J, Vincent A, Newsom-Davis J. Incidence of serum anti-P/Q-type and anti-N-type calcium channel autoantibodies in the Lambert-Eaton myasthenic syndrome. *J Neurol Sci* 1997;147:35–42.
62. Bain PG, Motomura M, Newsom-Davis J, et al. Effects of intravenous immunoglobulin on muscle weakness and calcium channel antibodies in the Lambert-Eaton myasthenic syndrome. *Neurology* 1996;47:678–683.
63. Mason WP, Graus F, Lang B, et al. Paraneoplastic cerebellar degeneration and small-cell carcinoma. *Brain* 1997;120:1279–1300.
64. Trivedi R, Mundanthanan G, Amyes L, Lang B, Vincent A. Which antibodies are worth testing in subacute cerebellar ataxia? *Lancet* 2000;356:565–566.
65. Sinha S, Newsom-Davis J, Mills K, et al. Autoimmune aetiology for acquired neuromyotonia (Isaacs' syndrome). *Lancet* 1991;338:75–77.

66. Sonoda Y, Arimura K, Kurono A, et al. Serum of Isaacs' syndrome suppresses potassium channels in PC-12 cell lines. *Muscle Nerve* 1996;19:1439–1446.
67. Arimura K, Watanabe O, Kitajima I, et al. Antibodies to potassium channels of PC12 in serum of Isaacs' syndrome: Western blot and immunohistochemical studies. *Muscle Nerve* 1997;20:299–305.
68. Nagado T, Arimura K, Sonoda Y, et al. Potassium current suppression in patients with peripheral nerve hyperexcitability. *Brain* 1999;122:2057–2066.
69. Harvey AL, Rowan EG, Vatanpour H, et al. Potassium channel toxins and transmitter release. *Ann NY Acad Sci* 1994;710:1–10.
70. Hart IK, Waters C, Vincent A, et al. Autoantibodies detected to expressed $K^+$ channels are implicated in neuromyotonia. *Ann Neurol* 1997;41:238–246.
71. Buckley C, Oger J, Clover L, et al. Potassium channel antibodies in two patients with reversible limbic encephalitis. *Ann Neurol* 2001;50:73–78.
72. Liguori R, Vincent A, Clover L, et al. Morvan's syndrome: peripheral and central nervous system and cardiac involvement with antibodies to voltage-gated potassium channels. *Brain* 2001;124:2417–2426.
73. Levy LM, Dalakas MC, Floeter MK. The stiff-person syndrome: an autoimmune disorder affecting neurotransmission of gamma-aminobutyric acid. *Ann Intern Med* 1999;131:522–530.
74. Dalakas, MC, Li M, Fujii M, Jacobowitz DM. Quantification, specificity, and intrathecal synthesis of $GAD_{65}$ antibodies. *Neurology* 2001;57:780–784.
75. Sohnlein P, Muller M, Syren K, et al. Epitope spreading and a varying but not disease-specific GAD65 antibody response in Type I diabetes. The Childhood Diabetes in Finland Study Group. *Diabetologia* 2000;43:210–217.
76. Schmierer K, Valdueza JM, Bender A, et al. Atypical stiff-person syndrome with spinal MRI findings, amphiphysin autoantibodies, and immunosuppression. *Neurology* 1998;51:250–252.
77. Butler MH, Hayashi A, Ohkoshi N, et al. Autoimmunity to gephyrin in stiff-man syndrome. *Neuron* 2000;26:307–312.

# 9

# Treatment of Myasthenia Gravis

## Henry J. Kaminski

## INTRODUCTION

In 1895, Jolly used the Greek terms for "muscle" and "weakness" to form *myasthenia* and the Latin *gravis* for "severe" to describe a condition manifesting with fatiguing strength that often led to death *(1,2)*. Treatment for myasthenia gravis (MG) began in the 1930s. Edgeworth *(3,4)*, a physician with MG, treated herself with ephedrine and described its benefit in a placebo-controlled trial. The drug is still used and advocated by some patients, but the primary effect is as a central nervous system stimulant with only minor influences on neuromuscular transmission *(5)*. Walker, as a house officer at St. Alfege's in the United Kingdom, appreciated the similarity of MG to curare poisoning, which was treated with physostigmine. She administered physostigmine to a patient with MG, and prompt improvement in ptosis was seen *(6,7)*.

In the late 1800s, it had been appreciated that MG patients often had pathology of the thymic gland *(8)*. Blalock, a cardiothoracic surgeon at Johns Hopkins, encountered a 19-year-old woman who had suffered for years with worsening relapsing and remitting weakness consistent with MG *(9,10)*. A chest radiograph demonstrated a mediastinal mass. After Blalock removed a thymic cyst, the patient improved significantly. He later reported on six patients who all improved postoperatively *(11,12)*. With these reports thymectomy became an established treatment, although its efficacy is debated *(13,14)*.

Initial results of adrenocorticotropic hormone treatment of MG were not impressive, and widespread use of prednisone did not occur until the 1970s *(13)*. Several immunosuppressive agents were used to treat MG in the 1960s, with azathioprine becoming an established treatment during the 1970s. In 1976, plasma exchange was identified as an effective acute treatment for severe MG and also served to support the presence of circulating factors as a cause of MG *(15)*. The current common treatments of intravenous immunoglobin (IVIg), cyclosporine, and mycofenilate mofetil came into use in the final two decades of the last century.

From: *Current Clinical Neurology: Myasthenia Gravis and Related Disorders*
Edited by: H. J. Kaminski © Humana Press Inc., Totowa, NJ

The rationale for all therapies for MG is compromised by the lack of well-designed investigations with appropriate statistical power to draw firm conclusions of efficacy. This situation results from the difficulty of studying a disease that has a variable presentation and course, a low incidence and prevalence, a lack of agreed-on clinical scales to measure outcome, and poor cooperation in clinical trials among major centers that care for patients with MG *(16,17)*. Treatment recommendations vary among experts in the field *(18–23)*. The discussion that follows therefore reflects the author's personal experiences and his interpretation of previous studies.

## PATIENT EDUCATION AND EVALUATION

In my experience, patient education is among the most important factors in allowing patients to adjust to a chronic illness with variable prognosis that often requires treatments with poor side effect profiles. Care of the MG patient begins with a thorough discussion of the natural history, treatment options, and disease pathogenesis. The patient, family, and other interested parties should all participate in this discussion. Psychological adjustment is difficult in an illness in which definite predictions of outcome cannot be made and patients fear the development of incapacitating weakness. These fears may limit functional improvement despite significant resolution of myasthenic weakness. The neurologist should attempt to strike a balance between the difficulties in treating MG and the hope of complete remission. Patients should be directed to the MG Foundation of America and other national MG organizations for additional information. The MG Foundation of America maintains an Internet site (www.myasthenia.org), which provides excellent resources on various aspects of the disease. Support group services provided by local chapters of the Foundation are of particular benefit to patients.

A list of medications that may exacerbate myasthenic weakness should be given to each patient. Those medications, which are particularly prone to compromise patient strength, are listed in **Table 1**. The MG Foundation of America maintains a complete and current list on their website. Counseling must indicate that these medications may be used, if indicated for other medical reasons, but that caution needs to be exercised. The patient should inform other health care professionals of the MG diagnosis. Because of these patients' special needs and the unfamiliarity of many therapists, physicians, and nurses with MG, the neurologist may wish to provide the patient's referring physicians with general information regarding MG. All patients should undergo certain evaluations at the time of diagnosis, as described below.

*Computed tomography* (CT) or magnetic resonance imaging (MRI) of the chest for detection of thymoma is indicated. Because CT is less expensive

**Table 1**
**Drugs That Frequently Exacerbate Myasthenia Gravis**

| | |
|---|---|
| **Antibiotics and antimicrobials** | **Central nervous system drugs** |
| Neomycin, kanamycin, streptomycin, gentamycin, tobramycin, amikacin, polymyxin B, colistins, tetracyclines, lincomycin, clindamycin, erythromycin, ampicillin, imipenem, clarithromycin, emetine, ciprofloxacin | Diphenylhydantoin (phenytoin), trimethadione[a] lithium, chlorpromazine, trihexyphenidyl |
| **Antirheumatic agents** | **Other drugs** |
| D-penicillamine[a], chloroquine[a], prednisone | Procaine/lidocaine, D,L-carnitine, lactate, methoxyflurane, magnesium, contrast agents, citrate anticoagulation, |
| **Cardiovascular drugs** | aprotinin (Trasylol®), ritonavir, |
| β-Blockers, quinidine, procainamide, verapamil, trimethaphan | levonorgestrel, desferrioxamine, interferon-α[a], pyrantel pamoate |

[a]Induction of autoimmune disorder.

and no indication exists that MRI is more sensitive or specific, I prefer CT *(24)*. Seybold *(25)* argues strongly that plain chest X-rays are best for the pediatric age group because of the extreme rarity of thymoma in this population. However, I would argue that the test with greater sensitivity is preferred when screening a population with a low likelihood of disease. It must be expected that false positives will occur, but since most patients undergo therapeutic thymectomy, a false-positive result is not of clinical significance. However, not identifying a thymoma in a patient who chooses not to undergo thymectomy is deleterious. Although striational antibodies are associated with thymoma, they are not of adequate sensitivity or specificity to eliminate the need for imaging *(26)*. Patients with positive striatonal antibodies who choose not to undergo thymectomy or are beyond the age typically treated with thymectomy may require serial imaging for the detection of a thymoma.

*Tuberculin skin tests* in anticipation of future corticosteroid treatment are performed because of the possibility that such treatment could activate dormant tuberculosis.

I routinely *screen for thyroid dysfunction* because of the high frequency of coincidence with MG and the benefit to myasthenic manifestations that patients may derive in treatment of thyroid abnormalities. Systemic lupus erythematosis, rheumatoid arthritis, and vitamin $B_{12}$ deficiency are associated with MG, and screening test should be performed if clinically indicated.

IgA deficiency is estimated to have a prevalence of 1 in 1000, and treatment of such patients with intravenous immunoglobulin (IVIg) may lead to life-threatening allergic reactions *(27)*. This has led to the recommendation that all patients be screened for the presence of IgA prior to IVIg treatment. Consideration may be given to screening for IgA deficiency in anticipation of IVIg therapy to avoid delay in initiation of treatment in emergency situations.

## TREATMENT

Treatment choices must be individualized based on the severity of the disease, the patient's lifestyle and career, associated medical conditions, and assessment of the risk and benefit of various therapies. For example, a young woman with an active career may require immunosuppressive treatment as long as she appreciates cosmetic and reproductive issues. An older individual with a sedentary lifestyle and mild general weakness may do well with cholinesterase inhibitors. The prognosis of MG is generally good. Generalized MG is no longer the grave disease it once was, and lifespans approach normal *(28)*, from a combination of modern critical care and immunosuppressive therapy. However, quality of life remains compromised *(29)*, in large part due to immunosuppressive therapies with poor side effect profiles. Formal studies are needed to assess the level of disability that MG patients suffer.

The complications of immunosuppressive treatment need thorough explanation, and the patient and physician must work together to optimize the care plan. In developed countries without comprehensive medical payment programs for their citizens, such as the United States, medication cost needs to be considered in making treatment choices (**Table 2**). If a patient has insurance with a drug benefit, the physician is not limited, and in my experience, all insurance companies approve use of the medications listed in **Table 2** for treatment of MG. Nearly all companies also have established programs to provide medications at reduced cost for patients who can demonstrate financial need. The website, www.needymeds.com, maintains contact information for such programs.

### *Cholinesterase Inhibitors*

Acetylcholinesterase (AChE) inhibitors, which retard the hydrolysis of acetylcholine at the neuromuscular junction, are the initial treatment for MG. Pyridostigmine bromide (Mestinon®) is the most commonly used agent. Initial therapy begins at doses of 30–60 mg of pyridostigmine, and dosing intervals of pyridostigmine are set at 3–6 h depending on symptoms (120 Mestinon 60-mg tablets typically cost $60 at the time of this writing.) Individual doses of >180 mg are rarely effective. Because of erratic absorption,

**Table 2**
**Cost Comparisons of Myasthenia Gravis Treatments**

| Treatment | Cost[a] |
|---|---|
| Prednisone 20 mg | 100 tablets $17.49 |
| Azathioprine (150 mg/day) | $122/month, generic; $198/month, brand name |
| Cyclosporine (200 mg/day) | $378/month, Neoral® |
| Mycophenolate mofetil (2 g/day) | $656/month, Cellcept® |

[a]From University Hospitals of Cleveland Outpatient Pharmacy.

**Table 3**
**Equivalent Doses of Cholinesterase Inhibitor Medications**

| Medication | Oral | Intramuscular | Intravenous |
|---|---|---|---|
| Pyridostigmine bromide | 60 mg | 2.0 mg | 0.7 mg |
| Neostigmine bromide | 15 mg | None | None |
| Neostigmine methylsulfate | None | 0.5 | 0.5 mg |
| Ambenonium | 7.5 mg | None | None |

variability in patient activity levels, severity of disease, and degrees of muscarinic side effects, strict dosing guidelines cannot be recommended. Once patients become aware of the effects of pyridostigmine on their symptoms and the adverse reactions to the medication, they should be able to modify the dose and timing of administration within limits set by the physician. Timed-release forms are available; they tend to have erratic absorption, but they may be useful in some patients, particularly when given at bedtime. An elixir form of pyridostigmine is available (although at the time of this writing its manufacture in the United States was temporarily discontinued). This preparation may be useful in some patients with difficulty swallowing and is easier to administer in patients with small nasogastric tubes. The manufacturer recommends crushing a tablet with a small amount of fruit juice or applesauce to provide a liquid or easy-to-swallow dose. (A Mestinon 60-mg tablet is a dose equivalent to 1 teaspoon of Mestinon syrup.) Neostigmine bromide (Prostigmin®) or ambenonium chloride (Mytelase®) are used but tend to have greater side effects and shorter periods of action (**Table 3**).

AChE inhibitor treatment is generally safe, but significant side effects may occur. If a patient has prominent bulbar muscle weakness, administration of AChE inhibitors will often not reverse weakness to an extent that a patient will be safe to swallow. Swallowing difficulties may be further worsened by excess and thick saliva, especially when concomitant treatment with antimuscarinic medications is used. Such apparent paradoxic responses should be appreciated, and a reduction of AChE inhibitors may improve symptoms. AChE inhibitors also cannot reverse respiratory muscle weakness reliably. Respiratory secretions may be increased, which complicates treatment of patients with pulmonary diseases and may actually worsen breathing. Reductions or discontinuation of AChE inhibitors may improve breathing difficulties *(30)*. Rare patients develop significant bradycardia necessitating discontinuation of the medication *(31)*.

Gastrointestinal complaints of nausea, vomiting, diarrhea, and abdominal cramps are most common but may be controlled with administration of atropine or glycopyrrolate. Muscle twitching, fasciculations, and cramps may be particularly bothersome to patients. Stretching exercises help cramps, while reassurance alleviates concerns regarding abnormal muscle movements. Rarely, patients may develop confusion from AChE inhibitor therapy.

AChE inhibitor-induced weakness ("cholinergic crisis") is frequently discussed but is rarely encountered now that effective immunosuppressive treatment is available. The use of intravenous edrophonium to determine whether muscle weakness is secondary to MG or AChE treatment is unreliable *(13,32, 33)*. If cholinergic weakness is seriously considered, then AChE therapy should be temporarily discontinued and the patient watched for improvement. In patients with myasthenic crisis, discontinuation of AChE inhibitors is recommended to limit secretions while patients are on artificial ventilation *(25)* (*see* Chap. 10).

### Corticosteroids

Corticosteroids are recommended for patients who are compromised by generalized weakness that limits their ability to function and that cannot be adequately improved by AChE inhibitors and moderation of activity *(21,22)*. Patients with respiratory or bulbar weakness generally require immunosuppression and usually will need corticosteroid therapy. Corticosteroids are the cheapest (**Table 1**), most reliable, and fastest acting of maintenance therapies for MG, but their use is complicated by a myriad of adverse effects (**Table 4**). Patients need to be made aware of expected complications and agree to institution of the medication. Some patients may not accept steroid therapy, and treatment with a slower onset of action (such as azathioprine or cyclosporine) may need to be used, often coupled with IVIg or plasma exchange.

The optimal manner of initiating corticosteroids depends on severity of weakness *(13,34–37)*. With initiation of 60–80 mg a day, 50% of patients

**Table 4**
**Immunodulating Drugs for Myasthenia Gravis and Adverse Effects**

| Treatment | Typical Dose | Major Adverse Effects |
|---|---|---|
| Prednisone | Initial doses 60–80 mg/day or 100 mg qod | Osteoporosis, weight gain with central obesity, glaucoma, cataracts, hypertension, peripheral edema, psychiatric changes (depression, mania, personality alterations), sleep disturbance, easy bruising, glucose intolerance |
| Azathioprine (Imuran®) | 1–3 mg/kg/day | Idiosyncratic flu-like reaction, leukopenia, hepatotoxicity, alopecia, teratogen, possible risk of neoplasia |
| Cyclosporine (Sandimmune®, Neoral®) | 2–3 mg/kg/day | Renal insufficiency, hypertension, gingival hyperplasia, numerous drug interactions |
| Mycophenolate mofetil (CellCept®) | 1 g bid | Anemia, leukopenia, gastrointestinal discomfort, diarrhea |

develop a worsening of strength in the first month, usually within the first few days of treatment. Sustained improvement usually begins within 2 weeks and in most patients within a month, but rare patients have a delay of 2 months. Maximal improvement usually occurs at 6 months. For patients with severe weakness, I admit the patient and institute a high-dose regimen or a rapidly increasing dosage coupled with an acute therapy, usually plasma exchange. In my opinion, the plasma exchange limits the severity of the corticoster-oid-associated increase in weakness, but this method has not been evaluated formally. Gradual initiation of corticosteroids beginning with 20 mg and increasing 5 mg every 3 days until a dose of 60–80 mg is reached decreases the frequency of exacerbation but delays the onset of improvement *(36,38, 39)*. Such a regimen may be considered in patients with moderate weakness and allows outpatient therapy. Regardless of treatment initiation, ultimately converting to a qod dosing schedule is desired to limit steroid complications *(34)*. Some advocate an every-other-day treatment with 100 mg of predni-sone at onset of therapy *(19)*. Regardless of regimen, the corticosteroid should be given as a single morning dose. High-dose solumedrol has been used, but there is no reason to believe such treatment is of greater benefit than stan-dard regimens *(40)*. Before common use of "steroid-sparing" adjunct therapy, slightly <20% of patients were able to stop corticosteroid treatment *(34)*.

During the time of corticosteroid treatment, patients often experience a lack of benefit to AChE inhibitors, and these may be tapered.

Monitoring of serum potassium and glucose as well as blood pressure and treatments to limit osteoporosis are usually necessary. Calcium, vitamin D, and bisphosphonates are indicated for most patients *(41)*. Ophthalmologic evaluation for cataracts and glaucoma should be performed on a yearly basis. Treatments for gastric ulcer prophylaxis need not be instituted unless patients have a previous history of ulcer disease or develop symptoms of gastric irritation.

## Mechanism of Action

Corticosteroids have numerous effects on the immune system leading to general immunosuppression *(27,42,43)*. The therapeutic effects for MG appear to be related to 1) reductions of lymphocyte differentiation and proliferation; 2) redistribution of lymphocytes from the circulation into tissues that remove them from sites of immunoreactivity; 3) alterations of lymphokine function (primarily tumor necrosis factor, interleukin-1, and interleukin-2); and 4) inhibition of macrophage function, in particular antigen processing and presentation. Acetylcholine receptor (AChR) antibody levels decrease in the first few months of therapy. Also, corticosteroids may exert their benefit in MG by increasing the muscle's AChR synthesis.

## Azathioprine

Azathioprine may be used alone or in combination with corticosteroids *(44–48)*. It is critical for the patient to receive a dose based on total body weight (1–3 mg/kg/day in divided doses) since underdosing may lead to the false impression of a lack of efficacy. Both the physician and patient need to be cognizant that improvement is gradual. Only after 3–9 months will improvement be appreciated, which may continue for 2 years after initiation of treatment. Improvement appears to correlate with elevations of mean red blood cell volume *(45)* and reduction of white blood cell count. If either of these is not observed, then the dose may be increased to its maximum. If white blood cell counts fall below 3000–3500 white blood cells/mm$^3$, the dose needs to be reduced and adjusted to maintain counts above 3500. Levels below 1000 white blood cells/mm$^3$ require discontinuation of the drug *(19,49)*.

In the United States 10% of patients in the first 2 weeks of initiation of azathioprine develop fever and flu-like symptoms necessitating discontinuation of the medication. This reaction is not prominently observed in Europe and perhaps is related to differences in formulation of the tablets. Mild hepatotoxicity may manifest with elevations of serum transaminase levels, but usually without clinically evident liver disease. Azathioprine needs to be discontinued if transaminase levels double. Monitoring of liver function tests and complete blood counts are necessary throughout the treatment course. Pancreatitis rarely occurs with azathioprine treatment. Allopurinol reduces metabolism of azathioprine necessitating reduction of dose by one-third to avoid complications. There is an increased risk of neoplasm, primarily lymphoma, in patients taking azathioprine for organ rejection and some autoimmune disorders *(50)*. This risk has not been confirmed among patients with MG, but it needs to be explained to the patient *(44)*. The agent also has teratogenic potential, and it is generally advised that women and men planning a pregnancy discontinue its use *(19)*. However, one report of MG patients receiving azathioprine during pregnancy did not note any birth defects *(51)*.

Azathioprine is a purine analog, which inhibits synthesis of nucleic acids. The drug is converted to 6-mercaptopurine and metabolized to 6-thioguanine nucleotides, which are the cytotoxic agents *(52,53)*. Thiopurine *S*-methyltransferase and xanthine oxidase oppose formation of 6-thioguanine nucleotides. Patients with thiopurine *S*-methyltransferase deficiency are at risk for severe reactions and should be identified by red cell thiopurine *S*-methyltransferase enzyme activity prior to initiation of azathioprine therapy.

## Mechanism of Action

The primary effect on the immune system is interference with T- and B-cell proliferation. Coupled with plasma exchange, azathioprine may offer relative selectivity for interference with the anti-AChR autoimmune response *(54)*. This is because depletion in blood immunoglobulin after plasma exchange would induce a compensatory increase in antibody-producing B-cells. Activated anti-AChR B-cells would respond vigorously and therefore may be preferentially affected by azathioprine.

## Cyclosporine

Cyclosporine has been used to treat MG patients with severe MG responding poorly to corticosteroids and thymectomy *(55,56)*. Doses of 5 mg/kg/day in two divided doses have been recommended. Although cyclosporine works more quickly than azathioprine, the patient and physician still cannot expect a response for several months after starting treatment. In a retrospective review, 55 of 57 patients who took cyclosporine for an average of 3½ years showed clinical improvement, usually occurring in <7 months. Corticosteroids were discontinued or decreased in nearly all the patients taking them *(56)*. Five percent could not afford or tolerate the drug *(56)*. I have found that lower doses may be initiated (2–3 mg/kg/day) with similar benefit. However,

**Table 5**
**Major Drug Interactions with Cyclosporine**

**Agents that increase cyclosporine levels**
  Erythromycin, ketoconazole, metoclopramide, cimetidine, diltiazem,
  nicardipine, verapamil, oral contraceptives, bromocriptine
**Agents that decrease cyclosporine levels**
  Rifampin, imipenem, nafcillin, trimethoprim, phenytoin, phenobarbital,
  carbamazepine
**Agents that may exacerbate renal insufficiency**
  Aminoglycoside antibiotics, trimethoprim, ciprofloxacin, amphotericin,
  ketoconazole, acyclovir, cimetidine, ranitidine, nonsteroidal antiinflammatory
  agents, captopril, furosemide (Lasix®)
**Special precautions**
  Elevation of serum potassium: angiotensin-converting enzyme inhibitors
  myopathy: statins (cholesterol-lowering agents)

such an approach requires rigorous evaluation. Cyclosporine may be used
alone, and this approach does have the advantage of avoiding corticosteroid
side effects *(22)*. Some advocate monitoring of drug levels to achieve a trough
level of 75–150 ng/mL *(49)*, but it is not clear that a specific level needs to be
maintained. Monitoring of drug levels may only be of benefit to ensure compliance and in patients on medications that affect cyclosporine metabolism.

The primary side effects of cyclosporine are renal insufficiency and hypertension. Creatinine measures need to be monitored throughout treatment
with cyclosporine. In the study of Ciafaloni et al. *(56)*, 16 patients had serum
creatinine elevations of 30–70% above pretreatment values (mean 48%). Five
patients required discontinuation of cyclosporine because the creatinine value
did not fall despite dose reduction. These patients were older than 62 years,
and the renal toxicity occurred 3–11 years after initiation of therapy. Cyclosporine has many drug interactions, which are reviewed in **Table 5**.

*Mechanism of Action*

Cyclosporine is derived from a fungus and is a cyclic undecapeptide with
actions directed exclusively toward T-cells. Cyclosporine blocks T-helper
cell synthesis of cytokines, in particular interleukin-2 and interleukin-2 surface receptors. The agent also interferes with transcription of genes critical
in T-cell function. Cyclosporine suppresses T-helper cell-dependent function, maintains tolerance in transplant patients, and prevents experimental
autoimmune MG *(50)*.

## Mycophenolate Mofetil

Two studies indicate that mycophenolate mofetil (MM; CellCept®) is an effective treatment for MG by reducing corticosteroid dose, improving strength, and reducing AChR antibody levels *(57,58)*. Greater experience is needed to define its role in the treatment of MG. MM is given at the standard dose of 1 g twice daily. In the patients reported, adverse effects were limited to gastrointestinal upset and anemia. Leukopenia may also occur. Although no information in humans regarding the risk of birth defects is available, animal studies indicate a teratogenic potential, and it is recommended that women of child-bearing years be informed of this and birth control offered. Experience from studies of transplant patients indicates that there is an increased risk of lymphoma with MM treatment *(59)*. Information regarding drug interactions is limited. Cholestyramine and antacids may reduce MM blood levels.

### Mechanism of Action

MM is another agent commonly used to treat transplant rejection with effects primarily on T- and B-cell proliferation through inhibition of guanosine nucleotide synthesis *(60,61)*. MM is hydrolyzed to mycophenolic acid, which inhibits inosine monophosphate dehydrogenase, the rate-limiting enzyme in synthesis of guanosine nucleotides. Mycophenolic acid is a more potent inhibitor of the dehydrogenase isoform expressed in activated lymphocytes, leading to its preferential immunosuppressant properties. Additional mechanism of immunosuppression include 1) apoptosis of activated T-lymphocytes; 2) alterations in cell adhesion molecule expression, decreasing recruitment of lymphocytes to sites of inflammation; and 3) reduction of inducible nitric oxide synthase activity.

### Plasma Exchange

Plasma exchange (plasmapheresis) produces rapid improvement in weakness regardless of whether patients are seronegative or -positive for anti-AChR antibody *(62,63)*. It is used in myasthenic crisis as well as to optimize muscle function prior to surgery, including thymectomy. The exchanges may be performed in an outpatient setting and (depending on the skill of the exchange technicians) often through peripheral venous catheters. Typically exchanges are done to remove 1–2 plasma volumes three times a week for up to six exchanges. In my experience, more than 6 exchanges during a single course are not beneficial, but others describe benefit after 14 exchanges *(49)*. Patients may show improvement within 48 h of the first or second exchange and continue to improve during an exchange course. Treatment reduces immunoglobulin levels rapidly; however, rebound may occur in weeks, leading to clinical worsening if concomitant immunosuppressive treatment is not used *(64)*. In rare patients, plasma exchange is used as a chronic therapy, but this has not been formally studied. The exchange is usually performed with resins that remove proteins at certain molecular weights, and studies of immuno-absorbent resins do not demonstrate any superiority to standard resins *(65,66)*.

The general usefulness of plasma exchange is limited by its restriction to major medical centers and the frequent need for large-bore intravenous catheters. During the infusion patients may complain of paresthesias from citrate-induced hypocalcemia, and hypotension may occur at initiation of the exchange. Some patients have nausea and vomiting related to fluid shifts and electrolyte alterations during the exchange. Infectious and thrombotic complications related to venous access occur *(67,68)*. The exchange process reduces coagulation factors, and concomitant use of heparin in the care of venous catheters may reduce platelet levels, leading to bleeding tendencies. Thrombotic complications also occur *(19)*.

*Mechanism of Action*

Removal of circulating pathogenic antibody, and in all likelihood other agents such as complement proteins, produces the clinical benefits of plasma exchange. The removal of antibodies that block AChR function may be primary in mediating the rapid improvement produced in some patients by plasma exchange. However, in patients with severe disease, the weakness is related to destruction of the endplate, which would not be expected to resolve in a few days. Therefore, it is likely that other mechanisms are important in mediating the therapeutic effect of plasma exchange.

**Intravenous Immunoglobulin**

IVIg is used in similar circumstances as plasma exchange *(69–71)*. The standard treatment regimen is a 4–6-h infusion of 400 mg/kg/day for 5 days, but some advocate a 1 g/kg/day dose for 2 days *(27,72)*. The latter can be administered without a higher rate of complications; however, in older patients with cardiac disease the lower dose regimen may be prudent. IVIg therapy improves strength rapidly, often within 5 days of initiation, and lowers AChR antibodies, but the response is short-lived and not uniformly observed *(73)*. A retrospective study comparing IVIg and plasma exchange for treatment of myasthenic crisis showed that patients had a better respiratory and functional outcome with plasma exchange, but IVIg had fewer complications *(67)*. A randomized trial compared three exchanges with either 3 or 5 days of IVIg (400 mg/kg/day) and showed a similar efficacy; again, IVIg had fewer adverse effects *(68)*. IVIg may also be used as maintenance therapy to limit corticosteroid dosage while other agents (such as cyclosporine or azathio-prine) are taking effect.

Adverse effects with IVIg occur commonly, but most are minor *(27,74, 75)*. Headache occurs frequently during infusion. Mild headaches may be treated with acetaminophen or nonsteroidal antiinflammatory drugs. (Since MG patients are frequently receiving corticosteroids, nonsteroidals should be used with caution to limit gastrointestinal irritation.) More severe migraine headaches occur, particularly in patients with a history of migraine. In appropriate individuals, triptan agents may be used. Aseptic meningitis may occur and recur with subsequent treatments. Some claim that prophylaxis with non-steroidal antiinflammatory drugs may be of benefit, but others disagree *(27, 74)*. Chills, myalgia, or chest discomfort may occur early during the infusion and usually resolves with stopping the infusion for 30 min and resuming at a slower rate. Flu-like symptoms may occur in the days following treatment, and some patients are described as having a transient worsening of strength *(76)*. Urticaria, lichenoid cutaneous lesions, pruritus of the palms, and pete-chiae may occur within days or weeks of treatment and may resolve over weeks to months *(77)*.

Rarely, significant complications occur with IVIg therapy. Anaphylactic reactions occur in patients with IgA deficiency, which may be present in 1 in 1000 people *(27)*. This deficiency should be screened for prior to infusion, and consideration may be given to provide an IVIg preparation depleted of IgA to deficient individuals *(78)*. Acute renal tubular necrosis, which is usually reversible, occurs in patients who have renal insufficiency. Age over 65, diabetes, and dehydration increase the risk of renal injury. Renal failure is associated with the high concentration of sucrose in one proprietary IVIg product but occurs with other preparations *(74)*. Diluting the IVIg preparation and slowing the rate of infusion decreases the chance of renal damage. Close monitoring of creatinine and blood urea nitrogen are essential if the agent needs to be given in patients with renal insufficiency. Deep vein thrombosis, cerebral infarction, and myocardial infarction may occur. For the immobilized MG patient, physicians should be vigilant for signs of deep vein thrombosis, and appropriate prophylactic treatments should be administered.

The choice of IVIg or plasma exchange for a particular patient with myasthenic exacerbation lies in assessment of the potential risks of each therapy. Since plasma exchange is offered only at specialized centers, IVIg has the advantage of being more accessible (one caveat is the shortage of the medication in the United States at the end of the 1990s and the beginning of this century), and vascular access is usually not difficult for administration of IVIg. In patients with renal insufficiency or risks for thrombotic complications, plasma exchange may be preferred. The cost of a single course of IVIg is on the order of $10,000; outpatient plasma exchange is slightly less *(19,21)*.

## Mechanism of Action

IVIg impacts on the autoimmune process by several mechanisms including inhibition of cytokines, competition with autoantibodies, inhibition of complement deposition, interference with Fc receptor binding on macrophages or the immunoglobulins on B-cells, and interference with antigen recognition by sensitized T-cells. The work of Samuelsson et al. *(79)* suggests that effects on Fc receptor binding are of primary importance.

## Other Immunosuppressive Treatments

Individual reports and small series have described the response of MG patients to various immunosuppressant treatments. Of course, these descriptions suffer from the tendency of physicians to report only positive results. All the treatment modalities described here should only be considered in special circumstances after the failure of the treatments described above. Intravenous and oral cyclophosphamide has been used to treat MG patients resistant to corticosteroids, and one study found that half the patients were asymptomatic after 1 year *(80,81)*. The drug, however, has a poor side effect profile. Nearly all patients develop alopecia. Additional complications include diarrhea, nausea, vomiting, and hemorrhagic cystitis, which may be severe. The drug has carcinogenic and teratogenic potential as well as a likelihood of producing infertility *(50)*. Rarely, interstitial pneumonitis and hepatic injury occur.

A case report documented a treatment-resistant MG patient improving with rituxmab, a monoclonal antibody against the B-cell surface membrane marker CD20 *(82)*. I have treated a clinically similar patient without benefit. Tacrolimus (FK-506, Prograf®) has been used in animal studies and anecdotally in MG patients to improve MG-related weakness *(83,84)*. Bone marrow transplantation has been performed for the treatment of severe MG; however, given the high morbidity and mortality, such treatment is warranted only in the rarest of patients *(85,86)*. Durelli et al. *(87)* treated 12 previously thymectomized patients with low-dose total body irradiation, and 5 had significant clinical improvement for 2 years after treatment.

## THYMECTOMY IN RELATION TO OTHER TREATMENTS

This section serves only to place thymectomy in the context of other therapies; Chapter 11 describes thymectomy in detail for treatment of MG. Critical assessments of appropriately performed studies and most MG experts recommend thymectomy to increase the chance of remission or improve the clinical course *(14,23,49,88)*. The present day mortality of thymectomy approaches zero, and morbidity is low. Generally thymectomy is restricted to patients who are young, which is often defined as <60 years, and otherwise healthy enough to withstand the operative procedure. Since older patients tend to have thymic atrophy, the argument can be made that these patients would be less likely to benefit from thymectomy. Seronegative patients may improve with thymectomy *(49)*; however, some think that these patients are less likely to have thymic hyperplasia and therefore would not be expected to improve with removal of the thymus *(23)*. It is also recommended that thymectomy be performed within the first years of diagnosis because of presumed better efficacy *(38)*. If a patient is willing to undergo a thymectomy, then I see no benefit in delay, and therefore surgery should be done close to the time of diagnosis. Clinical status should be optimized by preoperative plasma exchange (I usually perform two exchanges in the week prior to operation) and, if necessary, corticosteroids initiated. Thymectomy does not cause any long-term complications or have clinically important adverse effects on the immune system.

## SPECIFIC CLINICAL SITUATIONS

### Myasthenia Gravis and Pregnancy

MG preferentially affects women in the child-bearing years, leading to particular therapeutic issues. The effect of pregnancy on the clinical course of MG is highly variable among women, and each pregnancy may effect an individual woman differently *(51)*. A patient appears to have an equal probability of worsening, staying the same, or improving during the pregnancy or postpartum period *(51,89)*. The normal weight gain and other effects of pregnancy would be expected to exacerbate the fatigue of the MG patient. Labor is an exhausting event and should be expected to weaken the symptomatic MG patient; however, most women are able to deliver vaginally without complications *(51,90)*. If preeclampsia or eclampsia is present, then the obstetrician should be made aware that intravenous magnesium sulfate is contraindicated because of its deleterious effects on neuromuscular transmission. MG should not be considered a contraindication to pregnancy for most women.

MG treatments may affect the fetus. Azathioprine, MM, and cyclosporine are potential teratogens, and every attempt should be made to discontinue the medications prior to conception. Pyridostigmine and prednisone are safe.

There are no large studies of the effect of plasma exchange or IVIg in pregnant women, but they appear to be safe. Thymectomy should be delayed until after delivery, since there is no reason to believe the delay would be deleterious compared with the potential complications of performing a major surgical procedure during pregnancy.

Approximately a third of infants of MG patients have neonatal myasthenia. This is a transient disorder manifesting in general weakness, difficulty in feeding, and respiratory insufficiency in some. Such infants require supportive care and cholinesterase treatment. Weakness resolves over weeks without any permanent weakness or risk of development of MG later in life. Development of neonatal MG is independent of the clinical status of the mother, and the mother may be asymptomatic. AChR antibody levels of the mother also do not predict occurrence of MG. An increased ratio of antibodies against the fetal AChR compared with the antibodies directed only against the adult AChR isoform correlates with the development of neonatal myasthenia *(91)*. Commercial tests for this ratio are not available. Case reports exist of infants with arthrogryposis multiplex that were due to placental passage of antibodies against the fetal AChR, which severely compromised fetal muscle development *(92–94)*. If a women with MG has a history of children with arthrogryposis multiplex or recurrent fetal loss, consideration should be given to more intensive therapy of MG during pregnancy *(94)*.

## Treatment of the Myasthenia Gravis Patient with Thymoma

Ten percent of patients with MG have a thymoma; and Chapter 6 describes thymoma-associated MG in detail. The treatment of patients with thymoma does not differ from those patients without thymoma but is complicated by the necessity to treat the neoplasm. Some studies suggest that thymoma-associated MG has a more severe clinical picture *(95)*, but all do not confirm this *(96)*. Once a thymoma is detected, it should be removed, along with the remaining thymus, although the patient should be aware that the surgery is not to cure MG. If the tumor has broken through its capsule to involve adjacent tissue, local irradiation is necessary. Thymomas generally have good prognosis, with surgical resection being curative. However, some thymomas are aggressive and produce widespread metastases. In the elderly patient with a contraindication to surgery, consideration may be given to monitoring of tumor growth by CT, since many tumors are very slow growing.

## Juvenile Myasthenia Gravis

The pathophysiology of children younger than 18 years presenting with MG is no different from that of the adult disorder. Differential diagnosis and diagnostic methods are identical to those for adults; however, treatment considerations are more difficult. Prepubertal patients appear to have higher rates of spontaneous remission, and therefore thymectomy may delayed. Corticosteroids retard growth and increase the severity of osteoporosis in adulthood. Treatment with nonsteroidal immunosuppressive drugs involves the potential dose-dependent risk of neoplasia. As in adults, treatment must be individualized, and the parents need to appreciate the complications of therapy *(97)*.

## The Treatment-Resistant Patient

Patients referred to me for a poor treatment response come in three varieties: 1) those who never had MG; 2) those with complications related to treatment; and 3) those with severe MG.

When one is faced with a patient who continues to complain of weakness, it is imperative to confirm that the diagnosis of MG is based on unequivocal clinical manifestations and supported by serologic and electrophysiologic studies. Care is further complicated if the patients have been treated for MG with AChE inhibitors, or, worse, if they have been given immunosuppressive treatments and developed complications that produced weakness or fatigue. If, on review of previous evaluation, the physician concludes that MG is not present, then the patient must be informed of the determination using the utmost sensitivity; medications for MG need to be tapered and psychiatric support provided. Even if an alternate medical diagnosis is identified as a cause of symptoms, patients will have been traumatized and will require expert psychological counseling to assist them in recovering from misdiagnosis. In my experience, patients who have been misdiagnosed with MG often have a psychiatric condition as the cause of their symptoms.

Corticosteroids produce a legion of side effects that may lead patients to complain of "fatigue," "tiredness," and "weakness," that are often not distinguished by the patient from their presenting complaints of MG. Similar complaints could occur with immunosuppressants that produce anemia. Thus the neurologist must take a detailed history to determine that symptoms (corroborated by examination) are definitely related to MG. Sleep disturbances, including sleep apnea, may complicate MG and be exacerbated by weight gain related to steroid therapy, which leads to excessive somnolence, misinterpreted as fatigue *(98)*. I have seen several patients with MG who have developed steroid myopathy after several months of daily, high-dose therapy and who were also treated aggressively with plasma exchange and other immunosuppressive treatments. These patients have proximal muscle weakness and obvious systemic complications of steroids without MG manifestations

*(99)*. Taper of steroids, in particular to an every-other-day regimen, in concert with physical therapy, led to significant functional improvement after several months.

Fortunately, MG patients with persistent weakness despite prolonged therapy (usually this means thymectomy, corticosteroids, and at least one additional modality) are rare. Appropriate dosing of medications must be confirmed, and enough time from treatment initiation needs to pass to be sure an agent would be expected to have taken effect. If these are true, then alternative treatments need to be considered. If a patient has moderate to severe weakness, then I use IVIg or plasma exchange in the hopes of bringing about relatively rapid improvement; such treatment may then be provided monthly until oral medications take effect. If corticosteroids are at low doses, then an increase may also be helpful. Coincident with these treatments, a change to another immunosuppressant is made.

## EXPERIMENTAL TREATMENTS

In spite of the success of the current therapy for MG, there remains a need for specific treatments that will eliminate the autoimmune reaction, leave other immune functions intact, and present no systemic side effects. Various methods have been attempted: 1) administration of autoantigen, or the parts of its sequence to induce tolerance; 2) depletion of AChR-specific B-cells; 3) interruption of the MHC class II molecule, epitope peptide, T-cell receptor, and CD4$^+$ molecule complex; and 4) depletion of AChR-specific T-cells *(42,54,100)*.

Peripheral tolerance treatments may prove to be effective for MG treatment. Presentation of AChR epitopes by unsuitable cells or synthetic human AChR would lead to AChR-specific CD4$^+$ cells becoming anergic. For example, B-cells from naive rats incubated with AChR under conditions favoring the uptake and processing of the AChR were fixed and used as antigen-presenting cells *(100)*. They caused unresponsiveness of AChR-specific T-cells to any further stimulation with the AChR. This approach would present all epitopes produced upon AChR processing and anergize all AChR-specific T-cells. Thus, it might be useful for the treatment of MG, perhaps using as antigen biosynthetic subunits of the human AChR.

Oral, nasal, or subcutaneous administration of AChR to rodents prevents or delays the development of experimentally acquired MG (EAMG) *(101, 102)*. Use of the complete AChR molecule for peripheral tolerization procedures in MG, however, is problematic, since 1) a large amount of AChR is required, which is difficult to obtain; 2) the dose of AChR is critical. Although low doses are effective at reducing AChR-specific CD4$^+$ responses, they may stimulate the B-cells to produce antibody, and also synthesis of certain antibody classes may be stimulated, thereby worsening the disease. Subcutaneous administration to mice of soluble AChR or short peptides with AChR sequences prior to AChR immunization prevents EAMG, but its administration after development of EAMG occasionally leads to death *(101)*.

Administration to animals with EAMG of conjugates containing a toxic compound coupled to the AChR or to synthetic peptides simulating the AChR results in elimination of the B-cells producing anti-AChR antibody *(103, 104)*. AChR docks to the anti-AChR membrane-bound antibody expressed by the B-cells, and the toxic part of the conjugate specifically kills the anti-AChR B-cells. One problem with this is that the toxins may damage other cells. Another is that anti-AChR T-helper cells can rapidly recruit B-cells to synthesize more anti-AChR antibody.

Activation of CD4$^+$ T-helper cells requires interaction and stable binding of several proteins on the surfaces of the CD4$^+$ cell and the antigen-presenting cell; interference with formation of this complex usually reduces the activity of the autoimmune CD4$^+$ cells in experimental autoimmunity. This may be done by antibody that recognizes the T-cell receptor-binding site for the antigen. Such antibodies can be passively administered or induced by immunization with the pathogenic T-cells (T-cell vaccination) or with idiotypic peptide sequences of the T-cell receptor *(105,106)*. Another approach involves the use of altered peptide ligands (APLs), which are synthetic peptide analogs of epitopes recognized by the autoimmune CD4$^+$ T-cells. They are modified to bind to the MHC class II molecule and cannot stimulate the epitope-specific CD4$^+$ cells. The APLs compete with the peptide epitopes derived from the autoantigen and shut off the autoimmune response. The APLs might also stimulate modulatory antiinflammatory CD4$^+$ cells, or anergize the pathogenic CD4$^+$ cells, causing a global reduction of the pathogenic CD4$^+$ response. Approaches that interfere with T-cell activation such as these are compromised by the diverse epitope repertoire of anti-AChR CD4$^+$ cells of MG patients. Targeting of only a few epitopes may not significantly reduce the autoimmune response. The treatments are also likely to produce only transient improvement.

Wu et al. *(107,108)* developed a method to eliminate AChR-specific T-cells specifically. They genetically engineered antigen-presenting cells with relevant portions of the AChR, the Fas ligand (to eliminate the activated AChR-specific T-cells with which they interact), and a portion of FADD, which prevented self-destruction by the Fas ligand. It remains to be seen whether such a strategy can be used to modulate EAMG.

## REFERENCES

1. Keynes G. The history of myasthenia gravis. *Med Hist* 1961;5:313–326.
2. Pascuzzi R. The history of myasthenia gravis. *Neurol Clin* 1994;12:231–242.
3. Edgeworth H. The effect of ephedrine in the treatment of myasthenia gravis, second report. *JAMA* 1933;100:1401.
4. Edgeworth H. A report of progress on the use of ephedrine in a case of myasthenia gravis. *JAMA* 1930;94:1136.
5. Sieb J, Engel A. Ephedrine: effects on neuromuscular transmission. *Brain Res* 1993; 623:167–171.
6. Walker MB. Treatment of myasthenia gravis with physostigmine. *Lancet* 1934;1: 1200–1201.
7. Keesey JC. Contemporary opinions about Mary Walker: a shy pioneer of therapeutic neurology. *Neurology* 1998;51:1433–1439.
8. Bell ET. Tumors of the thymus in myasthenia gravis. *J Nerv Ment Dis* 1917;45: 130–143.
9. Blalock A, Mason MF, Morgan HJ, Riven SS. Myasthenia gravis and tumors of the thymic region. Report of a case in which the tumor was removed. *Ann Surg* 1939;110:544–561.
10. Kirschner PA. The history of surgery of the thymus gland. *Chest Surg Clin North Am* 2000;10:153–165.
11. Blalock A, Mason MF, Morgan HJ, Riven SS. Myasthenia gravis and tumors of the thymus region: report of a case in which the tumor was removed. *Am Surg* 1939;110:544–561.
12. Blalock A, Harvey AM, Ford FF, Lilienthal JL. The treatment of myasthenia gravis by removal of the thymus gland: preliminary report. *JAMA* 1941;117:1529–1533.
13. Rowland LP. Controversies about the treatment of myasthenia gravis. *J Neurol Neurosurg Psychiatry* 1980;43:644–659.
14. Gronseth GS, Barohn RJ. Practice parameter: thymectomy for autoimmune myasthenia gravis (an evidence-based review): report of the Quality Standards Subcommittee of the American Academy of Neurology. *Neurology* 2000;55:7–15.
15. Pinching AJ, Peters DK, Newsom-Davis J. Remission of myasthenia gravis following plasma exchange. *Lancet* 1976;2:1373–1376.
16. Jaretzki A, Barohn RJ, Ernstoff RM, Kaminski HJ, et al. Myasthenia gravis: recommendations for clinical research standards. Task Force of the Medical Scientific Advisory Board of the Myasthenia Gravis Foundation of America. *Neurology* 2000;55:16–23.
17. Kissel JT, Franklin GM. Treatment of myasthenia gravis: a call to arms. *Neurology* 2000;55:3–4.
18. Kaminski H. Myasthenia gravis. In: Katirji B, Kaminski H, Preston D, Ruff R, Shapiro B, eds. *Neuromuscular Disorders in Clinical Practice*. Boston, Butterworth Heinemann, 2002, pp. 916–930.
19. Seybold ME. Treatment of myasthenia gravis. In: Engel AG, ed. *Myasthenia Gravis and Myasthenic Disorders*. Oxford, Oxford University Press, 1999, pp. 167–204.
20. Keesey J. A treatment algorithm for autoimmune myasthenia in adults. *Ann NY Acad Sci* 1998;841:753–768.
21. Bedlack RS, Sanders DB. Steroids have an important role. *Muscle Nerve* 2002;25: 117–121.

22. Rivner MH. Steroids are overutilized. *Muscle Nerve* 2002;25:115–117.
23. Newsom-Davis J, Beeson D. Myasthenia gravis and myasthenic syndromes: auto-immune and genetic disorders. In: Karpati G, Hilton-Jones D, Griggs R, eds. *Disorders of Voluntary Muscle*. Cambridge, Cambridge University Press, 2001, pp. 660–675.
24. Emskotter T, Trampe H, Lachenmayer L. Magnetic resonance imaging in myasthenia gravis. An alternative to mediastinal computerized tomography? *Dtsch Med Wochenschr* 1988;113:1508–1510.
25. Seybold ME. Diagnosis of myasthenia gravis. In: Engel AG, ed. *Myasthenia Gravis and Myasthenic Disorders*. New York, Oxford University Press, 1999, pp. 146–166.
26. Kaminski HJ, Santillan C, Wolfe GI. Autoantibody testing in neuromuscular disorders. Neuromuscular Junction and Muscle Disorders. *J Clin Neuromusc Dis* 2000; 2:96–105.
27. Dalakas MC. Immunotherapies in the treatment of neuromuscular disorders. In: Katirji B, Kaminski H, Preston D, Ruff R, Shapiro B, eds. *Neuromuscular Disorders in Clinical Practice*. Boston, Butterworth Heinemann, 2002, pp. 364–383.
28. Phillips LH, Torner JC. Epidemiologic evidence for a changing natural history of myasthenia gravis. *Neurology* 1996;47:1233–1238.
29. Paul RH, Cohen RA, Goldstein JM, Gilchrist JM. Fatigue and its impact on patients with myasthenia gravis. *Muscle Nerve* 2000;23:1402–1406.
30. Liggett SB, Daughaday CC, Senior RM. Ipratropium in patients with COPD receiving cholinesterase inhibitors. *Chest* 1988;94:210–212.
31. Arsura EL, Brunner NG, Namba T, Grob D. Adverse cardiovascular effects of anticholinesterase medications. *Am J Med Sci* 1987;293:18–23.
32. Daroff RB. Ocular myasthenia: diagnosis and therapy. In: Glaser J, ed. *Neuroophthalmology*. St. Louis, CV Mosby, 1980, pp. 62–71.
33. Daroff RB. The office tensilon test for ocular myasthenia gravis. *Arch Neurol* 1986;43:843–844.
34. Pascuzzi RM, Coslett HB, Johns TR. Long-term corticosteroid treatment of myasthenia gravis: report of 116 patients. *Ann Neurol* 1984;15:291–298.
35. Beghi E, Antozzi C, Batocchi AP, et al. Prognosis of myasthenia gravis: a multicenter follow-up study. *J Neurol Sci* 1991;106:213–220.
36. Seybold M, Drachman D. Gradually increasing doses of prednisone in myasthenia gravis: reducing the hazards of treatment. *N Engl J Med* 1974;290:81–84.
37. Grob D, Arsura EL, Brunner NG, Namba T. The course of myasthenia gravis and therapies affecting outcome. *Ann NY Acad Sci* 1987;505:472–499.
38. Durelli L, Maggi G, Casadio C, et al. Actuarial analysis of the occurrence of remissions following thymectomy for myasthenia gravis in 400 patients. *J Neurol Neurosurg Psychiatry* 1991;54:406–411.
39. Drachman DB. Myasthenia gravis. *N Engl J Med* 1994;330:1797–1810.
40. Arsura E, Brunner N, Namba T, Grob D. High-dose intravenous methylprednisolone in myasthenia gravis. *Arch Neurol* 1985;42:1149–1153.
41. Lewis SJ, Smith PE. Osteoporosis prevention in myasthenia gravis: a reminder. *Acta Neurol Scand* 2001;103:320–322.
42. Conti-Fine BM, Kaminski HJ. Autoimmune neuromuscular transmission disorders: myasthenia gravis and Lambert-Eaton myasthenic syndrome. *Continuum* 2001;7:56–93.

43. Kaminski HJ. Myasthenia gravis. In: Katirji B, Kaminski HJ, Preston D, Shapiro B, Ruff RL, eds. *Neuromuscular Disorders in Clinical Practice*. Woburn, MA, Butterworth Heinemann, 2001, pp. 916–930.

44. Hohlfeld R, Michels M, Heininger K, Besinger U, Toyka KV. Azathioprine toxicity during long-term immunosuppression of generalized myasthenia gravis. *Neurology* 1988;38:258–261.

45. Witte AS, Cornblath DR, Parry GJ, Lisak RP, Schatz NJ. Azathioprine in the treatment of myasthenia gravis. *Ann Neurol* 1984;15:602–605.

46. Kuks J, Djojoatmodjo S, Oosterhuis H. Azathioprine in myasthenia gravis: observations in 41 patients and a review of literature. *Neuromusc Disord* 1991;1:423–431.

47. Group MGCS. A randomised clinical trial comparing prednisone and azathioprine in myasthenia gravis. Results of the second interim analysis. Myasthenia Gravis Clinical Study Group. *J Neurol Neurosurg Psychiatry* 1993;56:1157–1163.

48. Palace J, Newsom-Davis J, Lecky B. A randomized double-blind trial of prednisolone alone or with azathioprine in myasthenia gravis. Myasthenia Gravis Study Group. *Neurology* 1998;50:1778–1783.

49. Sanders D, Howard F Jr. Disorders of neuromuscular transmission. In: Bradley W, Daroff R, Fenichel G, Marsden C, eds. *Neurology in Clinical Practice*. Boston, Butterworth Heinemann, 2000, pp. 2167–2185.

50. Machkhas H, Harati Y, Rolak LA. Clinical pharmacology of immunosuppressants: guidelines for neuroimmunotherapy. In: Rolak LA, Harati Y, eds. *Neuroimmunology for the Clinician*. Boston, Butterworth Heinemann, 1997, pp. 77–104.

51. Batocchi AP, Majolini L, Evoli A, et al. Course and treatment of myasthenia gravis during pregnancy. *Neurology* 1999;52:447–452.

52. Stolk JN, Boerbooms AM, de Abreu RA, et al. Reduced thiopurine methyltransferase activity and development of side effects of azathioprine treatment in patients with rheumatoid arthritis. *Arthritis Rheum* 1998;41:1858–1866.

53. Armstrong VW, Oellerich M. New developments in the immunosuppressive drug monitoring of cyclosporine, tacrolimus, and azathioprine. *Clin Biochem* 2001;34:9–16.

54. Conti-Fine B, Bellone M, Howard JJ, Protti M. *Myasthenia Gravis. The Immunobiology of an Autoimmune Disease*. Austin, TX, Neuroscience Intelligence Unit, RG Landes, 1997.

55. Tindall RSA, Phillips JT, Rollins JA, Wells L, Hall K. A clinical therapeutic trial of cyclosporine in myasthenia gravis. *Ann NY Acad Sci* 1993;681:539–551.

56. Ciafaloni E, Nikhar NK, Massey JM, Sanders DB. Retrospective analysis of the use of cyclosporine in myasthenia gravis. *Neurology* 2000;55:448–450.

57. Ciafaloni E, Massey JM, Tucker-Lipscomb B, Sanders DB. Mycophenolate mofetil for myasthenia gravis: an open-label pilot study. *Neurology* 2001;56:97–99.

58. Chaudhry V, Cornblath DR, Griffin JW, O'Brien R, Drachman DB. Mycophenolate mofetil: a safe and promising immunosuppressant in neuromuscular diseases. *Neurology* 2001;56:94–96.

59. http://www.rocheusa.com/products/cellcept/pi.html#CLINICAL. CellCept. Vol. 2002: Roche Laboratories Inc, 2000.

60. Hood KA, Zarembski DG. Mycophenolate mofetil: a unique immunosuppressive agent. *Am J Health Syst Pharm* 1997;54:285–294.

61. Allison AC, Eugui EM. Mycophenolate mofetil and its mechanisms of action. *Immunopharmacology* 2000;47:85–118.
62. Assessment of plasmapheresis. Report of the Therapeutics and Technology Assessment Subcommittee of the American Academy of Neurology. *Neurology* 1996;47: 840–843.
63. Chiu HC, Chen WH, Yeh JH. The six year experience of plasmapheresis in patients with myasthenia gravis. *Ther Apher* 2000;4:291–295.
64. Seybold ME. Plasmapheresis in myasthenia gravis. *Ann NY Acad Sci* 1987;505: 584–587.
65. Haupt WF, Rosenow F, van der Ven C, Birkmann C. Immunoadsorption in Guillain-Barré syndrome and myasthenia gravis. *Ther Apher* 2000;4:195–197.
66. Grob D, Simpson D, Mitsumoto H, et al. Treatment of myasthenia gravis by immunoadsorption of plasma. *Neurology* 1995;45:338–344.
67. Qureshi AI, Choudhry MA, Akbar MS, et al. Plasma exchange versus intravenous immunoglobulin treatment in myasthenic crisis. *Neurology* 1999;52:629–632.
68. Gajdos P, Chevret S, Clair B, Tranchant C, Chastang C. Clinical trial of plasma exchange and high-dose intravenous immunoglobulin in myasthenia gravis. Myasthenia Gravis Clinical Study Group. *Ann Neurol* 1997;41:789–796.
69. Ferrero B, Durelli L, Cavallo R, et al. Therapies for exacerrbation of myasthenia gravis. The mechanism of action of intravenous high-dose immunoglobulin. *Ann NY Acad Sci* 1993;681:563–566.
70. Gajdos P, Outin H, Elkharray D, et al. High-dose intravenous gammaglobulin for myasthenia gravis. *Lancet* 1984;1:406–407.
71. Gajdos P, Outin HD, Morel E, Raphael JC, Goulon M. High-dose intravenous gamma globulin for myasthenia gravis: an alternative to plasma exchange. *Ann NY Acad Sci* 1987;505:842–844.
72. Howard JF. Intravenous immunoglobulin for the treatment of acquired myasthenia gravis. *Neurology* 1998;51:S30–S36.
73. Uchiyama M, Ichikawa Y, Takaya M, et al. High-dose gammaglobulin therapy of generalized myasthenia gravis. *Ann NY Acad Sci* 1987;505:868–871.
74. Kazatchkine MD, Kaveri SV. Immunomodulation of autoimmune and inflammatory diseases with intravenous immune globulin. *N Engl J Med* 2001;345:747–755.
75. Brannagan TH III, Nagle KJ, Lange DJ, Rowland LP. Complications of intravenous immune globulin treatment in neurologic disease. *Neurology* 1996;47:674–677.
76. Arsura EL, Bick A, Brunner NG, Namba T, Grob D. High-dose intravenous immunoglobulin in the management of myasthenia gravis. *Arch Intern Med* 1986;146: 1365–1368.
77. Dalakas MC. Meningitis and skin reactions after intravenous immunoglobulin therapy. *Ann Intern Med* 1997;127:1130.
78. Cunningham-Rundles C, Zhou Z, Mankarious S, Courter S. Long-term use of IgA-depleted intravenous immunoglobulin in immunodeficient subjects with anti-IgA antibodies. *J Clin Immunol* 1993;13:272–278.
79. Samuelsson A, Towers TL, Ravetch JV. Anti-inflammatory activity of IVIG mediated through the inhibitory Fc Receptor. *Science* 2001;291:484–486.
80. Niakan E, Harati Y, Rolak LA. Immunosuppressive drug therapy in myasthenia gravis. *Arch Neurol* 1986;43:155–156.

81. Perez M, Buot WL, Mercado-Danguilan C, Bagabaldo ZG, Renales LD. Stable remissions in myasthenia gravis. *Neurology* 1981;31:32–37.
82. Zaja F, Russo D, Fuga G, Perella G, Baccarani M. Rituximab for myasthenia gravis developing after bone marrow transplant. *Neurology* 2000;55:1062–1063.
83. Yoshikawa H, Iwasa K, Satoh K, Takamori M. FK506 prevents induction of rat experimental autoimmune myasthenia gravis. *J Autoimmun* 1997;10:11–16.
84. Evoli A, Di Schino C, Marsili F, Punzi C. Successful treatment of myasthenia gravis with tacrolimus. *Muscle Nerve* 2002;25:111–114.
85. Euler HH, Marmont AM, Bacigalupo A, et al. Early recurrence or persistence of autoimmune diseases after unmanipulated autologous stem cell transplantation. *Blood* 1996;88:3621–3625.
86. Marmont AM. Stem cell transplantation for severe autoimmune disorders, with special reference to rheumatic diseases. *J Rheumatol Suppl* 1997;48:13–18.
87. Durelli L, Ferrio MF, Urgesi A, et al. Total body irradiation for myasthenia gravis: a long-term follow-up. *Neurology* 1993;43:2215–2221.
88. Lanska DJ. Indications for thymectomy in myasthenia gravis. *Neurology* 1990;40: 1828–1829.
89. Plauché WC. Myasthenia gravis in mothers and their newborns. *Clin Obstet Gynecol* 1991;34:82–99.
90. Mitchell PJ, Bebbington M. Myasthenia gravis in pregnancy. *Obstet Gynecol* 1992; 80:178–181.
91. Gardnerova M, Eymard B, Morel E, et al. The fetal/adult acetylcholine receptor antibody ratio in mothers with myasthenia gravis as a marker for transfer of the disease to the newborn. *Neurology* 1997;48:50–54.
92. Dinger J, Prager B. Arthrogryposis multiplex in a newborn of a myasthenic mother —case report and literature. *Neuromuscul Disord* 1993;3:335–339.
93. Barnes PR, Kanabar DJ, Brueton L, et al. Recurrent congenital arthrogryposis leading to a diagnosis of myasthenia gravis in an initially asymptomatic mother. *Neuromuscul Disord* 1995;5:59–65.
94. Riemersma S, Vincent A, Beeson D, et al. Association of arthrogryposis multiplex congenita with maternal antibodies inhibiting fetal acetylcholine receptor function. *J Clin Invest* 1996;98:2358–2363.
95. Mygland A, Aarli J, Matre R, Gilhus N. Ryanodine receptor antibodies related to severity of thymoma associated myasthenia gravis. *J Neurol Neurosurg Psychiatry* 1994;57:843–846.
96. Bril V, Kojic J, Dhanani A. The long-term clinical outcome of myasthenia gravis in patients with thymoma. *Neurology* 1998;51:1198–1200.
97. Andrews I. A treatment algorithm for autoimmune myasthenia gravis in childhood. *Ann NY Acad Sci* 1998;841:789–802.
98. Van Lunteren E, Kaminski H. Perturbations of sleep and breathing during sleep in neuromuscular disease. *Sleep Breathing* 1999;3:23–30.
99. Al-Shekhlee A, Kaminski HJ, Ruff RL. Endocrine myopathies and muscle disorders related to electrolyte disturbance. In: Katirji B, Kaminski HJ, Preston D, Shapiro B, Ruff RL, eds. *Neuromuscular Disorders in Clinical Practice*. Boston, Butterworth Heinemann, 2002, pp. 1187–1204.
100. Drachman DB, McIntosh KR, Reim J, Balcer L. Strategies for treatment of myasthenia gravis. *Ann NY Acad Sci* 1993;681:515–528.

101. Karachunski PI, Ostlie NS, Okita DK, Garman R, Conti-Fine BM. Subcutaneous administration of T-epitope sequences of the acetylcholine receptor prevents experimental myasthenia gravis. *J Neuroimmunol* 1999;93:108–121.
102. Drachman DB, Okumura S, Adams RN, McIntosh KR. Oral tolerance in myasthenia gravis. *Ann NY Acad Sci* 1996;778:258–272.
103. Killen JA, Lindstrom JM. Specific killing of lymphocytes that cause experimental autoimmune myasthenia gravis by ricin toxin-acetylcholine receptor conjugates. *J Immunol* 1984;133:2549–2553.
104. Urbatsch I, Sterz R, Peper K, Trommer W. Antigen-specific therapy of experimental myasthenia gravis with acetylcholine receptor-gelonin conjugates in vivo. *Eur J Immunol* 1993;23:776–779.
105. Vandenbark AA, Vainiene M, Celnik B, Hashim G, Offner H. TCR peptide therapy decreases the frequency of encephalitogenic T cells in the periphery and the central nervous system. *J Neuroimmunol* 1992;39:251–260.
106. Vandenbark AA, Chou YK, Bourdette DN, et al. T cell receptor peptide therapy for autoimmune disease. *J Autoimmun* 1992;5(Suppl A):83–92.
107. Wu JM, Wu B, Miagkov A, Adams RN, Drachman DB. Specific immunotherapy of experimental myasthenia gravis in vitro: the "guided missile" strategy. *Cell Immunol* 2001;208:137–147.
108. Wu JM, Wu B, Guarnieri F, August JT, Drachman DB. Targeting antigen-specific T cells by genetically engineered antigen presenting cells. A strategy for specific immunotherapy of autoimmune disease. *J Neuroimmunol* 2000;106:145–153.

# 10
## Neurocritical Care
## of Myasthenia Gravis Crisis

## Jose Americo M. Fernandes Filho and Jose I. Suarez

### INTRODUCTION

Myasthenia gravis crisis (MGC) is defined as an exacerbation of myasthenia gravis (MG) weakness provoking an acute episode of respiratory failure that leads to institution of mechanical ventilation (MV). Weakness may involve respiratory muscles (altering respiratory mechanics) or bulbar muscles, which compromises airway protection and patency. MGC is the most dangerous complication of MG and is a life-threatening condition that requires immediate recognition and patient care in an intensive care unit setting for its optimal management *(1)*.

MGC usually occurs within the first 2 years after MG onset (74% of patients) *(2)*, and 15–20% of patients with MG will experience at least one episode of crisis. Its mortality has declined from 40% in the early 1960s to 5% in the 1970s, which probably reflects improvement in ventilatory and general medical management of these patients in intensive care units. However, despite the decrease in mortality, the duration of MGC has not changed much and continues to average 2 weeks *(2)*. This chapter reviews the most important aspects of MGC including its pathophysiology, etiology, and management.

### PATHOPHYSIOLOGY

*Precipitants*

MGC is usually precipitated by infections (30–40% of cases) *(3,4)*, the most frequent being respiratory tract infections caused by both viral and bacterial agents. Aspiration pneumonia accounts for about 10% of MGC cases *(3,4)* and may be more prevalent in patients with oropharyngeal weakness, manifested by difficulty in swallowing and chewing, altered facial expression, and dysarthria *(5)*. Certain medications may exacerbate MG and lead to

From: *Current Clinical Neurology: Myasthenia Gravis and Related Disorders*
Edited by: H. J. Kaminski © Humana Press Inc., Totowa, NJ

**Table 1**
**Drugs That Exacerbate Myasthenia Gravis**

| Association | Drugs |
|---|---|
| Definite | Corticosteroids |
| Probable | Antibiotics: |
| |   aminoglycosides |
| |   ciprofloxacin |
| |   clindamycin |
| | Antiarrhythmics: |
| |   procainamide |
| |   propranolol |
| |   timolol |
| | Neuropsychiatric: |
| |   phenytoin |
| |   trimethadione |
| |   lithium |
| Possible | Antibiotics: |
| |   ampicillin |
| |   imipenen/cilastatin |
| |   erythromycin |
| | Antiarrhythmics: |
| |   propafenone |
| |   verapamil |
| |   quinidine |
| | Miscellaneous: |
| |   trihexyphenidyl |
| |   chloroquine |
| |   neuromuscular-blocking drugs |
| |   carbamazepine |
| |   oral contraceptives |
| |   transdermal nicotine |

MGC (**Table 1**) *(6)*. It is crucial to obtain a reliable history of current medication use including specific inquiry of the patient, family, and friends for nonprescription drugs, including so-called alternative medicines. When treatment of MG was limited to anticholinesterase medications, overdose could lead to MGC, but this is not encountered frequently now, and its importance may have been overstated previously *(3,7)*. Other factors that may lead to MGC include botulinum toxin injection *(8)*, recent surgical procedures (including thymectomy), and trauma. In 30–40% of the patients no trigger can be identified *(4)*. The presence of thymoma seems to be a risk factor for

MGC. MG patients with thymoma may have a more severe disease course (*see* Chap. 6), and thymoma patients are identified twice as often among patients in crisis compared with myasthenia patients in general (30% vs. 15%) *(3)*.

## Respiratory Abnormalities

The major muscle groups included in MGC are oropharyngeal and respiratory muscles. As weakness of respiratory muscles progresses, there is a decrease in lung expansion, along with inefficiency of the cough reflex to clear the airway. Patients' forced vital capacity (FVC) progressively decreases, making them prone to the development of atelectasis and, eventually, respiratory failure *(3)*. It is proposed that patients follow a stereotyped sequence of events leading to MGC directly related to their FVC *(9)*:

1. Normal respiratory function is present with FVC of 65 mL/kg.
2. Poor cough is evident with accumulation of secretions and with FVC of 30 mL/kg.
3. With FVC of 20 mL/kg, the sigh mechanism is impaired, with development of atelectasis and hypoxia.
4. Sigh is lost with FVC of 15 mL/kg, and atelectasis and shunting appear.
5. Hypoventilation starts with FVC of 10 mL/kg.
6. Hypercapnia develops with FVC between 5 and 10 mL/kg.

## Oropharyngeal Dysfunction

The oropharyngeal muscles maintain the patency of the upper airway by regulation of its cross-sectional area, and their dysfunction increases resistance to airflow *(10)*. Weakness of laryngeal muscles causes the vocal cords to remain adducted during inspiration, instead of the normal abduction *(10, 11)*. This creates the so-called sail phenomenon. Paralyzed vocal cords, because of their position and curvature, catch the airflow during inspiration and are pulled inward to the midline like the sail of a boat *(10)*. Weakness of the tongue obstructs the oropharyngeal cavity. In addition to the mechanical obstruction of the airway, oropharyngeal dysfunction leads to an inability to protect from aspiration *(5,10)*.

## CLINICAL PRESENTATION AND EVALUATION

MGC may occur in patients previously diagnosed but also may be the presenting event of MG. Patients with the definite diagnosis of MG who complain of worsening weakness or shortness of breath need to be assessed for dysphagia, stridor, and adequacy of ventilation. During the examination, the respiratory pattern requires assessment. Rapid, shallow breathing indicates respiratory muscle fatigue, which should not be confused with psychogenic hyperventilation *(3)*. Diaphragmatic function is assessed by observation of abdominal movements during the respiratory cycle. With severe weakness, a paradoxic respiratory pattern develops with inward movement of the abdomen during inspiration. The strength of neck muscles correlates with diaphragm strength, and weakness of these muscles should alert the clinician to possible respiratory compromise. A simple way to evaluate ventilatory reserve is by asking the patient to count from 1 to 25 in a single breath *(3)*. Patients with significant limitation should undergo measures of respiratory parameters.

Assessment of oropharyngeal muscles begins with inquiries about difficulty swallowing, episodes of choking, or coughing while eating. A wet, gurgling voice or stridor may indicate the need for intubation for airway protection *(3)*. Swallowing may be tested at the bedside by observing the patient swallow 3 oz of water and watching for coughing or choking *(12)*. However, caution should be observed in performing this assessment, and it need not be done in patients with clear signs of oropharyngeal weakness.

Patients may present with worsening of respiratory status because of vocal cord paralysis. In these patients, flexible laryngoscopy or flow volume loops should be performed *(10,11)*. The finding of vocal cords in the adducted position should alert the physician to the possible need for a cricothomy in case conventional endotracheal intubation is not feasible *(11)*.

In one series of 63 MGCs, initial manifestations were generalized weakness in 76% of patients, focal bulbar weakness in 19%, and weakness of respiratory muscles in 5%. Most patients (68%) required mechanical ventilation between 1 and 3 days after initial myasthenic exacerbation *(1)*. Some patients may present with respiratory failure without any evidence of generalized weakness *(2,10)*.

The respiratory status of patients at risk for MGC should be monitored closely. Bedside measurements of FVC (normal $\geq$ 60 mL/kg), negative inspiratory force (NIF; normal > 70 cm $H_2O$), and positive expiratory force (PEF; normal > 100 cm $H_2O$) should be done serially. Arterial blood gases are also important, and pulse oximetry is not a substitute for this measurement. Blood gas assessments are abnormal (showing hypoxia and hypercarbia) with advanced respiratory dysfunction, but patients may have normal oxygenation by pulse oximetry while arterial blood gases show developing hypercarbia, a sign of impending respiratory arrest.

Values of FVC $\leq$ 1.0 L (<15 mL/kg body weight), NIF < 20 cm $H_2O$, and PEF < 40 cm $H_2O$ are indications for institution of mechanical ventilation *(3, 4,13)*. However, each patient should be considered individually, with assessment of comfort level, heart rate, respiratory rate, arterial blood gas values, and the ability to protect and maintain the airway. Respiratory dysfunction may progress rapidly and should be promptly recognized. Some independent predictors of the need to institute mechanical ventilation include abnor-

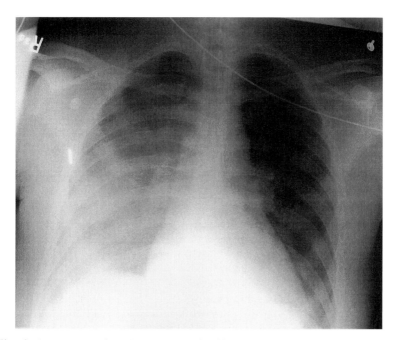

**Fig. 1.** Anteroposterior chest X-ray of a 33-year-old man with known MG for 1 year, who presented with worsening of generalized weakness and dysphagia, followed by tachypnea and fever. The X-ray on admission revealed right lower lung pneumonia and left lower lobe atelectasis. The patient required mechanical ventilation within 12 h of admission.

mal chest roentgenogram on hospital admission (pneumonia or atelectasis; **Fig. 1**) and complications during hospitalization such as atelectasis, cardiac arrhythmia, and anemia requiring transfusion *(14)*. Early mechanical ventilation is preferable to prevent worsening atelectasis. Patients with low FVC (but not to a level warranting prompt intubation) and those with independent predictors of mechanical ventilation should be admitted to an intensive care unit for serial measurements of the spirometry parameters. Cardiac arrhythmias are common among patients with MGC (14–17% of patients) and are an additional reason for intensive care monitoring of patients with MG exacerbation and evidence of impending MGC *(1,15)*.

## DIFFERENTIAL DIAGNOSIS

In any patient who is difficult to wean from a ventilator, MG should be considered; other possible disorders are Lambert-Eaton syndrome, botulism, Guillain-Barré syndrome, polymyositis, motor neuron disease, critical illness

**Table 2**
**Neuromuscular Disorders in Critical Care Patients**[a]

| Condition | Key presenting features |
| --- | --- |
| Acute intermittent porphyria | Asymmetric limb weakness progressing to quadriplegia after several attacks |
| Botulism | Nausea and vomiting preceding muscle weakness Blurred vision, dysphagia, dysarthria, descending muscle paralysis, dilated pupils, dry mouth, constipation, and urinary retention |
| Critical illness myopathy | Patient with COPD or asthma requiring mechanical ventilation and use of neuromuscular blockers and corticosteroids |
| Critical illness polyneuropathy | Patient with sepsis and difficulty weaning from the ventilator, diminished or absent reflexes |
| Electrolyte imbalance | Generalized muscle weakness, cardiac arrhythmias with or without rhabdomyolisis |
| Guillain-Barré syndrome | Preceded by upper respiratory or gastrointestinal infection; ascending paralysis, arreflexia |
| Lambert-Eaton syndrome | Symmetric proximal muscle weakness, hypoactive or absent deep tendon reflexes, dry mouth, blurred vision, orthostatic hypotension |
| Lead poisoning | Pure motor weakness, initially of extensors muscles, fasciculations, abdominal pain, constipation, anemia, renal failure |
| Motor neuron disease | Weakness, wasting, fasciculations |
| Organophosphate poisoning | Exposure to insecticides, petroleum additives, and modifiers of plastics followed by acute cholinergic crisis (muscle weakness, myosis, abdominal cramping) |
| Polymyositis | Proximal, symmetrical muscle weakness, elevated creatine kinase |
| Prolonged neuromuscular blocking | Patient with impaired renal function or hepatic failure who had been on continuous neuromuscular blocking agents |

[a]COPD = chronic obstructive pulmonary disease.

polyneuropathy, and organophosphate poisoning, among others (**Table 2**) *(16–20)*. Electrodiagnostic studies (*see* Chap. 7) are instrumental in differentiating among these conditions and may guide additional specific evaluation as well as provide prognostic information *(16)*.

## MANAGEMENT

To ensure recovery of patients from MGC, it is important that their overall medical condition be optimized. Identified trigger factors should be removed or corrected. All patients should undergo extensive evaluation for infection including cultures of sputum, urine, and blood as well as other sites as clinically indicated. Empiric use of antibiotics needs to be carefully tailored to the clinical situation because of the potential for some antibiotics to impair neuromuscular transmission further as well as the development of bacterial resistance. Avoidance of unnecessary antibiotics is further emphasized by the observation that *Clostridium difficile* colitis has been associated with prolonged crisis *(2,3)*. Nutritional assessment needs to be made early in the course of MGC. A determination is made for the necessity of short-term nasogastric tube feeding, peripheral hyperalimentation, or a gastrostomy tube with the expectation that myasthenic weakness is not expected to resolve rapidly. Electrolyte imbalance will compromise neuromuscular function, and close monitoring with appropriate correction is required. Intermittent positive pressure breathing may be useful in preventing development of atelectasis; if the patient is already intubated or has a respiratory tract infection, aggressive pulmonary toilet is necessary. Deep venous thrombosis prophylaxis measures should be undertaken with the use of compression stockings, sequential compression devices, and subcutaneous heparin. Coagulation status may be deranged from heparin use when plasma exchange is performed, and intravenous immunoglobulin therapy may predispose to hypercoagulation. Gastrointestinal prophylaxis is given either with sucralfate or histamine receptor blockers to prevent stress ulcers and gastrointestinal bleeding. Psychological support for the patient and family is also important, with an emphasis on the ultimate ability to return most patients to an excellent functional level.

## Ventilatory Management

Rapid sequence intubation should be performed once the decision for mechanical ventilation is made *(13)*. This entails bag-masking the patient to obtain arterial oxygen saturation of >97%, administration of free running intravenous normal saline, continuous blood pressure monitoring, and bolus infusion of sedative medications (usually etomidate at 0.2–0.3 mg/kg). If short-acting muscle relaxants are needed (preferably they are to be avoided), then non-depolarizing agents like vecuronium should be used. Oral intubation should be undertaken whenever possible.

Once the patient is intubated, a mode of ventilation needs to be chosen, but no mode is perfect. Assist-control (AC) and synchronized intermittent mandatory ventilation (SIMV) are commonly used; each has advantages and disadvantages. Muscle fatigability with weakness and poor lung expansibility are the main determinants in the development of MGC. Thus, the initial objectives of mechanical ventilation should be to promote rest and expand the lungs *(3)*. It was previously thought that, as long as the patient does not have primary lung disease compromising lung compliance, large tidal volumes (15 mL/kg) combined with lower rates to maintain a normal minute ventilation, with positive end-expiratory pressure (PEEP) at levels of 5–15 could be used, provided that peak airway pressures are maintained within acceptable limits (<40 cm $H_2O$) *(3)*. However, the recent literature suggests that smaller tidal volumes (7–8 mL/kg) with faster respiratory rates (12–16 breaths/min) should be used to avoid lung injury, adding intermittent sighs (1.5 × tidal volume, 3–4 times every hour) to avoid atelectasis *(21)*.

## Ventilator Weaning

Several parameters may be helpful in determining when to initiate weaning from mechanical ventilation: FVC > 15 mL/kg, NIF < −30 cm $H_2O$, PEF ≥ 40 cm $H_2O$, and minute ventilation <15 L/min *(3,13,22)*. However, these parameters have limited predictive power, and other general conditions should be satisfied before weaning is attempted *(13)*:

1. The patient needs to be adequately oxygenating, with a $PaO_2$ > 60 mmHg, with fractional oxygen concentration in inspired gas ($FiO_2$) 40%, and PEEP < 5 cm $H_2O$.
2. The patient also needs to have an intact respiratory drive [in MG patients, respiratory drive was found not to be impaired *(23)*], to be able to protect the airway, and have an adequate cough reflex.
3. The hemodynamic status should be stable, electrolyte levels normal, and nutritional status adequate.
4. The patient should be free of infection or other significant medical complications.
5. The need for airway suctioning should be less than every 2–3 h.

For MG patients, one major and initial indicator of timing for mechanical ventilation weaning is the improvement of general muscle strength by objective physical examination. The rapid shallow breathing index is thought to be the best predictor of successful weaning *(13)*; it is calculated by division of the tidal volume by the respiratory rate of the patient while temporarily off the ventilator. Patients with index values >100 have a 95% likelihood of failing a weaning trial *(22)*.

Once patients meet criteria for extubation, the method chosen for a weaning trial varies according to an individual physician's clinical experience. One method is a daily trial of continuous positive airway pressure (CPAP) and pressure support levels of 5–15 cm $H_2O$. If the patient remains comfortable after 1–4 h, the level of pressure support can be decreased by 1–3 cm $H_2O$ each day. Patients should be returned to the original ventilatory mode overnight or when signs of fatigue appear *(3)*.

The SIMV mode can also be used for weaning. It is accomplished by decreasing the ventilatory rate by 2–3 breaths once or more times a day based on patient comfort level *(13)*. An increase in respiratory rate, fall in tidal volume, agitation, and tachycardia may all be indicators of fatigue *(3)*. Once a patient has demonstrated good endurance (the number of hours the patient tolerates the weaning mode with minimal support, usually more than 2 h) and general conditions are adequate, the patient may be extubated.

Extubation should be performed early in the day. Stridor may occur immediately to 1 h after extubation, and aerosolized racemic epinephrine may reverse the condition, but reintubation might be necessary. Laryngospasm is less common but is a life-threatening condition. Lidocaine administered intravenously (2 mg/kg) may significantly reduce laryngospasm, if used several minutes prior to extubation *(22)*.

## Treatment of Neuromuscular Dysfunction

Therapies may be divided into those that improve strength rapidly with a short duration of action and those that improve strength slowly with a more permanent response. The first category includes acetylcholinesterase inhibitors, plasmapheresis, and intravenous immunoglobulin (IVIg) (*see* Chap. 9). The second category comprises immunosuppressive agents such as corticosteroids, azathioprine, cyclophosphamide, and cyclosporine *(24)*. The latter are not used in rescuing patients from MGC but in the long-term management of MG patients. The use of corticosteroids during MGC is debated. Some advocate their use during crisis in patients only with refractory weakness; others suggest that they be started while the patient is treated with IVIg or plasmaphereis *(3,4,25)*.

Cholinesterase inhibitors provide symptomatic improvement in myasthenic patients by decreasing the degradation of ACh at the neuromuscular junction. The continuous intravenous infusion of pyridostigmine is reported to be an effective treatment in MGC compared with plasmapheresis as measured by mortality, duration of ventilation, and outcome. Its use has been defended, especially when MGC is triggered by an infection *(1)*. However, it is common practice to discontinue these agents in mechanically ventilated patients because of their propensity for promoting excess respiratory secretions and mucus plugging *(3)*. Another concern is the reported occurrence of cardiac arrhythmias in MGC patients, including those receiving intravenous pyridostigmine *(1,15)*. Cholinesterase inhibitors could increase cholinergic activity at cardiac muscarinic synapses, leading to arrhythmias *(15)*.

Plasmapheresis is the preferred treatment in managing MCG, with a reported efficacy of 75% *(3)*. Its mechanism of action is related to the removal of circulating factors, such as acetylcholine receptor (AChR) antibodies. Even though AChR antibody titers do not correlate with MG severity, the decrease in AChR antibodies titers has correlated with clinical improvement. There is no standard protocol for plasmapheresis. The usual regimen is exchange of 1–1.5 plasma volumes every day or every other day for 5–6 treatments. Clinical improvement may be seen as early as 24 h, but in most patients the first effect appears after 2–3 sessions of plasmapheresis. Some patients may have an initial worsening thought to be due to reduction in plasma concentration of cholinesterase. The duration of effect is usually <10 weeks if other immunosuppressive treatment is not instituted *(24,26)*.

The most frequent complications of plasmapheresis are hypotension, electrolyte imbalance (reduction of calcium, potassium, and magnesium), depletion of clotting factors, and thrombocytopenia. Obtaining vascular access may at times be difficult and may be complicated by pneumothorax, thrombosis, and infection *(3,24,26)*. When a large volume of plasma is removed, intravascular volume should be replaced with albumin in saline solution *(26)*. Any electrolyte imbalance should be corrected to prevent exacerbating muscle weakness. The coagulopathy is usually mild but should be kept in mind when utilizing subcutaneous heparin for deep venous thrombosis prophylaxis. Reducing antihypertensive drug dosages and administering intravenous fluids before the procedure may avoid hypotension.

Another option for specific treatment of MGC is IVIg. A standard course consists of 400 mg/kg/day of IVIg for 5 days *(24)*. Response to IVIg is usually observed 5 days after treatment initiation. Some report IVIg to have a similar efficacy and tolerance as plasmapheresis *(27)*. However, others find that patients treated with plasmapheresis have a superior respiratory status at 2 weeks (ability to extubate) and a better functional outcome at 1 month compared with IVIg *(28)*. Furthermore, some patients may not respond to IVIg but may have improvement after subsequent plasmapheresis *(29)*. IVIg may be a better choice in patients with hemodynamic instability, vascular access problems, or a poor response to plasmapheresis. Adverse effects occur in <10% of patients and most commonly include headache, chills and fever, fluid overload, and (rarely) renal failure *(30,31)*. Anaphylaxis may occur to IgA components in patients with IgA deficiency *(31)*. IgA levels and baseline renal function should be obtained before treatment is initiated.

## OUTCOME OF MYASTHENIC CRISIS

One study identified three main independent predictors of prolonged mechanical ventilation: age > 50 years, preintubation serum bicarbonate ≥ 30, and peak vital capacity < 25 mL/kg on days 1–6 post intubation. The proportion of patients intubated for >2 weeks was 88% in patients with three risk factors, 46% in those with two, 21% in those with one, and zero for patients with no risk factors. The same study also revealed that atelectasis, anemia requiring transfusion, *Clostridium difficile* infection, and congestive heart failure were complications associated with prolonged intubation *(2)*. Tracheostomy is usually performed after 2 weeks of intubation, but early tracheosthomy is recommended for patients expected to require prolonged mechanical ventilation. Tracheostomy is more comfortable for the patient, reduces the risk of tracheolaryngeal stenosis, permits more effective suctioning of tracheal secretions, and facilitates weaning from mechanical ventilation owing to reduction in dead space and resistance to air flow from the endotracheal tube *(3,22)*. In general, 25% of patients will be extubated by 1 week, 50% by 2 weeks, and 75% by 1 month. Intubation and mechanical ventilation for >2 weeks is associated with a threefold increase in hospital stay (median 63 days) and a twofold increase in likelihood of functional dependency at discharge *(2)*. One-third of patients who survive the first crisis will have a second episode *(3)*.

Although myasthenic crisis is a potentially lethal event and is always devastating for the patient and loved ones, optimizing critical care and long-term treatment of MG has prevented the event from being "grave," as it once was.

## REFERENCES

 1. Berrouschot J, Baumann I, Kalischewski P, Sterker M, Schneider D. Therapy of myasthenic crisis. *Crit Care Med* 1997;25:1228–1235.
 2. Thomas CE, Mayer SA, Gungor Y, et al. Myasthenic crisis: clinical features, mortality, complications, and risk factors for prolonged intubation. *Neurology* 1997; 48:1253–1260.
 3. Mayer SA. Intensive care of the myasthenic patient. *Neurology* 1997;48(Suppl 5): S70–S75.
 4. Bedlack RS, Sanders DB. How to handle myasthenic crisis. *Postgrad Med* 2000; 107:211–214, 220–222.
 5. Weijnen FG, Van Der Bilt A, Wokke JHJ, Wassenberg MWM, Oudenaarde I. Oral functions of patients with myasthenia gravis. *Ann NY Acad Sci* 1998;841:773–776.
 6. Wittbrodt, ET. Drugs and myasthenia gravis. *Arch Intern Med* 1997;157:399–408.
 7. Grob D. Natural history of myasthenia gravis. In: Engel AG, ed. *Myasthenia Gravis and Myasthenic Disorders.* New York, Oxford University Press, 1999, pp. 131–145.
 8. Borodic G. Myasthenic crisis after botulinum toxin. *Lancet* 1998;352:1832.
 9. Ropper AH. The Guillain-Barré syndrome. *N Engl J Med* 1992;326:1130–1136.
10. Putman MT, Wise RA. Myasthenia gravis and upper airway obstruction. *Chest* 1996;109:400–404.
11. Cridge PB, Allegra J, Gerhard H. Myasthenic crisis presenting as isolated vocal cord paralysis. *Am J Emerg Med* 2000;18:232–233.
12. DePippo KL, Holas MA, Reding MJ. Validation of the 3 oz water swallow test for aspiration after stroke. *Arch Neurol* 1992;49:1259–1261.

13. Suarez JI. Ventilatory management in the neurosciences critical care unit. In: *Brazilian Academy of Neurology Minimonograph: Proceedings of the 19th Brazilian Congress of Neurology,* 2000, Salvador, Brazil.
14. Suarez JI, Boonyapisit K, Zaidat OO, Kaminski HJ, Ruff RL. Predictors of mechanical ventilation in patients with myasthenia gravis exacerbation [abstract]. *J Neurol Sci* 2001;187:S464.
15. Mayer SA, Thomas CE. Therapy of myasthenic crisis. *Crit Care Med* 1998;26: 1136.
16. Maher J, Rutledge F, Remtulla H, et al. Neuromuscular disorders associated with failure to wean from the ventilator. *Intensive Care Med* 1995;21:737–743.
17. Vita G, Girlanda P, Puglisi RM, Marabello L, Messina C. Cardiovascular-reflex testing and single fiber eletromyography in botulism. *Arch Neurol* 1987;44:202–206.
18. Suarez JI, Cohen ML, Larkins J, et al. Acute intermittent porphyria. Clinicopathologic correlation. Report of a case and review of the literature. *Neurology* 1997;48: 1678–1683.
19. Anzueto A. Muscle dysfunction in the intensive care unit. *Clin Chest Med* 1999;20: 435–452.
20. Bosch EP, Smith BE. Disorders of peripheral nerves. In: Bradley WG, Daroff RB, Fenichel GM, Marsden CD, eds. *Neurology in Clinical Practice*, 3rd ed., vol. 2. Boston, Butterworth-Heineman, 2000, pp. 2045–2130.
21. The acute respiratory distress syndrome network. Ventilation with lower tidal volumes as compared with traditional tidal volumes for acute lung injury and the acute respiratory distress syndrome. *N Engl J Med* 2000;342:1301–1308.
22. Wijdicks FM. Management of airway and mechanical ventilation. In: Wijdicks FM, ed. *The Clinical Practice of Critical Care Neurology*. Philadelphia, Lippincott-Raven, 1997, pp. 25–45.
23. Borel CO, Teitelbaum JS, Hanley DF. Ventilatory drive and carbon dioxide response in ventilatory failure due to myasthenia gravis and Guillain-Barré syndrome. *Crit Care Med* 1993;21:1717–1726.
24. Kokontis L, Gutmann L. Current treatment of neuromuscular diseases. *Arch Neurol* 2000;57:939–943.
25. Seybold ME. Treatment of myasthenia gravis. In: Engel AG, ed. *Myasthenia Gravis and Myasthenic Disorders*. New York, Oxford University Press, 1999, pp. 167–191.
26. Batocchi AP, Evoli A, Di Schino C, Tonali P. Therapeutic apheresis in myasthenia gravis. *Ther Apher* 2000;4:275–279.
27. Gajdos P, Chevret S, Clair B, Tranchant C, Chastang C. Clinical trial of plasma exchange and high-dose intravenous immunoglobulin in myasthenia gravis. *Ann Neurol* 1997;41:789–796.
28. Qureshi AI, Choudhry MA, Akbar MS, et al. Plasma exchange versus intravenous immunoglobulin treatment in myasthenic crisis. *Neurology* 1999;52:629–632.
29. Stricker RB, Kwiatkowska BJ, Habis JA, Kiprov DD. Myasthenic crisis. Response to plasmapheresis following failure of intravenous γ-globulin. *Arch Neurol* 1993;50: 837–840.
30. Drachman, DB. Myasthenia gravis. *N Engl J Med* 1994;330:1797–1810.
31. Dalakas, MC. Intravenous immunoglobulin in the treatment of autoimmune neuromuscular diseases: present status and practical therapeutic guidelines. *Muscle Nerve* 1999;22:1479–1497.

# 11
# Thymectomy

## Alfred Jaretzki III

## INTRODUCTION

Many physicians caring for patients with myasthenia gravis (MG) are convinced that thymectomy plays an important role in treatment, even though the operation has not been proved effective. I share their conviction, believe there is supporting evidence, and recommend total thymectomy as the cornerstone of therapy for adult patients with generalized MG.

Unfortunately, proof of the effectiveness of thymectomy has been hampered by serious problems. There are no satisfactory prospective studies, no accepted objective definitions of severity of the illness or response to therapy, and no consensus regarding patient selection or timing, type, and results of surgery. There is a lack of recognition that all thymectomies are not equal in extent and possibly, if not probably, not equal in effectiveness. A surprisingly pervasive but improper analysis of the data has resulted in incorrect conclusions. Without resolution of these issues, there can be no unequivocal determination of the effectiveness of thymectomy or a valid comparison of the several operative techniques. In this review I attempt to clarify these issues.

A Task Force of the Myasthenia Gravis Foundation of America (MGFA) was formed to address these issues. Their recommendations for clinical research standards were published simultaneously in neurologic and thoracic surgical journals (1–3). The recommendations include clinical classification, quantitative scoring, therapy status, thymectomy type and extent, postintervention staus, clinical trials, and outcomes analysis. The Medical/Scientific Advisory Board of the MGFA subsequently formed two additional task forces, one on Thymic Pathology to develop guidelines for the evaluation of the nonthymomatous thymus in MG and a Pediatric Task Force to develop standards for the evaluation of children with MG (4,5). If the concepts delineated in these series of recommendations are incorporated in future studies of thymectomy for MG, many of the current conflicts should be resolved.

From: *Current Clinical Neurology: Myasthenia Gravis and Related Disorders*
Edited by: H. J. Kaminski © Humana Press Inc., Totowa, NJ

## AN ACCOUNT
## OF THE AUTHOR'S INVOLVEMENT WITH MG

The following is a brief account of my initiation into the treatment of patients with MG. I believe it will help to clarify the complexities involved in the evaluation of thymectomy.

I am a general thoracic surgeon with many years of experience in general surgery, including thyroid surgery. In 1973 I was asked to perform transcervical thymectomies on patients with MG. I reviewed the work of Kirschner, Kark, and Papatestas *(6,7)*, observed Dr. Papatestas perform several transcervical resections at Mt. Sinai Hospital in New York, and naively accepted the view that the thymus was *invariably* bilobed, was *readily* accessible through the neck, and could be *totally* removed by a transcervical *intracapsular* extraction. I also accepted *uncorrected crude data* as an appropriate method of analysis of results. As will be seen, I was wrong on all *four* counts.

I then performed four trans*cervical* resections with the understanding that a total thymectomy was indicated. At the time of the first operation, I discovered that the cervical portion of the right thymic lobe extended behind the thyroid to the level of the angle of the jaw, requiring an additional high cervical incision for its removal. In the fourth operation, after the distal end of the *right* lobe broke off deep in the mediastinum, a median sternotomy was performed to retrieve it. A separately encapsulated accessory lobe on the *left,* which had been missed during the transcervical portion of the operation, was also discovered. The anatomic variants uncovered in these two operations would have been overlooked had the additional incisions not been made.

It was therefore clear that the anatomy of the thymus was more extensive in both the mediastinum and the neck than was described by advocates of the transcervical approach or in surgical texts. Accordingly, in an attempt to understand the true extent of the thymus in the mediastinum and the neck, the embryology of the thymus was reviewed, and over the next several years I removed increasing amounts of mediastinal and cervical tissue followed by meticulous anatomic and pathologic studies of the specimens by Marianne Wolfe, MD. As more and more tissue was removed, more and more thymus was found. This experience led to a detailed study of the surgical anatomy of the thymus in patients with MG and the design of the *transcervical-transsternal maximal thymectomy* technique *(8).*

Although this extensive resection seemed to produce remission rates higher than previously reported, this impression was not supported by the uncorrected crude data analyses that were universally employed at that time. It was not until 1987, when Papatestas employed life table analysis *(9),* and later, when I analyzed controversies *(10)* and learned more about statistical analysis *(3)*, that I finally recognized the false conclusions developed from use of uncorrected crude data.

This account demonstrates the progress of my enlightenment. I hope it will help others become similarly enlightened in less than the 27 years it took me.

## TOTAL THYMECTOMY IS INDICATED

From the beginning, even before the role of the thymus in MG was understood, "total" thymectomy was considered the goal of surgery. In 1941 Blalock wrote, "complete removal of all thymus tissue offers the best chance of altering the course of the disease" *(11)*, and most leaders in the field have reiterated this *(6,12–24)*. The thymus plays a central role in the autoimmune pathogenesis of MG. Pathologic and immunologic studies support this thesis *(25–27)*. Complete neonatal thymectomy in rabbits prevents experimental autoimmune MG, whereas incomplete removal does not *(28)*.

Incomplete trans*cervical or* trans*sternal* resections have been followed by persistent symptoms that were later relieved by a more extensive reoperation with the finding of residual thymus *(29–35)*. Removal of as little as 2 g of residual thymus has been therapeutic *(33)*. In addition, several studies comparing aggressive with limited resections support the premise that the entire thymus should be removed *(10,36,37)*.

## SURGICAL ANATOMY OF THE THYMUS

Since complete removal of the thymus appears to be indicated when a thymectomy is performed in the treatment of nonthymomatous MG, thymic anatomy should be understood by all those involved in the treatment of these patients and in the analysis of the results of the surgery. The thymus is not "two well-defined lobes that appear almost as distinct as do the two lobes of the thyroid," as described by Blalock *(11)*, and still depicted in surgical texts *(38,39)*.

Detailed surgical-anatomic studies (**Fig. 1**) demonstrate that the thymus frequently consists of multiple lobes, often separately encapsulated, in both the neck and mediastinum, and these may not be contiguous. In addition, unencapsulated lobules of thymus and microscopic foci of thymus may be *widely* and *invisibly* distributed in the pretracheal and anterior mediastinal fat from the level of the thyroid to the diaphragm and bilaterally from beyond each phrenic nerve *(8,40)*. Occasionally, microscopic foci of thymus are found in subcarinal fat *(41)*.

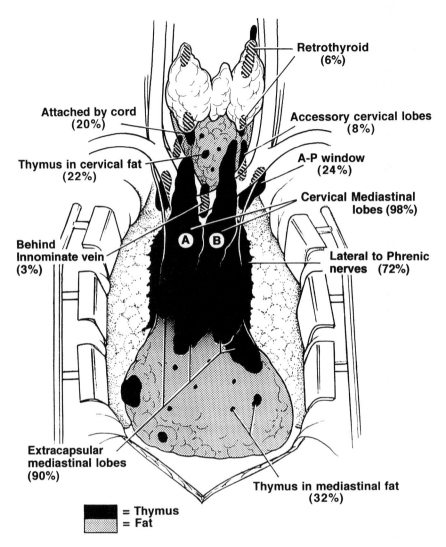

**Fig. 1.** Composite anatomy of the thymus. This illustration represents what is now accepted as the surgical anatomy of the thymus *(8)*. The frequencies (percentages of occurrence) of the variations are noted. Thymus was found outside the confines of the two classical cervical-mediastinal lobes (**A** and **B**) in the neck in 32% of the specimens and in the mediastinum in 98%. Black = thymus; gray = fat, which may contain islands of thymus and microscopic thymus. (Reproduced with permission from ref. *10*.)

## RESECTIONAL POTENTIAL
## OF THE SURGICAL TECHNIQUES

If total thymectomy is the goal of surgery and gross and microscopic extra-lobar thymus should be removed, an understanding of how much thymus each resectional technique removes is necessary. The following discussion presents estimates based on published reports, drawings, and photographs of resected specimens, videos of the procedures when available, and my personal experience. The illustrations, photographs, and videos of the resected specimens are frequently the most revealing. A review of the potential of each thymectomy technique strongly suggests that all resections are not equal in extent (**Fig. 2**) *(10)*.

### *Combined Transcervical and Transsternal Thymectomy*

*Transcervical-transsternal maximum thymectomy (8)* is also known as *extended cervico-mediastinal thymectomy (42)*. Under direct vision, these procedures employ wide exposure in the neck and a complete median sternotomy. An *en bloc* resection is used, removing in a single specimen all gross thymus, suspected thymus, and cervical-mediastinal fat. The resections include removal of both sheets of mediastinal pleura and sharp dissection on the pericardium. They are exenteration in extent and are "performed as if it were an en bloc dissection for a malignant tumor" *(43)*. Extreme care is taken to protect the recurrent, left vagus, and phrenic nerves. A photograph of a typical specimen illustrates the extent of these resections (**Fig. 3**). A video illustrating the details of this procedure is available *(44)*. Lennquist et al. *(45)* described a similar procedure, with a less extensive resection in the neck and mediastinum.

### *Comment*

The maximal resection has been considered the benchmark against which the other resectional procedures should be measured *(19)*. Its design is based on the surgical anatomy of the thymus. It predictably removes all surgically available thymus in the neck and mediastinum, including the unencapsulated lobes, and the lobules of thymus and microscopic thymus in the precervical and anterior mediastinal fat that are not visible to the naked eye. The *en bloc* technique serves to ensure that islands of thymus are not missed and to guard against the potential of seeding of thymus in the wound. Piecemeal removal of the thymus may "herald a poorer prognosis than clean removal" *(46)*. The sharp dissection on the pericardium (with division of the fingers of pericardium that enter the thymus) and the removal of the mediastinal pleural sheets

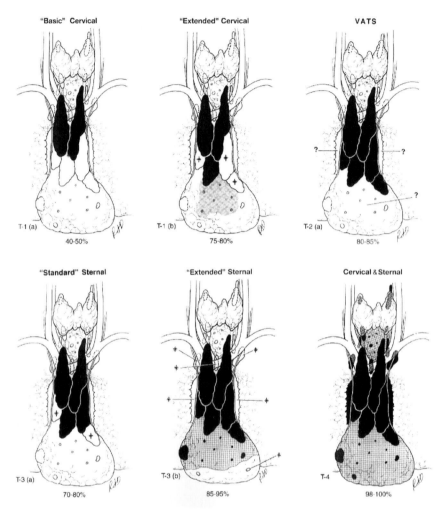

**Fig. 2. (a–f)** Estimated resectional extent of six thymectomy techniques. See text for details. The VATET resection is not illustrated. Black = thymus; gray = fat removed by the designated operation, possibly containing islands of thymus and microscopic thymus; * = thymic lobes or thymo-fatty tissue that may or may not be removed; white = tissue not removed by the designated procedure; and ? = thymo-fatty tissue that may or may not be removed by the designated procedure. (Modified with permission from ref. *10.*)

with the specimen (with the confirmed adherent microscopic thymus) are an integral part of the procedure. Blunt dissection has been demonstrated to leave microscopic foci of thymus on the pericardium and pleura.

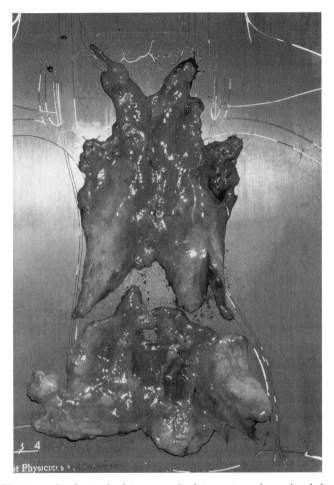

**Fig. 3.** Photograph of a typical transcervical-transsternal maximal thymectomy specimen. The specimen consists of the *en bloc* resected cervical and mediastinal thymus, suspected thymus, and pretracheal and anterior mediastinal fat from thyroid isthmus to diaphragm with adherent mediastinal pleural sheets bilaterally. The specimen was divided *after* removal to indicate the division between the grossly visible thymus and the distal anterior mediastinal fat. (Reproduced with permission from ref. *39*.)

## Transsternal Thymectomies

The *extended transsternal thymectomy (15,36,47–55)* is also known as *aggressive transsternal thymectomy (56)* or *transsternal radical thymectomy (57)*. The extent of these resections in the mediastinum varies and may or may not include all the mediastinal tissue removed by the combined transcervical-transsternal techniques. The cervical extensions are removed from below, with or without additional tissue, but without a formal neck dissection. Mulder describes in detail an aggressive mediastinal dissection approximating the dissection of the maximal technique *(55,58)*. A video illustrating the details of this aggressive mediastinal dissection is also available *(59)*.

*Comment.* These aggressive transsternal resections are identical in the mediastinum to the mediastinal dissection of the maximal procedure *when* they are exenteration in extent, use sharp dissection on the pericardium, *include* removal of the mediastinal pleural sheets, and remove the other tissue in the mediastinum defined in the maximal technique. They do, however, remove less tissue in the neck, where thymus may persist. Mulder has expressed the view that the risk to the recurrent laryngeal nerves in performing the aggressive neck dissection of the combined transcervical-transsternal thymectomy is not justified by the small potential gain *(58)*.

The *standard transsternal thymectomy* used by Blalock, Keynes, and Clagett *(11,12,60,61)*, was originally limited to removal of the well-defined cervical-mediastinal lobes that were thought to be the entire gland *(62)*. Currently, although a complete *(63)* or partial *(64–66)* sternotomy may be performed, the resection is more extensive than originally described and includes removal of all visible mediastinal thymic lobes. Mediastinal fat, varying in extent, may or may not be removed. The cervical extensions of the thymus are removed from below, with or without some adjacent cervical fat. Variations of this technique include a video-assisted technique using a complete median sternotomy via a limited lower sternal transverse skin incision *(67)*.

*Comment.* This resection, as recently illustrated in surgical textbooks *(68–71)*, falls short of total thymectomy. Residual thymus may be found in the neck and in the mediastinum at reoperation following a standard trans*sternal* thymectomy *(32–34)*. This fact is often overlooked, it being assumed that residual thymus is found only after the basic trans*cervical* resections. Accordingly, most major centers since the early 1980s *(33,42,47–53,56,57,72)*, with some exceptions *(70,73)*, consider it incomplete and have abandoned it.

## Transcervical Thymectomies

The *extended transcervical thymectomy (74,75)* employs a special manubrial retractor for improved exposure of the mediastinum. The mediastinal dissection is extracapsular and includes resection of the visible mediastinal thymus and mediastinal fat. Sharp dissection may or may not be performed on the pericardium. The mediastinal pleural sheets are usually not included in the specimen. The neck exploration and dissection vary in extent and may or may not be limited to exploration and removal of the cervical-mediastinal extensions. Variations of this procedure include the addition of a partial median sternotomy without an additional skin incision *(76)* and the associated use of mediastinoscopy *(77)*.

*Comment.* This resection, as Cooper et al. *(74)* warned, as described in a textbook *(78)*, and as photographed *(79)*, is usually less extensive than that described by Cooper. Although the incision is in the neck, the resection does not routinely include the accessory thymic lobes in the neck, retrothyroid thymus, or thymus in the pretracheal fat.

The *basic transcervical thymectomy* employs an *intra*capsular *extraction* of the mediastinal thymus via a small cervical incision and is limited to the removal of the *intracapsular* portion of the central cervical-mediastinal lobes. *No other tissue* is removed in the neck or mediastinum *(7,13)*.

*Comment.* This resection, although touted as a "total thymectomy" *(13)*, is unequivocally a limited resection, incomplete in both the neck and mediastinum. The limited extent is evident in descriptions of the technique *(7,80)*, the surgical anatomy of the thymus *(8)*, and findings of many reoperations for MG after an initial trans*cervical* resection *(29–35)*. Henze *(31)* reoperated on 27% of his basic transcervical series of 95 patients, because of persistent or progressively severe MG manifestations, finding 10–60 g of residual thymus in all. A computer-matched study, comparing the basic transce*rvical* with the standard trans*sternal* operation, demonstrated that twice as much thymus was removed by the trans*sternal* than in the trans*cervical* procedure, even though the trans*sternal* operation was the more limited standard type *(37)*.

This technique routinely fails to remove not only accessory thymus present in the neck and mediastinum but also encapsulated thymic lobes in the mediastinum. I recommend that it be abandoned.

## Videoscopic-Assisted Thymectomies

Variations in videoscopic thymectomy are being developed. Their resectional potential and the results are still in the investigative phase. Two basic techniques dominate.

The *video-assisted thoracic surgery* (VATS) thymectomy employs unilateral videoscopic exposure of the mediastinum (right or left) with removal of the grossly identifiable thymus and variable amounts of anterior mediastinal fat. Sharp dissection is not routinely performed on the pericardium, and the mediastinal pleural sheets are not routinely removed with the specimen, blunt dissection being performed at these sites. The cervical extensions of the thymus are usually removed from below *(24,81–85)*. Illustrations and photographs of the technique and specimens are available *(24,84–86)*.

The *video-assisted thoracoscopic extended thymectomy* (VATET) uses bilateral thoracoscopic exposure of the mediastinum for improved visualization of both sides of the mediastinum. Extensive removal of the mediastinal thymus and perithymic fat is described, the thymus and fat being removed separately. Sharp dissection may or may not be used on the pericardium. The mediastinal pleural sheets are not usually removed. A cervical incision is performed with exposure of the recurrent laryngeal nerves and removal of the cervical thymic lobes and pretracheal fat under direct vision *(87,88)*.

*Comment.* The VATS resections, based on the published reports, vary in extent in the mediastinum. They appear to be more extensive than the standard transsternal but less than the extended transsternal operations. Although some photographs of the specimens confirm the described extent *(85)*, others show a more limited resection. No attempt is made to remove the accessory thymus in the neck.

As Mack *(85)* warned, "thymectomy is an advanced VATS procedure that should only be undertaken by surgeons…well versed in simpler VATS operations and who have the enthusiasm and patience to pursue minimally invasive techniques."

The VATET operation is conceptually more complete than the VATS. The undated video I reviewed, however, does not confirm the reported extent in the neck or mediastinum.

## STATISTICAL ANALYSIS

Inappropriate statistical analysis, in many instances, if not most, has led to incorrect conclusions concerning the relative merits of the thymectomy techniques. The following is a brief review of material previously concisely reviewed *(3)* and analyzed *(10)*.

Life table analysis using the Kaplan-Meier method is considered the preferred statistical technique for the analysis of remissions following thymectomy *(89)*. It provides comparative analysis using all follow-up information accumulated to the date of assessment, including information on patients subsequently lost to follow-up and on those who have not yet reached the date of assessment *(76,90)*. This analysis should be supplemented by multivariable analysis to identify and correct for significant variables. Hazard rates (remissions per 1000 patient-months) correct for length of follow-up and censor patients lost to follow-up. However, these rates depend on the "risk" (remissions per unit of time) being constant *(91)*, which may not be the case in MG.

Unfortunately, uncorrected crude rates (the number of remissions divided by the number of patients operated on *or* divided by the number of patients followed) have been the primary form of analysis in the comparative evaluation of remissions and improvement following thymectomy. This form of analysis does not include in the evaluation all the follow-up information accumulated to the date of assessment. In addition, patients evaluated many years after surgery may appear to do as well or better than patients with a shorter follow-up. Also, even the differing denominators in the two subsets (*patients operated on vs. patients followed*) are not comparable but have frequently been compared without comment. Accordingly, uncorrected crude data should have no place in the comparative analysis of results of thymectomy; conclusions based on this type of analysis should be ignored.

## RESULTS OF THYMECTOMY

Ordinarily the results of an operation are presented *after* the recommendations for the performance of the procedure. Here, the results are presented first because an understanding of the effectiveness of the several techniques is necessary to make decisions on whether to operate, when to operate, and what type of operation to use.

### Pitfalls of the Thymectomy Literature

Unfortunately, in addition to the problems with statistical analysis, most of the reports are flawed because of the "absence of standardized methods for assessing patient status both before and after surgery" *(57)*. The following is a brief review of these issues *(10)*.

The studies are primarily retrospective and therefore do not address the variability and unpredictability of MG, the differing response to treatment among patients with different subtypes of MG, or the bias inherent in the selection of patients for thymectomy. Clinical classifications are used to stratify patients and evaluate results, yet there have been at least 15 (often conflicting) classifications. These systems are not quantitative, do not accurately describe changes in disease severity, and are not a reliable measure of response.

Although "remission" is the measurement of choice in defining results following thymectomy*(92–94)*, there has been no uniform definition. "Improvement" and changes in "mean grade," widely used as determinants of success, are unreliable measurements; objective criteria, such as a quantitative scoring system, have not been applied. In addition, in the studies evaluating combinations of thymectomy and immunosuppression, the patients are not compared with a control group and do not follow a predefined schedule of medications and dose reduction that is required to assess the additive benefit from thymectomy and immunosuppression. When patients continue to take immunosuppressive medications after thymectomy, it is not possible to infer retrospectively the effects of thymectomy itself *(95)*.

In comparing results of different techniques, other confounding factors are also frequently ignored and may conceal the disadvantages of the procedure being touted *(10)*. These include 1) failure to assess or define the length of illness preoperatively; 2) failure to account for the length of postoperative follow-up; 3) muddying the analysis by inclusion of multiple surgical techniques and combining two or more series with differing definitions and standards; 4) including patients with and without thymoma; 5) including reoperations when most patients at the time of the reoperation had severe symptoms of long duration and may have failed earlier thymectomy for reasons unknown; 6) use of metaanalysis based on mixed and uncontrolled data; 7) failure to report relapses; and 8) failure to consider the rate of spontaneous remissions.

## Thymectomy vs. Medical Management

There is a paucity of data and no prospective randomized studies comparing medical management of MG and thymectomy. The data available, however, do suggest a significant thymectomy benefit.

In 1976 a computer-assisted retrospective matched study of patients with nonthymomatous MG, aged 17 to over 60 years, demonstrated better results following thymectomy than with medical management *(96)*. Eighty of 104 surgical patients were matched "satisfactorily" from the files of 459 medically treated patients. Using crude data corrected for length of follow-up, *complete remission was experienced in 35% of the surgical patients (at an average of 19.5 years of follow-up) compared with 7.5% of the medical group (at an average of 23 years of follow-up)*, even though presumably only a limited standard transsternal thymectomy was performed. The relative mortality from MG was 14% surgical vs. 34% medical. However, the study was done before modern immunomodulatory treatments and more sophisticated intensive care.

An evidence-based review of thymectomy in nonthymomatous MG included 21 controlled but nonrandomized studies published between 1953 and 1998 *(97)*. The authors found positive associations in most studies between thymectomy and MG remission. After thymectomy, patients were twice as likely to attain medication-free remission than nonoperated patients. However, as the authors noted, there were multiple confounding factors between the thymectomy and nonthymectomy patient groups, with differences in baseline characteristics that were expected to be of prognostic importance. It was not emphasized by the authors that the thymectomy techniques in most instances were the limited basic trans*cervical* and the limited standard trans*sternal* operations. Thus, if this metaanalysis is otherwise valid, a total thymectomy should produce a higher remission rate than demonstrated in this analysis of incomplete thymic resections.

Wolfe, Newsom-Davis, and associates are undertaking a prospective randomized multiinstitutional international study, in which the Myasthenia Gravis Foundation of America clinical research standards are employed *(1)*, to establish in generalized autoimmune nonthymomatous myasthenia gravis whether an extended trans*sternal* thymectomy for patients receiving immunosuppressive medication confers added benefits to treatment by immunosuppressive medication alone *(98)*. If the results are better with the addition of a thymectomy, it should demonstrate conclusively that thymectomy does play a role in the treatment of MG.

Although in 1977 and 1980 McQuillen and Rowland expressed doubts about the effectiveness of thymectomy *(92,99)*, Rowland stated in a 2001 letter to Newsom-Davis: "I should have known that you would be behind such a good idea. A trial of thymectomy is only about 50 years late. The citations to McQuillen and me from 20 years ago should be labeled as obsolete" (L.P. Rowland, personal communication, 2001). It is of note that from 1978, when we started performing maximal thymectomies at the Columbia Presbyterian Medical Center in New York, until my retirement from surgery in 1992, Rowland recommended a maximal thymectomy for adult patients with generalized MG.

## Maximal Thymectomy Results

We evaluated the results of the transcervical-transsternal maximal thymectomy in a cohort of 72 patients (27 men and 45 women) with generalized MG, aged 16–66 years (68% younger than 35) *(33)*. Fifteen additional patients with thymoma and eight reoperations were analyzed separately. The statement in the original report "Of the 124 thymectomies, 95 were evaluated 6 to 89 months after operation" was poorly phrased and resulted in misinterpretation *(24,100)*. The 29 patients not analyzed were operated on after the study had been concluded. Eighty percent of the patients had had moderately severe or severe weakness, and 12.5% had a history of crisis. The mean duration of preoperative symptoms was 2.8 (range 0.1–20) years. The mean follow-up was 3.4 (range 0.5–7.4) years. Remission was defined as "no signs, no symptoms, and no medication" for at least 6 months.

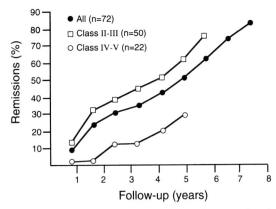

**Fig. 4.** Remission rates (life table analysis) following maximal thymectomy for nonthymomatous MG. The predicted remission rate is 81% when all patients will have been followed for 7.5 years. The remission rate is greater for patients with mild and moderate manifestations compared with those with severe manifestations and crisis; the differences are statistically significant ($p = 0.04$). (Modified with permission from ref. *33*.)

Life table analysis (**Fig. 4**) for this cohort predicted 81% remissions at 7.5 years. The milder the disease and the longer the patients were followed postoperatively, the better the results. The crude remission rate *(remission divided by number of patients operated on)* corrected for length of follow-up was 62% at 7.4 years (**Fig. 5**). Two patients who achieved a remission had a relapse (3%), one temporary and one prolonged. The *hazard* rate was 13.6 remissions per 1000 patient-months of follow-up (**Table 1**). Age, sex, the presence or absence of microscopic hyperplasia, or the presence or absence of measurable acetylcholine receptor antibodies in this cohort of patients did not influence the results *(101)*. However, the presence of a thymoma, invasive or not, influenced results unfavorably.

Until a suitably designed prospective study demonstrates otherwise, these results should be the benchmark for evaluation of techniques.

### Comparison of Results Based on Type of Thymectomy

In a review of the published reports of thymectomy from 1970 to 1996, 49 studies had sufficient data to compare with maximal thymectomy. Only four included life table analysis, 43 used *uncorrected* crude data analysis alone, and only two of the latter included hazard analysis *(10)*. Three meta-analyses of this information (life table, hazard, and crude corrected for length of follow-up) support the premise that the more aggressive the resection the

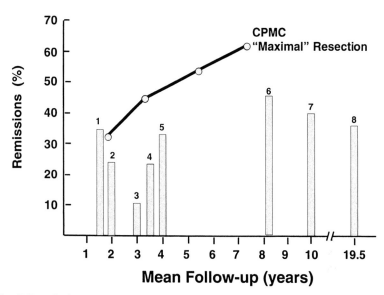

**Fig. 5.** Remission rates (crude corrected for mean follow-up) following five thymectomy techniques for nonthymomatous MG. This analysis compares crude data corrected for mean length of follow-up. The corrected data, although not recommended as mechanism to replace life table analysis, provide a mechanism for a rough comparison of uncorrected crude data, which otherwise *cannot* be compared. Although a number of baseline characteristics were not constant, this analysis supports the premise of a direct relation between extent of resection and results and refutes statements, based on uncorrected crude data, that the results of the various thymectomy techniques are comparable. 1, Maximal thymectomy of Ashour et al. *(131)*; 2, VATS thymectomy of Mack and Scruggs *(85)*; 3, Basic transcervical thymectomy, collected series *(37,114)*; 4, Standard transsternal thymectomy, collected series *(17,37,132, 133)*; 5, Extended transsternal thymectomy, collected series *(43, 49,51,57)*; 6, Extended transcervical thymectomy of Cooper and colleagues *(75)*; 7, Standard transsternal thymectomy of Wilkins *(73)*; 8, Standard transsternal thymectomy of Buckingham and colleagues *(96)*. CPMC, Columbia Presbyterian Medical Center (Modified with permission from ref. *10*.)

better the result and refute the assertion by some that results are comparable regardless of the type of resection. However, these analyses suffer from differences in baseline characteristics that are of prognostic importance. Accordingly, prospective studies with control of the variables are required to determine unequivocally the relative merits of the various resectional techniques.

*Life table analyses* of remissions of four resectional techniques were compared (**Fig. 6**). The results favor the "maximal" resection even though the

**Table 1**
**Remission Rates (Hazard) of Three Transsternal**
**Thymectomy Techniques for Nonthymomatous MG**

| Thymectomy Technique | Hazard Rate |
|---|---|
| Maximal* | 13.6 |
| Extended sternal[+] | 9.95 |
| Standard sternal[0] | 6.13 |

This analysis supports the premise of a direct relation between extent of resection and results. The patient cohorts, however, are not comparable since the "extended" and "standard" trans*sternal* resections include patients with thymoma. * = maximall thymectomy *(33)*; [+] = extended transsternal thymectomy *(105)*; and [0] = standard transsternal thymectomy *(49)*.

baseline characteristics of prognostic significance favor the others. The trans*sternal* thymectomy of Lindberg is a more extensive resection than the standard trans*sternal* but less than the extended trans*sternal* resection *(102)*. The extended trans*cervical* resection of Durelli employs an upper partial sternotomy *(76)*. The basic trans*cervical* resection of Papatestas is the most limited resection *(9)*. A study of standard trans*sternal* resections limited to children under the age of 17 was not included in this analysis, although the results are similar to those of adults with this type of resection *(103)*. Statistical confirmation of this metaanalysis requires that the data be available for co-analysis.

*Hazard analyses* of three trans*sternal* resections are compared (**Table 1**). The results also favor the maximal resection compared with the extended trans*sternal (49)* and the standard trans*sternal* thymectomies *(104)*, although the cohorts are not entirely comparable

*Crude data corrected for length of follow-up* of 13 of the 49 reports qualified for this metaanalysis. Correcting for length of follow-up allows a rough comparison of uncorrected crude data remission rates. This analysis indicates a direct relationship between the extent of the thymic resection and results, again favoring the "maximal" resection (**Fig. 5**). The criteria for selecting the 13 reports *(10)* were nonthymomatous patients only, "remission" strictly defined, use of a single surgical technique, and available mean follow-up data. However, other baseline characteristics were not constant. This analysis also indicates the folly of comparing *uncorrected crude data*, a common practice used by all of us for many years, and even used now *(24,38,75,105,107)*.

The less aggressive resections have been defended; however, Mack suggested that "the goal of thymectomy should be removal of all *gross* thymic

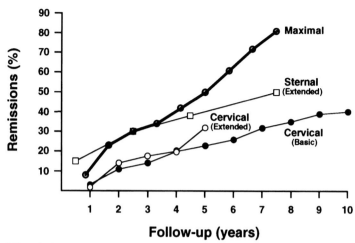

**Fig. 6.** Remission rates (life table analysis) following four thymectomy techniques for nonthymomatous MG. This analysis compares the results of the maximal thymectomy *(33)*, Lindberg's resection, which is slightly less extensive than the extended trans*sternal* thymectomy *(102)*, Durelli's modified extended trans*cervical* thymectomy *(76)*, and the limited basic trans*cervical* thymectomy of Papatestas *(9)*. The difference in results supports the premise of a direct relationship between the extent of the resection and results. Statistical confirmation requires that the data be available for co-analysis.

tissue…. it has not been demonstrated that microscopic foci are clinically relevant" *(107)*. The evidence suggests otherwise, and these comments suggest that the procedures being advocated may not remove as much thymus as the aggressive resections. Similarly, a Papatestas report is frequently quoted as evidence that trans*cervical* resections produce results equivalent to trans*sternal* resections *(9)*. Although the results were equivalent in that study, the generalization is not valid since the trans*sternal* resections cited were early standard *limited* trans*sternal* resections that removed approximately the same amount of thymus as was removed by the trans*cervical* resections.

## INDICATIONS FOR THYMECTOMY

Neurologists hold differing views *(108)* as to when, and even if, a thymectomy is indicated in the course of treatment of autoimmune nonthymomatous MG. A better understanding of the indications for surgery awaits prospective studies.

Keesey's algorithm in reference to moderate generalized MG *(109)* represents a centrist position in the treatment of adult patients:

Thymectomy is recommended for those relatively healthy patients whose myasthenic symptoms interfere with their lives enough for them to consider undergoing major thoracic surgery. While it is expensive and invasive, thymectomy is the only treatment available that offers a chance of an eventual drug-free remission. This chance seems to be better earlier in the disease than later. The potential benefit of thymectomy also decreases as the adult patient gets older and as the thymus naturally involutes with time. Further, the risk of surgery increases with age. The age at which the risks outweigh the potential benefits must be individualized for every patient.

Keesey's group routinely performs the extended transsternal thymectomy *(55)*.

My recommendations, based on our experience with the maximal thymectomy described above, are that at the least an aggressive trans*sternal* thymectomy be considered for most adult patients with more than very mild generalized autoimmune nonthymomatous MG, *regardless* of the duration of symptoms or age of the patient. The patient's medical condition has to be satisfactory for the planned surgery, and patients over age 65 have to be selective.

In our series *(33)*, the remission rate was independent of the duration of symptoms or age of the patient. Contrary to the belief that the thymus disappears with age, we found thymus in all patients we operated on (to age 75), and thymus was also found in all 10 specimens in an autopsy study of aging individuals without MG (ages 60–90) *(33)*. Seronegative patients with convincing clinical evidence of MG should have a thymectomy *(110)*. The results of "maximal" thymectomy were equally good for these patients, possibly because seronegative patients harbor antibodies to other proteins of the neuromuscular junction *(101)*. Thymectomy may be appropriate for some patients with purely ocular manifestions that interfere with lifestyle or work when immunosuppressive therapy is contraindicated or not effective *(111)*. Thymectomy within the first year of the illness in adults (early thymectomy) has been recommended *(112–114)* but lacks prospective documentation.

The indication for thymectomy in children is a separate issue addressed by others *(103,115–118)* and by a recently appointed Pediatric Task Force *(5)*.

## SELECTING THE THYMECTOMY TECHNIQUE FOR THE PATIENT

In view of the available evidence and our experience, transcervical-transsternal maximal thymectomy remains my choice when thymectomy is undertaken for MG. This recommendation is supported by Bulkley and Drachman

*(42).* In the previously quoted letter to Newsom-Davis, Rowland commented: "I have no idea why surgeons are unwilling to do maximal thymectomies" (L.P. Rowland, personal communication, 2001). There are some caveats, however. This recommendation is only applicable if the surgeon is willing to take the time to remove all available thymus and do this safely. It may be appropriate to request the assistance of a surgeon experienced in surgery of the neck.

However, since thoracic surgeons usually are not experienced in exposing and protecting the recurrent laryngeal nerves in the neck, until such time as prospective studies prove otherwise, for the reasons expressed by Mulder *(55)* it is reasonable to accept an aggressive extended trans*sternal* thymectomy as an alternative. The VATS technique, or preferably the more extensive VATET technique, has appeal, with the caveats expressed by Mack and Scruggs *(85)* if and when the extent of the resections and the rates of remission are demonstrated to equal the maximal or at least the extended trans*sternal* operations. However, the remission rates reported to date are not equivalent to the aggressive transsternal procedures *(24,38,85).* Based on the anatomy of the thymus, the specimens removed, and the available results, I do not recommend the lesser trans*sternal* and the trans*cervical* resections. Certainly, the basic trans*cervical* procedure should be abandoned.

Regardless of the surgical approach, surgical expertise is required. The surgeon should be convinced of the importance of complete removal of the thymus, willing to commit the necessary time, and avoid injury to the phrenic, recurrent laryngeal, and left vagus nerves. It is preferable to leave behind a small amount of thymus rather than injure the nerves. Injury to these structures, especially in a patient with MG, can be devastating. The review and recommendations noted above are supported by many of the experts in the field, although clearly not all. In view of the lack of unambiguous prospective studies, however, it is not possible to be dogmatic. Hopefully, these recommendations will, at the least, be seriously considered in the decision-making process. In addition to the Newsom-Davis prospective randomized study under way *(98)*, properly controlled prospective studies, comparing the results of the benchmark procedure with the less aggressive resections, are required to resolve the many issues discussed.

## REOPERATION

The concept of reoperation for an unsatisfactory result after one of the more limited resections should be accepted. This recommendation appears to be straightforward when applied to a patient who still has, or progresses to, an incapacitating and poorly controlled illness, especially if repeated hospitalizations and ICU stays have been required 3 or more years after a basic trans*cervical* or a standard trans*sternal* thymectomy.

It is more difficult to recommend reoperation for less severe disease manifestations or after more aggressive operations, but it is appropriate in selected instances. Unfortunately, at this time, it is not possible to predict the presence or location of even moderate amounts of residual thymus; chest X-rays, computed tomography, magnetic resonance imaging, and aceytylcholine receptor antibody studies are usually not helpful *(35)*. However, a review of the operative note and pathologic report of the original surgery, which is mandatory in any case, makes it clear that an incomplete resection had been performed. The timing of reoperation is also a difficult decision. Although a 3–5-year wait seems prudent, occasionally earlier surgery may be appropriate, and reoperation should be considered even in patients many years after original thymectomy.

If reoperation is undertaken for persistent or recurrent disease, it should be as aggressive as the maximal technique in both the neck and mediastinum, regardless of the earlier procedure. This recommendation is supported by the findings following reoperations using the maximal technique (**Table 2**). It seems illogical to limit the reoperation procedure, as some have done, to a repeat trans*cervical* approach *(9,19,20)*, a limited trans*sternal* approach *(19,32)*, or even an extended transsternal resection without a formal neck dissection *(29)*. Thoracoscopic surgery also seems inappropriate for reoperations. Incomplete resections at reoperations may explain the occasional failure to find thymus or lack of benefit *(20)*.

Obviously, reoperation is more difficult and time-consuming than a primary resection, and the risk to the nerve damage is greater. Wide exposure in the neck and mediastinum is mandatory, and a T incision is indicated. In our experience with 15 patients whose original thymectomy was a basic trans*cervical* or a standard trans*sternal* resection, residual thymus was found in all (**Table 2**), and all patients subsequently benefited, some dramatically *(33)*. Striking examples included: 1) a patient 1 year after a previous basic trans*cervical* thymectomy (the patient was on a respirator and the original resection was predictably incomplete); 2) a patient 5 years after a basic trans*cervical* resection (confined to a wheelchair, unable to care for her baby, and on large doses of steroids); and 3) a patient 30 years after a standard trans*sternal* resection (the patient was having repeated hospitalizations and ICU stays prior to the reoperation). Residual thymus was present in all, and at the time of the relatively short follow-up, although not in remission, the three patients had markedly improved.

**Table 2**
**Reoperation for Nonthymomatous MG Following Previous**
**Basic Transcervical and Standard Transsternal Thymectomy**[a]

| Parameter | No. of Patients |
|---|---|
| Disease extent | |
|     Moderate-severe | 3 |
|     Severe | 7 |
|     Crisis | 5 |
| Residual thymus (2–23 g) | |
|     Previous transcervical (9) | In neck (1 of 4) |
| | In mediastinum (9 of 9) |
|     Previous transsternal | In neck (6 of 6) |
| | In mediastinum (4 of 6) |
| Results | |
|     Remission | 1 |
|     Pharmacologic remission | 5 |
|     Minimal manifestations | 3 |
|     Improved | 4 |
|     Unchanged | 2 |

[a]Employing the maximal thymectomy technique, residual thymus was found in all cases. Thymus was found in the previously unopened compartment (neck or mediastinum) in 100% of the cases. It was also found in the neck in one-fourth of the previous trans*cervical* cases and in the mediastinum in two-thirds of the previous trans*sternal* cases.

## TRACHEOSTOMY: *TIMING AND TECHNIQUE*

Although tracheostomy is no longer necessary on a routine basis in the perioperative management of these patients, sometimes it is either mandatory or desirable (to make the care easier and safer). If the patient has a tracheostomy in place at the time of any of the trans*sternal* resections, anesthesia is given via an oral endotracheal tube, and the sternal wound is sealed from the tracheostomy site. To complete the maximal thymectomy, a formal neck dissection must be performed after the tracheostomy tube has been removed and the wound is well healed. If a tracheostomy is required within the first 2–3 weeks after a trans*cervical* or trans*sternal* resection, it must be a two-stage procedure, the stages separated by at least 4–5 days. If the need for a tracheostomy postoperatively is anticipated at the time of the thymectomy, the first stage can be performed at the time of the initial surgery.

## SURGICAL MANAGEMENT OF THYMOMA

In the resection of thymic neoplasms (regardless of size, lack of preoperative evidence of invasion, or presence of MG), it is inappropriate to use any approach that circumvents complete sternotomy *(119,120)*. To avoid tumor seeding and late recurrences, these tumors require wide local resection with as good tumor margins as practical, including the removal of adherent pericardium or wedges of lung. In most instances the phrenic nerves can be preserved. Chest computed tomography is indicated prior to thymectomy in all patients with MG and should identify most thymomas *(121)*. Antibodies to striated muscle antigens when present predict the presence of a thymoma *(23)*. However, small thymomas may first be discovered at surgery, and we had a case in which two histologically distinct thymomas were present in separate lobes of the thymus; this raises additional concern about the use of minimally invasive surgery in MG. Total thymectomy should always be performed, whether or not MG is present preoperatively, because MG may follow removal of a thymoma (6–10% after removal of an asymptomatic thymoma without removal of the coexisting thymus) *(122)*.

## PERIOPERATIVE PATIENT MANAGEMENT

Patients undergoing thymectomy for the treatment of MG require the care of a team of neurologists, pulmonogists, respiratory therapists, intensive care specialists, anesthesiologists, and surgeons who have had appropriate experience. Regardless of the surgical technique, the surgeons should be totally conversant with the special problems of MG patients and committed to their sometimes difficult postoperative care. To accomplish these goals, these operations should be performed at centers where such teams exist.

The special problems associated with perioperative care are directly related to the severity of the MG at the time of surgery. The major risks are oropharyngeal and respiratory muscle weakness with the potential for aspiration of oral secretions, inability to cough effectively postoperatively, and respiratory failure. If oropharyngeal and respiratory weakness is eliminated preoperatively, the risks are those of any patient without MG. Accordingly, the patient should be as strong as possible at the time of surgery and should especially be free of signs and symptoms of oropharyngeal and respiratory weakness, using plasmapheresis and immunosuppression when necessary. The concern about wound healing and infection associated with corticosteroids is valid, but I believe overemphasized and much less of a concern than performing an operation on an inadequately prepared patient. One should not rely on cholinesterase inhibitors in the preoperative preparation of these patients because these medications only temporarily mask weakness, which may then flare up in the early postoperative period.

The preoperative preparation must include a detailed evaluation of the pulmonary function. Vital capacity (VC) and respiratory muscle force measurements are recommended, both before and after cholinergic inhibitors (1.5–2 mg neostigmine im for adults in association with 0.4 mg atropine), if the patient is receiving this medication and can tolerate its withdrawal for 6–8 h. The dual before and after measurements give an indication of the deficits that may be masked by the cholinesterase medication and the potential need for preoperative plasmapheresis or immunosuppression. Measurement of maximum expiratory force (MEF) is as easy to perform as the VC, is an excellent measure of cough effectiveness (an important determination), and is much more sensitive and reliable than the VC in the evaluation of these patients, both preoperatively and in the early postoperative period *(123)*. An MEF of <40–50 cm $H_2O$ indicates a potential for postoperative respiratory complications and respiratory failure. Accordingly, it should be corrected with immunomodulatory treatment before proceeding to surgery as well as before extubation in the postoperative period.

Many believe that muscle relaxants should be avoided if possible. However, it is preferable to face the potential need for postoperative ventilation than to have the patient suffer the consequences of hypoxia. Accordingly, should intubation be difficult, whether during anesthesia induction or at any time intubation is required, immediate muscle paralysis may be mandatory to achieve intubation successfully. Curare can be employed, using 10% of the standard dose. The use of succinylcholine is somewhat controversial and can usually be avoided; in emergencies, ordinary doses can also be used.

Postoperatively, these patients should be managed in an intensive care setting *(124)* where they can be closely observed by experienced personnel. An institutional protocol for the management of the postoperative MG patient is helpful and can include details of the ventilatory support management, the role of MEF measurements in deciding when to extubate, the role of physical therapy and bronchoscopy in maintaining a clear airway, pain control techniques, immunosuppression if indicated, the use of cholinergic medication, and timing and technique of a two-stage tracheostomy if necessary. A copy of a protocol, although outdated in some respects, is available as a guideline *(125)*.

If the patient is well prepared preoperatively and the preoperative MEF off cholinergic medication is satisfactory, regardless of the incision, extubation may be acceptable immediately postoperatively. However, emergency reintubation and respiratory support should be instituted immediately at any time for *early* signs of fatigue, progressive weakness, or impending respir-

atory failure. The use of cholinergic medication at this time is usually ineffective and may delay needed intubation. The need for intubation may even
occur after discharge from a special care unit. Under these circumstances
the temptation is to await the availability of an ICU bed. To delay may, however, be catastrophic; reintubation may have to be performed as a true emergency before an ICU bed can be arranged or even considered.

## HOSPITAL MORBIDITY AND MORTALITY

If the MG patient is well prepared preoperatively, thymectomy should be
a safe procedure and the mortality should be that of a similar operative procedure in a patient without MG. The recent operative mortality for thymectomy has been reported to be 0–2%. In 250 maximal thymectomies for MG,
we were able to avoid nerve injury and had 1 death (0.04%; 2 months postoperatively following complications of severe MG in a 65-year-old patient
receiving immunosuppression).

Clearly the transcervical and thoracoscopic approaches avoid the postoperative pain and unpleasant scar of the sternotomy. However, the sternotomy
pain is now usually well controlled and the intercostal pain of the VATS procedures may persist for some time. In the evaluation of therapeutic options,
determination is required of the remission-improvement status, postoperative
morbidity, complications directly related to each form of therapy, quality of
life and cost-benefit assessment *(3)*, and number and duration of subsequent
hospitalizations and ICU stays *(1)*.

If it is determined by prospective studies that the combined cervical-mediastinal or aggressive transsternal operations produce significantly improved
results, especially if they avoid multiple subsequent hospitalizations and the
need for prolonged immunosuppressive therapy with its inherent risks, the
initial disadvantages of the combined and aggressive transsternal procedures
may well be outweighed by their subsequent advantages.

## OUTCOMES RESEARCH

Well-designed, controlled, prospective studies are required to begin to
resolve the many conflicts and unanswered questions that exist concerning
thymectomy in the treatment of MG. This goal must be achieved if patient
protocols and operative techniques are to be properly evaluated. In this era
of outcome analyses, these steps are not only desirable, but also mandatory.

The ideal method of such evaluation is to undertake a prospective randomized clinical trial *(126)*. However, when this is not feasible, a prospective
risk-adjusted outcome analysis of nonrandomly assigned treatment *(127)* is
an acceptable and achievable method of study that (if properly controlled

and monitored) should resolve many of the unresolved issues. It is strongly recommended that these steps be undertaken.

In addition to a prospective study, the use of clinical research standards (which include definitions of clinical classification, *quantitative* assessment of disease severity, grading systems of postintervention status, and approved methods of analysis) is required. The data bank concept, appropriately developed and rigorously monitored *(1)*, should be particularly useful and practical for multiple institutions to compare the relative value of the various thymectomy techniques.

The primary focus of comparative analysis of thymectomy for MG should remain complete stable remission. Survival instruments, which are used in the analysis of remissions, are the most reliable determinant. Kaplan-Meier life table analysis is the technique of choice. Different levels of clinical improvement should also be *quantitatively* evaluated *(1,128)*. The use of uncorrected crude data to compare results *must* be discontinued.

Qualify of life instruments should be employed because therapy for MG is usually not innocuous and frequently does not produce a completely stable remission. These measures evaluate the impact of intermediate levels of clinical improvement and morbidity of therapy, and they complement information provided by survival and clinical improvement analysis. They should not, however, replace survival instrument evaluation. Although a functional status instrument assessing activities of daily living has been developed for MG *(129)*, there are no disease-specific quality of life instruments for MG at this time. They are needed, and it is recommended that they be developed *(130)*.

Experts in the fields of biostatistics and outcomes analysis should be consulted in the design of all studies and in the collection and evaluation of the data. An outcomes analysis guideline *(3)* and a diagram defining interrelationships between instruments (**Fig. 7**) give background information on the available analytical techniques.

## EPILOGUE

Although arguments can undoubtedly be made to refute some of the statements given here, I hope that this presentation will lead to a better understanding of the thymectomy controversies and improved results following thymic resection for MG. I also hope, and expect, the day will come when some form of targeted immunosuppression or other nonsurgical therapy (with no significant side effects) will produce long-term remissions in patients with autoimmune nonthymomatous MG. At that time, thymectomy in any form, especially the procedure that arguably produces the most complete resection, will be considered barbaric. Until such time, however, a thymectomy, *properly performed*, should be considered an integral part of the therapy of MG.

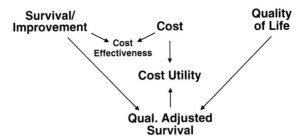

**Fig. 7.** The interrelationship between outcomes instruments. The interrelationship among survival-improvements instruments, quality of life instruments, and quality adjusted survival-cost effective instruments is demonstrated. Remissions are a survival function. Reproduced with permission from Weinberg A, Gelijns A, Moskowitz A, Jaretzki A. Myasthenia gravis: outcomes analysis. 2000. www.neurology.org. Reprints available via Myasthenia Gravis Foundation of America, Inc., 5841 Cedar Lake Road (Suite 204), Minneapolis, MN 55416.

Twenty-six years ago, Buckingham et al. *(96)* made basically the same statement: "It seems likely that future discoveries will permit the management of myasthenia gravis without surgical intervention but, for the present, the beneficial role of thymectomy for these unfortunate patients has been clearly demonstrated." Amen.

I am indebted to Lewis (Bud) P. Rowland, MD, and Audrey S. Penn, MD, for the opportunity of joining them in the care of patients with MG at the Columbia Presbyterian Medical Center in New York, for the experience of collaboration on clinical reports, for their patience and tolerance, and, most importantly, their friendship. I am especially grateful to Bud for his review and detailed editing of this chapter. I am also indebted to Alan D. Weinberg, MS, Director of Biostatistics, and Annetine Gelijns, PhD, Director of the International Center for Health Outcomes and Innovation Research, Department of Surgery, Columbia Presbyterian Medical Center, New York, NY, for helping me understand statistical techniques and outcomes analyses. However, to quote Bud Rowland again: "To all of them I am indebted, but none of them is responsible for any errors, intemperate comments, or apparent lapses of judgement in this essay" *(99)*.

## REFERENCES

1. Task Force of the Myasthenia Gravis Foundation of America, Inc. Myasthenia gravis: recommendations for clinical research standards. *Neurology* 2000;55:16–23.
2. Jaretzki A III, Barohn RB, Ernstoff RM, et al. Myasthenia gravis: recommendations for clinical research standards. *Ann Thorac Surg* 2000;70:327–334.

3. Weinberg A, Gelijns A, Moskowitz A, Jaretzki A. Myasthenia gravis: outcomes analysis. 2000. www.neurology.org. Reprints available via Myasthenia Gravis Foundation of America, Inc., 5841 Cedar Lake Road (Suite 204), Minneapolis, MN 55416.

4. Melms A. Guidelines for the Evaluation of the Non-Thymomatous Thymus in Myasthenia Gravis. Report of the Thymic Pathology Task Force of the Medical Scientific Advisory Board of the Myasthenia Gravis Foundation of America, Inc., 2001, in preparation.

5. Andrews PI. Standards for the Evaluation of Children with Myasthenia Gravis. Report of the Pediatric Task Force of the Medical Scientific Advisory Board of the Myasthenia Gravis Foundation of America, Inc., 2001, in preparation.

6. Kirschner PA, Osserman KE, Kark AE. Studies in myasthenia gravis: transcervical total thymectomy. *JAMA* 1969;209:906–910.

7. Kark AE, Papatestas AE. Some anatomic features of the transcervical approach for thymectomy. *Mt Sinai J Med* 1971;38:580–584.

8. Jaretzki A III, Wolff M. "Maximal" thymectomy for myasthenia gravis: surgical anatomy and operative technique. *J Thorac Cardiovasc Surg* 1988;96:711–716.

9. Papatestas AE, Genkins G, Kornfield P, et al. Effects of thymectomy in myasthenia gravis. *Ann Surg* 1987;206:79–88.

10. Jaretzki A III. Thymectomy for myasthenia gravis: an analysis of the controversies regarding technique and results. *Neurology* 1997;48(Suppl 5):S52–S63.

11. Blalock A, Harvey AM, Ford FF, Lilienthal J Jr. The treatment of myasthenia gravis by removal of the thymus gland. *JAMA* 1941;117:1529–1533.

12. Keynes G. The surgery of the thymus gland. *Br J Surg* 1946;32:201–214.

13. Kark AE, Kirschner PA. Total thymectomy by the transcervical approach. *Br J Surg* 1971;56:321–326.

14. Faulkner SL, Ehyai AS, Fisher RD, Fenichel GM, Bender HW. Contemporary managment of myasthenia gravis: the clinical role of thymectomy. *Ann Thorac Surg* 1977;23:348–352.

15. Olanow CW, Wechsler AS, Roses AD. A prospective study of thymectomy and serum acetylcholine receptor antibodies in myasthenia gravis. *Ann Surg* 1982;196:113–121.

16. Vincent A, Newsom-Davis J, Newton P, Beck N. Acetylcholine receptor antibody and clinical response to thymectomy in myasthenia gravis. *Neurology* 1983;33:1276–1282.

17. Hankins JR, Mayer RF, Satterfield JR, et al. Thymectomy for myasthenia gravis: 14 year experience. *Ann Surg* 1985;201:618–625.

18. Otto TJ, Strugalska H. Surgical treatment for myasthenia gravis. *Thorax* 1987;42:199–204.

19. Cooper J, Jaretzki A III, Mulder DG, Papatestas AS. Symposium: thymectomy for myasthenia gravis. *Contemp Surg* 1989;34:65–86.

20. Papatestas AE, Cooper J, Jaretzki A III, Mulder DG. Symposium: thymectomy for myasthenia gravis. *Contemp Surg* 1989;34:65–85.

21. Verma P, Oger J. Treatment of acquired autoimmune myasthenia gravis: a topic review. *Can J Neurol Sci* 1992;19:360–375.

22. Drachman DB. Myasthenia gravis. *N Engl J Med* 1994;330:1797–1810.

23. Penn AS. Thymectomy for myasthenia gravis. In: Lisak RP, ed. *Handbook of Myasthenia Gravis and Myasthenic Syndromes.* New York, Marcel Dekker, 1994, pp. 321–339.

24. Mack MJ, Landreneau RD, Yim AP, Hazelrigg SR, Scruggs GR. Results of video-assisted thymectomy in patients with myasthenia gravis. *J Thorac Cardiovasc Surg* 1996;112:1352–1360.

25. Penn AS, Jaretzki A III, Wolff M, Chang HW, Tennyson V. Thymic abnormalities: antigen or antibody? Response to thymectomy in myasthenia gravis. *Ann NY Acad Sci* 1981;377:786–803.

26. Wekerle H, Muller-Hermelink HK. The thymus in myasthenia gravis. *Curr Top Pathol* 1986;75:179–206.

27. Younger DS, Worrall BB, Penn AS. Myasthenia gravis: historical perspective and overview. *Neurology Suppl* 1997;48:S1–S17.

28. Penn AS, Lovelace RE, Lange DJ, et al. Experimental myasthenia gravis in neonatally thymectomized rabbits. *Neurology* 1977;27:365.

29. Masaoka A, Monden Y, Seike Y, Tanioka T, Kagotani K. Reoperation after transcervical thymectomy for myasthenia gravis. *Neurology* 1982;32:83–85.

30. Rosenberg M, Jauregui WO, Vega MED, Herrera MR, Roncoroni AJ. Recurrence of thymic hyperplasia after thymectomy in myasthenia gravis: its importance as a cause of failure of surgical treatment. *Am J Med* 1983;74:78–82.

31. Henze A, Biberfeld P, Christensson B, Matell G, Pirskanen R. Failing transcervical thymectomy in myasthenia gravis, an evaluation of transsternal re-exploration. *Scand J Thorac Cardiovasc Surg* 1984;18:235–238.

32. Rosenberg M, Jauregui WO, Herrera MR, et al. Recurrence of thymic hyperplasia after trans-sternal thymectomy in myasthenia gravis. *Chest* 1986;89:888–891.

33. Jaretzki A III, Penn AS, Younger DS, et al. "Maximal" thymectomy for myasthenia gravis: results. *J Thorac Cardiovasc Surg* 1988;95:747–757.

34. Miller RG, Filler-Katz A, Kiprov D, Roan R. Repeat thymectomy in chronic refractory myasthenia gravis. *Neurology* 1991;41:923–924.

35. Kornfeld P, Merav A, Fox S, Maier K. How reliable are imaging procedures in detecting residual thymus after previous thymectomy. *Ann NY Acad Sci* 1993;681: 575–576.

36. Masaoka A, Monden Y. Comparison of the results of transsternal simple, transcervical simple and extended thymectomy. *Ann NY Acad Sci* 1981;377:755–764.

37. Matell G, Lebram G, Osterman PO, Pirskanen R. Follow up comparison of suprasternal vs transsternal method for thymectomy in myasthenia gravis. *Ann NY Acad Sci* 1981;377:844–845.

38. Yim AP, Izzat MB. VATS approach to the thymus. In: Yim AP, Hazelrigg SR, Izzat B, et al., eds. *Minimal Access Cardiothoracic Surgery.* Philadelphia, WB Saunders, 1999, pp. 209–215.

39. Kirby TJ, Ginsberg RJ. Transcervical thymectomy. In: Shields T, LoCicero J, Ponn R, ed. *General Thoracic Surgery,* 5th ed. Philadelphia, Lippincott Williams & Wilkins, 2000, pp. 2239–2242.

40. Masaoka A, Nagaoka Y, Kotake Y. Distribution of thymic tissue at the anterior mediastinum: current procedures in thymectomy. *J Thorac Cardiovasc Surg* 1975; 70:747–754.

41. Fukai I, Funato Y, Mizuno Y, Hashimoto T, Masaoka A. Distribution of thymic tissue in the mediastinal adipose tissue. *J Thorac Cardiovasc Surg* 1991;101:1099–1102.

42. Bulkley GB, Bass KN, Stephenson R, et al. Extended cervicomediastinal thymectomy in the integrated management of myasthenia gravis. *Ann Surg* 1997;226: 324–335.
43. Clark RE, Marbarger JP, West PN, et al. Thymectomy for myasthenia gravis in the young adult. *J Thorac Cardiovasc* 1980;80:696–701.
44. Jaretzki A III. Transcervical-transsternal "maximal" thymectomy for myasthenia gravis (Video). Society of Thoracic Surgeons' Film Library, 1996; P.O. Box 809285, Chicago, IL 60680–9285.
45. Lennquist S, Andaker L, Lindvall B, Smeds S. Combined cervicothoracic approach in thymectomy for myasthenia gravis. *Acta Chir Scand* 1990;156:53–61.
46. Andersen M, Jorgensen J, Vejlsted H, Clausen PP. Transcervical thymectomy in patients with non-thymomatous myasthenia gravis. *Scand J Thorac Cardiovasc Surg* 1986;20:233–235.
47. Kagotani K, Monden Y, Nakaha K, et al. Anti-acetylcholine receptor antibody titer with extended thymectomy in myasthenia gravis. *J Thorac Cardiovasc Surg* 1985;90:7–12.
48. Monden Y, Nakahara K, Fujii Y, et al. Myasthenia gravis in elderly patients. *Ann Thorac Surg* 1985;39:433–436.
49. Mulder DG, Graves M, Hermann C Jr. Thymectomy for myasthenia gravis: recent observations and comparison with past experience. *Ann Thorac Surg* 1989;48:551–555.
50. Fujii N, Itoyama Y, Machi M, Goto I. Analysis of prognostic factors in thymectomized patients with myasthenia gravis: correlation between thymic lymphoid cell subsets and postoperative clinical course. *J Neurol Sci* 1991;105:143–149.
51. Nussbaum MS, Rosenthal GJ, Samaha FJ, et al. Management of myasthenia gravis by extended thymectomy with anterior mediastinal dissection. *Surgery* 1992;112: 681–688.
52. Frist WH, Thirumalai S, Doehring CB, et al. Thymectomy for the myasthenia gravis patient: factors influencing outcome. *Ann Thorac Surg* 1994;57:334–338.
53. Masaoka A, Yamakawa Y, Niwa H, et al. Extended thymectomy for myasthenia gravis: a 20 year review. *Ann Thorac Surg* 1996;62:853–859.
54. Detterbeck FC, Scott WW, Howard JF, et al. One hundred consecutive thymectomies for myasthenia gravis. *Ann Thorac Surg* 1996;62:242–245.
55. Mulder DG. Extended transsternal thymectomy. *Chest Surg Clin North Am* 1996;6: 95–105.
56. Fischer JE, Grinvalski HT, Nussbaum MS, et al. Aggressive surgical approach for drug-free remission from myasthenia gravis. *Ann Surg* 1987;205:496–503.
57. Hatton P, Diehl J, Daly BDT, et al. Transsternal radical thymectomy for myasthenia gravis: a 15-year review. *Ann Thorac Surg* 1989;47:838–840.
58. Mulder DM. Extended transsternal thymectomy. In: Shields TW, ed. *General Thoracic Surgery*, 5th ed. Philadelphia, Lippincott Williams & Wilkins, 2000, pp. 2233–2237.
59. Steinglass KM. Extended transsternal thymectomy for myasthenia gravis (Video) 2001. Available from the Myasthenia Gravis Foundation of America, Inc., 5841 Cedar Lake Road (Suite 204), Minneapolis, MN 55416.
60. Blalock A, Mason MF, Morgan HJ, Riven SS. Myasthenia gravis and tumors of the thymus region: report of a case in which the tumor was removed. *Am Surg* 1939; 110:544–561.

61. Clagett OT, Eaton LM. Surgical treatment of myasthenia gravis. *J Thorac Surg* 1947;16:62–80.
62. Blalock A. Thymectomy in the treatment of myasthenia gravis: report of 20 cases. *J Thorac Surg* 1944;13:1291–1308.
63. Olanow CW. The surgical management in myasthenia gravis. In: Sabiston DC Jr, Spencer FC, eds. *Surgery of the Chest*, 6th ed. Philadelphia, WB Saunders, 1995, pp. 1100–1122.
64. LoCicero J III. The combined cervical and partial sternotomy approach for thymectomy. *Chest Surg Clin North Am* 1996;6:85–93.
65. Trastek VF. Thymectomy. In: Kaiser LR, Krin IL, Spray TL, eds. *Mastery of Cardiothoracic Surgery*. Philadelphia, Lippincott-Raven, 1998, pp. 105–111.
66. deCampos JRM, Filomeno LTB, Marchiori PE, Jatene FB. Partial sternotomy approach to the thymus. In: Yim AP, Hazelrigg SR, Izzat B, Landreneau RJ, Mack MJ, Naunheim KS, eds. *Minimal Access Cardiothoracic Surgery*. Philadelphia, WB Saunders, 1999, pp. 205–208.
67. Granone P, Margaritora S, Cesario A, Galetta D. Thymectomy (transsternal) in myasthenia gravis via video assisted infra-mammary cosmetic incision. *Eur J Cardiothorac Surg* 1999;15:861–863.
68. Olanow CW, Wechsler AS. The surgical management of myasthenia gravis. In: Sabiston DC, Spencer FC, eds. *Gibbon's Surgery of the Chest*, 4th ed. Philadelphia, WB Saunders, 1983, pp. 849–869.
69. Olanow CW, Wechsler AS. The surgical management in myasthenia gravis. In: Sabiston DC Jr, ed. *Textbook of Surgery*, 14th ed. Philadelphia, WB Saunders, 1991, pp. 1801–1814.
70. Trastek VF, Pairolero PC. Standard thymectomy. In: Shields TW, ed. *Mediastinal Surgery*. Philadelphia, Lea & Febiger, 1991, pp. 365–368.
71. Trastek VF, Pairolero PC. Surgery of the thymus gland. In: Shields TW, ed. *General Thoracic Surgery*, 4th ed. Baltimore, William & Wilkins, 1994, pp. 1770–1781.
72. Olanow CW, Wechsler AS, Sirotkin-Roses M, Stajich J, Roses AD. Thymectomy as primary therapy in myasthenia gravis. *Ann NY Acad Sci* 1987;505:595–606.
73. Wilkins EW Jr. Thymectomy. *Mod Techn Surg* 1981;38:1–13.
74. Cooper J, Al-Jilaihawa A, Pearson F, Humphrey J, Humphrey HE. An improved technique to facilitate transcervial thymectomy for myasthenia gravis. *Ann Thorac Surg* 1988;45:242–247.
75. Bril V, Kojic S, Ilse W, Cooper J. Long-term clinical outcome after transcervical thymectomy for myasthenia gravis. *Ann Thorac Surg* 1998;65:1520–1522.
76. Durelli L, Maggi G, Casadio C, et al. Actuarial analysis of the occurrence of remission following thymectomy for myasthenia gravis in 400 patients. *J Neurol Neurosurg Psychiatry* 1991;54:406–411.
77. Klingen G, Johansson L, Westerholm CJ, Sundstroom C. Transcervical thymectomy with the aid of mediastinoscopy for myasthenia gravis: eight years' experience. *Ann Thorac Surg* 1977;23:342–347.
78. Kirby TJ, Ginsberg RJ. Transcervical thymectomy. In: Shields TW, ed. *Mediastinal Surgery*. Philadelphia, Lea & Febiger, 1991, pp. 369–371.
79. Hagan JA, Patterson GA. Surgery of myasthenia gravis. In: Pearson FG, ed. *Thoracic Surgery*. New York, Churchill Livingstone, 1995, pp. 1511–1521.
80. Papatestas AE, Genkins G, Kornfeld P, Horowitz S, Kark AE. Transcervical thymectomy in myasthenia gravis. *Surg Gynecol Obstet* 1975;140:535–540.

81. Sugarbaker DJ. Thoracoscopy in the management of anterior mediastinal masses. *Ann Thorac Surg* 1993;56:653–656.
82. Roviaro G, Rebuffat C, Varoli F, et al. Vidiothoracoscopic excision of mediastinal masses: indications and technique. *Ann Thorac Surg* 1994;58:1679–1684.
83. Sabbagh MN, Garza JJS, Patten B. Thoracoscopic thymectomy in patients with myasthenia gravis. *Muscle Nerve* 1995;18:1475–1477.
84. Yim APC, Kay RLC, Ho JKS. Video-assisted thoracoscopic thymectomy for myasthenia gravis. *Chest* 1995;108:1440–1443.
85. Mack MJ, Scruggs GR. Video-assisted thymectomy. In: Shields T, LoCicero J, Ponn R, eds. *General Thoracic Surgery*, 5th ed. Philadelphia, Lippincott Williams & Wilkins, 2000, pp. 2243–2249.
86. Mineo TC, Pompeo E, Ambrogi V, et al. Adjuvant pneumomediastinum in thoracoscopic thymectomy for myasthenia gravis. *Ann Thorac Surg* 1996;62:1210–1212.
87. Novellino L, Longoni M, Spinelli L, et al. "Extended" thymectomy, without sternotomy, performed by cervicotomy and thoracoscopic technique in the treatment of myasthenia gravis. *Int Surg* 1994;79:378–381.
88. Scelsi R, Ferro MT, Scelsi L, et al. Detection and morphology of thymic remnants after video-assisted thoracoscopic thymectomy (VATET) in patients with myasthenia gravis. *Int Surg* 1996;81:14–17.
89. Lawless JF. Statistical Models and Methods for Life Table Data. New York, John Wiley & Sons, 1982, pp. 52–99.
90. Olak J, Chiu RCJ. A surgeon's guide to biostatistical inferences. Part II. ACS Bull 1993;78:27–31.
91. Blackstone EH. Outcome analysis using hazard function methodology. *Ann Thorac Surg* 1996;61:S2–S7.
92. McQuillen MP, Leone MG. A treatment carol: thymectomy revisited. *Neurology* 1977:1103–1106.
93. Viet HR, Schwab RS. Thymectomy for myasthenia gravis. In: Veit HR, ed. *Records of Experience of Massachusetts General Hospital*. Springfield, Charles C. Thomas, 1960, pp. 597–607.
94. Oosterhuis HJ. Observations of the natural history of myasthenia gravis and the effect of thymectomy. *Ann NY Acad Sci* 1981;377:678–689.
95. Sanders DS, Kaminski HJ, Phillips LH, JR, Jaretzki A III. Letter to the editor. *J Am Coll Surg* 2001;193:340–344.
96. Buckingham JM, Howard FM, Bernatz PE. The value of thymectomy in myasthenia gravis: a computer-assisted matched study. *Ann Surg* 1976;184:453–458.
97. Gronseth S, Barohn RJ. Practice parameters: thymectomy for autoimmune myasthenia gravis (an evidence base review). *Neurology* 2000;55:7–15.
98. Newsom-Davis J. Thymectomy trial in non-thymomatous myasthenia gravis patients receiving immunosuppressive therapy. 2001, in preparation.
99. Rowland LP. Controversies about the treatment of myasthenia gravis. *J Neurol Neurosurg Psychiatry* 1980;43:644–659.
100. Mulder DG. Thymectomy for myasthenia gravis: reply to letter to editor. *Ann Thor Surg* 1990;49:688–689.
101. Hoch W, McConville J, Melms A, Newsom-Davis J, Vinvent A. Autoantibodies to the receptor tyrosine kinase MuSK in patients with myasthenia gravis without acetylcholine receptor antibodies. *Nat Med* 2001;7:365–368.

102. Lindberg C, Andersen O, Larsson S, Oden A. Remission rate after thymectomy in myasthenia gravis when the bias of immunosuppressive therapy is eliminated. *Acta Neurol Scand* 1992;86:323–328.
103. Rodriguez M, Gomez MR, Howard F, Taylor WF. Myasthenia gravis in children: long term follow-up. *Ann Neurol* 1983;13:504–510.
104. Mulder DG, Herrmann C Jr, Keesey J, Edwards H. Thymectomy for myasthenia gravis. *Am J Surg* 1983;146:61–66.
105. Kirschner PA. Myasthenia gravis. In: Shields T. ed. *General Thoracic Surgery,* 5th ed. Philadelphia, Lippincott Williams & Wilkins, 2000, pp. 2207–2218.
106. Budde JM, Morris CD, Gal AA, Mansour KA, Miller JI. Predictors of outcome in thymectomy for myasthenia gravis. *Ann Thorac Surg* 2001;72:197–202.
107. Mack MJ. Commentary on minimally access thymectomy for myasthenia gravis. In: Yim AP, Hazelrigg SR, Izzat B, et al., eds. *Minimal Access Cardiothoracic Surgery.* Philadelphia, WB Saunders, 1999, pp. 218–219.
108. Lanska D. Indications for thymectomy in myasthenia gravis. *Neurology* 1990;40: 1828–1829.
109. Keesey JC. A treatment algorithm for autoimmune myasthenia in adults. *Ann NY Acad Sci* 1998;841:753–768.
110. Soliven BC, Lange DJ, Penn AS, Younger DS III. Seronegative myasthenia gravis. *Neurology* 1988;38:514–517.
111. Schumm F, Wietholter H, Fateh-Mogbadan A, Dichgans J. Thymectomy in myasthenia with pure ocular symptoms. *J Neurol Neurosurg Psychiatry* 1985;48:332–337.
112. Rubin JW, Ellison RG, Moore HV, Pai GP. Factors affecting response to thymectomy for myasthenia gravis. *J Thorac Cardiovasc Surg* 1981;82:720–728.
113. Monden Y, Nakahara K, Kagotani K, et al. Effects of preoperative duration of symptoms on patients with myasthenia gravis. *Ann Thorac Surg* 1984;38:287–291.
114. DeFilippi VJ, Richman DP, Ferguson MK. Transcervical thymectomy for myasthenia gravis. *Ann Thorac Surg* 1994;57:194–197.
115. Adams C, Theodorescu D, Murphy E, Shandling B. Thymectomy in juvenile myasthenia gravis. *J Child Neurol* 1990;5:215–218.
116. Andrews PI, Massey JM, Howard JF, Sanders DB. Race, sex, and puberty influence onset, severity, and outcome in juvenile myasthenia gravis. *Neurology* 1994; 44:1208–1214.
117. Andrews PI. A treatment algorithm for autoimmune myasthenia gravis in children. *Ann NY Acad Sci* 1998;841:789–802.
118. Seybold ME. Thymectomy in childhood myasthenia gravis. *Ann NY Acad Sci* 1998; 841:731–741.
119. Lovelace RE, Younger DS. Myasthenia gravis with thymoma. *Neurology* 1997;48: S76–S81.
120. Shields TW. Thymic tumors. In: Shields TW, ed. *General Thoracic Surgery,* 5th ed. Philadelphia, Lippincott Williams & Wilkins, 2000, pp. 2181–2205.
121. Ellis K, Austin JHM, Jaretzki A III. Radiologic detection of thymoma in patients with myasthenia gravis. *Am J Radiol* 1988;151:873–881.
122. Namba T, Brunner NG, Grob D. Myasthenia gravis in patients with thymoma, with particular reference to onset after thymectomy. *Medicine* 1978;57:411–433.
123. Younger DS, Braun NMT, Jaretzki A III, Penn AS, Lovelace AE. Myasthenia gravis: determinants for independent ventilation after transsternal thymectomy. *Neurology* 1984;34:336–340.

124. Mayer SA. Intensive care of the myasthenbic patient. *Neurology* 1997;48:S70–S81.
125. Jaretzki A III, Penn AS, Rowland LP, Sanborn K, Hyman A. Thymectomy for myasthenia gravis: a guideline for pre- and post-operative care. 1987. Available from Myasthenia Gravis Foundation of America, Inc., 5841 Cedar Lake Road (Suite 204), Minneapolis, MN-55416.
126. Miller RG, Rosenberg JA, Force APPT. Care of patient with ALS: report of the Quality Standards Subcommittee of the AAN. *Neurology* 1999;52:1311–1323.
127. Kirklin JW, Blackstone EH. Clinical studies with nonrandomly assigned treatment. In: Kirklin JW, Barrett-Boyes BG, eds. *Cardiac Surgery,* 2nd ed. New York, Churchill-Livingstone, 1993, pp. 269–270.
128. Haegerty PJ, Zeger SL. Marginal regression models for clustered ordinal measurements. *J Am Stat Assoc* 1996;91:1024–1036.
129. Wolfe GI, Herbelin L, Nations SP, et al. Myasthenia gravis activities of daily living profile. *Neurology* 1999;52:1487–1489.
130. Jaeschke R, Guyatt GH. How to develop and validate a new quality of life instrument. In: Spilker B, ed. *Quality of Life Assessments in Clinical Trials.* New York, Raven, 1990, pp. 47–57.
131. Ashour MH, Jain SK, Kattan KM, et al. Maximal thymectomy for myasthenia gravis. *Eur J Cardiothorac Surg* 1995;9:461–464.
132. Emeryk B, Strugalska MH. Evaluation of results of thymectomy in myasthenia gravis. *J Neurol* 1976;211:155–168.
133. Hayat G, Mohyuddin YA, Naunheim K. Efficacy of thymectomy in myasthenia gravis. *Miss Med* 1995;92:252–257.

# 12
# Lambert-Eaton Syndrome

*DEDICATED TO DR. EDWARD H. LAMBERT*
*ON THE OCCASION OF HIS 87TH BIRTHDAY*

## C. Michel Harper and Vanda A. Lennon

## INTRODUCTION

The Lambert-Eaton syndrome* (LES) is an autoimmune presynaptic disorder of peripheral cholinergic neurotransmission characterized by proximal myasthenic weakness and mild autonomic dysfunction. Approximately 60% of cases are associated with small cell lung carcinoma (SCLC), and LES can appear before or after the clinical diagnosis of cancer. The P/Q-type voltage-gated calcium channel in motor nerve terminals [classified by structure and function as $Ca_V2.1$ *(1)*] is the presumptive target of autoantibodies that mediate LES. This channel is related antigenically to calcium channels expressed on surface membranes of SCLC tumor cells. When the neuronal $Ca_V2.1$ channel's function is impaired, nerve-stimulated quantal release of the neurotransmitter acetylcholine (ACh) is reduced. This lowers the safety margin for synaptic transmission at the neuromuscular junction and in certain autonomic nerve terminals.

## HISTORY

The first reported association of a myasthenic syndrome with lung cancer is commonly attributed to Anderson, Churchill-Davidson, and Richardson, in 1953 *(2)*. This trio of English clinicians described a patient with bronchial carcinoma who presented with generalized weakness that was worse in proximal muscles and in the evening and was accompanied by transient diplopia

---

*The authors prefer *Lambert-Eaton syndrome*, rather than the more commonly used *Lambert-Eaton myasthenic syndrome*, to designate this disorder.

From: *Current Clinical Neurology: Myasthenia Gravis and Related Disorders*
Edited by: H. J. Kaminski © Humana Press Inc., Totowa, NJ

and dysphagia. No electrophysiologic abnormality was found. A neurologic diagnosis of myasthenia gravis was made on the basis of a positive edrophonium (Tensilon®) test and the therapeutic benefit of neostigmine. The case may indeed have been myasthenia gravis *(3,4)*. Churchill-Davidson, who was the electromyographer of the 1953 report, wrote 10 years later *(5)*: "Originally it was thought that there was a close relationship between cases of bronchial carcinoma and myasthenia gravis" *(2)*. This view is now known to be wrong. Lambert *(6)* was the first to describe (the paraneoplastic) "myasthenic syndrome." Beginning in 1956, Lambert and his colleagues at the Mayo Clinic described the clinical and electrodiagnostic features of a unique "myasthenic syndrome associated with malignant tumors" *(7–10)*. Characteristic findings were facilitation of both muscle strength and the amplitude of the compound muscle action potential (CMAP) after exercise or high-frequency electrical stimulation. Elmqvist and Lambert *(11,12)* demonstrated the presynaptic origin of LES by using microelectrodes to study biopsied intercostal nerve-muscle preparations of these patients. They documented a severe reduction in endplate potential (EPP) amplitude and quantal content, with preservation of miniature endplate potential (MEPP) amplitude. Further advances in understanding the pathogenesis of LES were the recognition that patients with this syndrome have a heightened frequency of autoimmune disorders and autoantibodies *(13,14)*, the demonstration that active zone particles in the presynaptic nerve terminals of affected patients are disorganized and reduced in number *(15)*, the recognition of the pivotal role of $Ca_v$ channels in ACh release *(16)*, the transfer of LES to mice using IgG from serum of LES patients *(17–20)*, evidence for the interaction of LES serum antibodies with a $Ca_v$ channel expressed in cultured lung cancer cells *(21)*, the development of $Ca_v$ channel subtype-specific ligands and sensitive radioimmunoassays that aid the serologic diagnosis of LES *(22–26)*, and the improvement in neuromuscular transmission in LES after successful treatment of the underlying malignancy *(27)*, or immunomodulatory therapy *(28–31)*, or administration of drugs that promote the quantal release of ACh *(32–35)*.

## PATHOGENESIS

### Physiology of Neuromuscular Transmission

Normal neuromuscular transmission ensures the generation of a single muscle fiber action potential in response to each motor nerve action potential at firing rates up to 40–50 Hz. The safety margin of neuromuscular transmission refers to the amplitude of the EPP above that required to reach threshold for activating a muscle action potential. Postsynaptic factors that affect the size of the EPP (and therefore the size of the safety margin of neuromuscular transmission) are the number and function of acetylcholine receptors (AChRs), the presence of acetylcholinesterase, and the three-dimensional configuration of the synapse *(36)*. The EPP is affected by two important pre-synaptic factors as well. The first is the presence of adequate quanta within the readily releasable pool of ACh vesicles adjacent to the active zones of the nerve terminal membrane *(37)*. The second is the number and function of nerve terminal $Ca_v$ 2.1 channels. In normal as well as diseased endplates, the EPP amplitude falls with slow rates of repetitive nerve stimulation (2–5 Hz) owing to depletion of immediately available stores of ACh *(38)*. When the EPP amplitude drops below threshold, the muscle fiber action potential is blocked. The safety margin of neuromuscular transmission is large enough to prevent blocking at normal endplates *(39)*. The characteristic pathophysiologic finding in neuromuscular junction diseases of either presynaptic or postsynaptic origin is blocking at multiple endplates. This correlates with blocking observed by single-fiber electromyography (EMG), motor unit potential (MUP) amplitude variation observed by standard concentric needle EMG, decrement of the CMAP observed at slow rates of repetitive stimulation in nerve conduction studies, and the patient's weakness worsening with exertion *(40)*.

During exercise or rapid rates of repetitive nerve stimulation, mobilization of the recycling pool of ACh vesicles during influx of $Ca^{2+}$ into the nerve terminal through $Ca_v2.1$ channels temporarily improves the safety margin of neuromuscular transmission (postactivation facilitation). This is followed by several minutes of a worsened safety margin (postactivation exhaustion). A CMAP decrement observed at slow rates of repetitive nerve stimulation is usually repaired by brief exercise or by a rapid rate of repetitive stimulation, but it returns and may worsen several minutes later. In the patient who has a severe defect of neuromuscular transmission, the EPP fails to reach threshold in a majority of fibers. This results in objective weakness and a low-amplitude CMAP at rest. Brief exercise or rapid rates of repetitive stimulation produce a transient increase in the EPP above threshold and temporary facilitation of the CMAP.

The mechanism by which $Ca^{2+}$ facilitates release of ACh from the motor nerve terminal has been partially elucidated *(16)*. The $Ca_v2.1$ channels are arranged within the terminal membrane in double arrays that lie immediately adjacent to the crests of the postsynaptic folds. This brings the point of ACh release in close proximity to the area of postsynaptic membrane where AChR concentration is the greatest. Entry of $Ca^{2+}$ through the $Ca_v2.1$ channel is triggered by nerve terminal depolarization. Prolongation of the time constant of depolarization [e.g., by blockade of nerve terminal potassium ($K_v$)

channels using 3,4-diaminopyridine] increases the amount of $Ca^{2+}$ influx. The abrupt local rise in $Ca^{2+}$ concentration in the nerve terminal is "sensed" by active zone proteins exemplified by synaptotagmin, a vesicular membrane (v-soluble N-ethylmaleimide-sensitive factor attachment protein receptor [SNARE]) protein. The resulting fusion of the readily releasable (docked) vesicle and nerve terminal membranes culminates in exocytosis of ACh. The $Ca_v2.1$ channel itself is a target membrane (t-)SNARE protein and plays a central role in docking and fusion of the neurotransmitter vesicle by interacting noncovalently with synaptobrevin in the vesicle membrane and with syntaxin and synaptic vesicle-associated protein (SNAP)-25 in the nerve terminal membrane, in concert with soluble cytoplasmic factors, including N-ethylmaleimide-sensitive factor (NSF) and $\alpha$-SNAP *(16,38)*. Following exocytosis, vesicles are recycled from the plasma membrane by clathrin-dependent and -independent processes. Synaptotagmin plays a role in the former, which involves sequential interactions of clathrin adaptor proteins, dynamin, amphiphysin, and other highly conserved cytoplasmic proteins *(37)*.

Neuronal $Ca_v$ channels consist of five subunits *(41,42)*. The $\alpha1$-subunit is the largest and contains the voltage sensor and cation pore. It has four homologous domains, each with six transmembrane segments. The M4 segments contribute the voltage sensor, and loops between M5 and M6 segments in each domain form the ion channel and determine $Ca^{2+}$-selective permeability. $\alpha1$ also bears high-affinity binding sites for channel antagonists, including $\omega$-conopeptides, and for regulatory G proteins and SNARE proteins. Its sequence determines the family and subfamily of the $Ca_v$ channel complex (**Table 1**). The auxiliary subunits, $\beta$, $\alpha2\delta$ and $\gamma$, influence insertion and stability of $\alpha1$ in the plasma membrane and modify the conductance and kinetics of the channel.

## *Pathophysiology of Neuromuscular Transmission in LES*

LES was initially recognized as a disorder of neuromuscular transmission because of its clinical similarities to myasthenia gravis, including fatigable weakness that is improved with cholinesterase inhibitors. The characteristic electrophysiologic findings described by Lambert and colleagues were established by standard electrodiagnostic studies, and by microelectrode studies *(7,9,12)*. The microelectrode findings are normal amplitude and frequency of the MEPP, with reduction of the EPP amplitude secondary to a low quantal content of the nerve action potential *(12)*. The quantal content and the size of the EPP increase during high-frequency nerve stimulation and with addition of extracellular $Ca^{2+}$. Biochemical studies of nerve-muscle preparations from LES patients have revealed a reduction in the amount of ACh released and normal function of acetylcholinesterase *(43)*.

**Table 1**
**Classification of Voltage-Gated Calcium (Ca$_v$) Channels[a]**

| Class | Type | α1-Subunit | Antagonists | Effector Function | Predominant Cell Expression |
|---|---|---|---|---|---|
| Ca$_v$1.1 | L | S | Dihydropyridines, phenylalkylamines, benzothiazepines | Contraction | Skeletal muscle |
| Ca$_v$1.2 | | C | | Contraction | Heart |
| Ca$_v$1.3 | | D | | Secretion; gene transcription | Neuron soma; pancreatic islet; kidney; ovary; cochlea |
| Ca$_v$1.4 | | F | | Gene transcription | Retina |
| Ca$_v$2.1 | P/Q | A | ω-Conotoxin M$_{VIIC}$, ω-agatoxin$_{IIIA}$ and $_{IVA}$ | Neurotransmitter release | Central, autonomic, and peripheral motor neurons |
| Ca$_v$2.2 | N | B | ω-Conotoxin G$_{VIA}$ | Neurotransmitter release | Central sensory and motor, and autonomic neurons |
| Ca$_v$2.3 | R | E | SNX-482, ω-agatoxin$_{IIIA}$ | Neurotransmitter release | Central neurons, cochlea, retina, heart, pituitary |
| Ca$_v$3.1 | T | G | ω-Agatoxin$_{IIIA}$, succinimides | Pacemaker activity | Central and peripheral neuron soma |
| Ca$_v$3.2 | | H | | Neurotransmitter release | Central neurons, heart, kidney, liver |
| Ca$_v$3.3 | | I | | Neurotransmitter release | Central neurons |

[a]Channels of Ca$_v$1 and Ca$_v$2 classes are activated by high voltage; class Ca$_v$3 (T-type) channels are activated by low voltage.

273

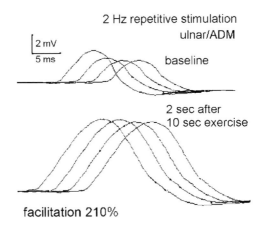

Fig. 1. Repetitive stimulation study in a patient with moderate-severe weakness caused by LES. *x*-axis = time (milliseconds); *y*-axis = CMAP amplitude (millivolts); ADM = abductor digiti minimi.

The fully developed defect of neuromuscular transmission in LES is typically severe, reducing the EPP amplitude below threshold in the majority of fibers in resting muscle. The patient is weak at rest, and CMAP responses to initial supramaximal nerve stimuli are low in amplitude (**Fig. 1**). Brief exercise produces transient clinical improvements in strength and tendon reflex responses and EMG facilitation of the CMAP amplitude. If exercise is impractical for the patient, repetitive stimulation at 20–50 Hz can be used to elicit facilitation of the CMAP amplitude. At this stage, standard concentric needle EMG shows MUP amplitude variation, and stimulated single-fiber EMG shows increased jitter and blocking, both of which improve at higher rates of stimulation *(44)*.

The patient with early LES may have a relatively mild defect of neuromuscular transmission, in which the safety margin is not reduced sufficiently to drop the EPP below threshold at rest. This ensures relatively preserved strength at rest and a normal CMAP amplitude (**Fig. 2**). During repetitive stimulation at slow rates (2–5 Hz), there is decrement of the CMAP, which improves with exercise or higher rates of repetitive stimulation. Thus, when LES is mild, the results of electrophysiologic tests of neuromuscular transmission are very similar to those of myasthenia gravis or other postsynaptic disorders of neuromuscular transmission *(44)*. The abnormalities revealed by standard clinical electrophysiologic testing (nerve conduction studies, repetitive stimulation, and needle EMG) sometimes reflect the severity more than the synaptic element responsible for the defect of neuromuscular transmission.

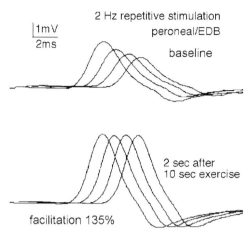

**Fig. 2.** Repetitive stimulation study in a patient with mild weakness caused by LES. *x*-axis = time (milliseconds); *y*-axis = CMAP amplitude (millivolts); EDB = extensor digitorum brevis.

## Immunopathophysiology of LES

LES may occur as a paraneoplastic syndrome or as an idiopathic organ-specific autoimmune disease *(31,45)*. Thyrogastric autoimmune diseases, which include thyroiditis, pernicious anemia, and type 1 diabetes, and their serologic markers are frequent in LES patients, particularly in those without evidence of lung cancer *(13,14,45,46)*. The P/Q-type ($Ca_v2.1$) calcium channel in the presynaptic membrane at the neuromuscular junction is strongly implicated but not yet proved definitively to be the target of pathogenic autoantibodies. It is also implicated in autonomic manifestations of LES *(47)*. The finding of P/Q-type calcium channel antibody in the serum of more than 90% of nonimmunosuppressed LES patients *(25)* is compelling but circumstantial evidence for this antibody being the effector of neuromuscular transmission impairment. The capacity of serum IgG from LES patients to produce the clinical, electrophysiologic, and ultrastructural lesions characteristic of LES to mice *(18–20)* is also circumstantial for, and not proof, of the pathogenicity of P/Q-type calcium channel antibodies. No monoclonal antibody or affinity-purified antibody of P/Q-type calcium channel specificity has been reported to transfer the neuromuscular or autonomic transmission defect to laboratory animals. This long-awaited evidence will definitively prove the pathogenicity of P/Q-type calcium channel antibodies. The Takamori laboratory has reported electrophysiologic abnormalities consistent with LES in rats immunized with a peptide corresponding to an extracellular segment of the $\alpha_{1A}$ subunit of the $Ca_v2.1$ channel complex *(48)*. This important report awaits independent confirmation.

SCLC is the most common neoplasm associated with paraneoplastic LES. It is usually occult when neurologic manifestations appear. The $Ca_v2.1$ channel at the neuromuscular junction is related antigenically to the $Ca_v$ channels in SCLC and other neuroendocrine cells *(21,22,49)*. Reports that the prognosis of SCLC is better when associated with LES *(50)* and that successful treatment of SCLC leads to remission of LES in 70% of patients *(27,31)* support the hypothesis that paraneoplastic LES arises as an immune response initiated by antigens expressed in the patient's neoplasm. The antigen that initiates and perpetuates $Ca_v$ channel autoimmunity in the idiopathic form of LES has not been identified.

The pathophysiology of LES is entirely reproducible in mice with antibodies as effectors. As we reviewed above, IgG isolated from LES patients' sera confers electrophysiologic and morphologic characteristics of LES at the motor nerve terminal *(17–19)*. Mice receiving IgG from serum of individually selected patients can become profoundly weak and die from respiratory failure *(20)*. The IgG in those cases presumably has high affinity for mouse $Ca_v2.1$ channel epitopes. The reduction of $Ca_v$ channel function is independent of complement *(20)* and is attributed to IgG-mediated acceleration of $Ca_v$ channel degradation through bivalent crosslinking of adjacent channels, a phenomenon known as antigenic modulation *(51,52)*. LES IgG reduces $Ca^{2+}$ influx through multiple $Ca_v$ channel subtypes in cultured SCLC cells and motor neurons *(21,53–57)*, as well as reducing neurotransmitter release in mice *(47,57)*. The benefit of immunotherapy in LES patients is plausibly explained by increased clearance of antibodies [plasmapheresis, intravenous immunoglobulin *(58)*] or reduced production of antibodies (immunosuppressive medications). Effector T-lymphocytes have not been implicated in the pathophysiology of LES, but the production of antigen-specific IgG by B-lymphocytes requires continuing helper T-lymphocyte activity.

## EPIDEMIOLOGY

The incidence and prevalence of LES are unknown, but the frequency of new LES diagnoses in the Mayo Clinic EMG laboratory, excluding referral cases, approximates 1 for every 10 cases of acquired myasthenia gravis (C.M. Harper, unpublished observations). The incidence of myasthenia gravis is estimated to be 4–6/million/yr in the United States, and its prevalence 40–60/million. Females predominate in idiopathic LES *(31)*, and the age of onset varies from the first decade to old age. Patients with idiopathic LES are frequently nonsmokers and tend to have a personal and family history of organ-specific autoimmune diseases as well as a higher prevalence of certain HLA gene products than patients with paraneoplastic LES *(59,60)*. It has been estimated that the frequency of LES in patients with newly diagnosed SCLC is 3% *(61)*. In its earliest descriptions, paraneoplastic LES predominantly affected men. This sex bias was attributed to cigarette smoking habits. Lung cancer epidemiology has paralleled the sociology of smoking, with a two-decade lag. Thus, in 1987, lung cancer became the leading cause of cancer death in North American women *(62)*. Men still outnumber women in lung cancer prevalence. It is therefore not surprising that among cases of SCLC-related LES identified serologically in the Mayo Clinic Neuroimmunology Laboratory since 1987, and not complicated by other autoimmune neurologic disorders, men marginally outnumber women (authors' unpublished observation; $N > 100$ patients).

By contrast, in that same period women account for 66% of patients diagnosed with SCLC-related paraneoplastic neurologic disorders recognized serologically by the type 1 anti-neuronal nuclear autoantibody (ANNA-1, or anti-Hu) *(63,64)*. Unlike LES, disorders associated with the ANNA-1 autoantibody are generally inflammatory and affect both the peripheral and central nervous system. The immunologic outcome of an immune response, i.e., whether inflammatory or not, is determined by the cytokine milieu at the level of helper T-lymphocyte activation. It is conceivable that this is influenced both by sex hormones and by onconeural antigen dominance among proteins released to lymph nodes by necrosing tumor cells. A proinflammatory response would yield cytotoxic T-cell effectors, for which nuclear and cytoplasmic-directed antibodies serve as a surrogate marker *(65)*, whereas a noninflammatory response may favor production of plasma membrane ion channel antibodies.

Cancer is diagnosed in about 45% of contemporary LES cases, and SCLC accounts for 90% of paraneoplastic LES *(45)*. Overall, 18% of patients who have SCLC without clinical evidence of LES are seropositive for P/Q-type calcium channel antibodies *(25)*. When multiple paraneoplastic disorders coexist, particularly with severe peripheral neuropathy and subacute cerebellar ataxia, the diagnosis of LES tends to be overlooked (authors' unpublished observations). Other cancers have been reported with LES, including thymoma, lymphoma, reproductive tract tumors, and renal cell cancer *(45,66–71)*, but the likelihood of the patient having a coexisting occult SCLC is high *(22,64)*. Anticipation of SCLC in these cases is supported by observations that the diagnosis of LES can antedate the detection of SCLC by 5–8 years *(45*; and unpublished observations of E.H. Lambert). Primary small cell carcinoma in an extrapulmonary site, such as skin (Merkel cell carcinoma), tongue, larynx, breast, cervix, or prostate *(72,73)* should also be considered in patients presenting with LES, particularly in the absence of known risk factors for lung cancer.

## CLINICAL PRESENTATION

### Symptoms and Signs

Subacute progressive fatigue, weakness, and unaccustomed injurious falls are the most common presenting manifestations of LES. The weakness increases with exertion and improves transiently with rest. Sometimes a history of transient clinical facilitation of strength following brief exercise is elicited, but more commonly there are complaints of increased weakness with exercise. Aching pain in the hip and posterior thigh region is common in paraneoplastic LES, but significant myalgia and other sensory symptoms are rare. Muscle atrophy is rare, and fasciculations and cramps are not observed. The distribution of weakness is characteristic. Starting in hip flexors and other proximal lower limb muscles, it leads to complaints of difficulty arising from low chairs or a squatting position or trouble climbing stairs and inclines. In one series of 50 LES patients, weakness began in the lower limbs in 65% and was generalized in 12% of patients *(45)*. Even after weakness is more generalized, the hip girdle muscles are involved disproportionately in most patients. Proximal muscles of the upper limb and neck as well as interossei muscles of the hand are also preferentially affected in LES.

Contrary to common belief, approximately 25% of patients have cranial muscle involvement at some point. Ptosis, facial weakness, dysphagia, dysarthria, and difficulty chewing are usually milder than in myasthenia gravis and may occur later *(35,45)*. When it occurs, respiratory involvement is usually mild, with a restrictive functional pattern, unless complicated by emphysema related to smoking, in which case respiratory failure can occur terminally. In rare cases respiratory failure is the presenting manifestation of LES *(74;* authors' unpublished observation). Deep tendon reflexes are characteristically reduced or absent in LES, but it is important to note that reflexes may be relatively preserved early in the course of the illness. Facilitation of the reflex after brief exercise is an important sign supporting the diagnosis of LES and is easier to demonstrate at the bedside than facilitation of muscle strength.

Approximately 80% of LES patients have symptoms of autonomic dysfunction, and in 6% of patients these may be the presenting symptoms *(45)*. Most common autonomic symptoms are impotence in men and xerostomia in both sexes, and most common abnormalities of autonomic testing are in sweating, cardiovagal reflexes, and salivation *(46)*. Slowing of pupillary reflexes, gastrointestinal dysmotility, orthostatic hypotension, and urinary retention are sometimes noted, but these signs usually indicate a coexisting paraneoplastic autonomic neuropathy in the setting of SCLC and are often accompanied by one or more marker autoantibodies specific for neuronal nuclear or cytoplasmic antigens *(65,75,76)*, particularly collapsin response mediator protein (CRMP)-5 IgG, ANNA-1, ANNA-2, ANNA-3, Purkinje cell antibody (PCA)-2 or amphiphysin autoantibody (V.A. Lennon, unpublished observations).

The sensory system is spared in LES, but sensory symptoms and signs may be present if there is an associated paraneoplastic sensory neuronopathy, peripheral neuropathy, or myelopathy. Constitutional symptoms of anorexia and weight loss are attributable to an underlying malignancy and may be evidence of paraneoplastic gastroparesis for which autoantibodies of ANNA-1, N-type calcium channel, and ganglionic AChR specificities are valuable serologic markers *(77,78)*. Symptoms of lung cancer itself, particularly hemoptysis and chest pain, are very uncommon. On the other hand, manifestations of other organ-specific autoimmune disorders (e.g., pernicious anemia, hyperthyroidism, or hypothyroidism) are very common in association with LES. The authors have personally encountered two patients with idiopathic LES in whom weight loss was explained by concurrent but initially unrecognized Graves' disease.

## Natural History

The course of LES is more varied among patients who have lung cancer or are at high risk for it, than in those without lung cancer risk. LES frequently presents several months or years prior to the diagnosis of cancer. If sputum cytology, chest X-ray, and computed tomography are negative in LES patients at risk for SCLC, the diagnostic yield is increased by performing magnetic resonance imaging or positron emission tomography scanning of the chest, bronchoscopy, and transbronchial biopsy or thoracoscopy if imaging studies suggest a neoplasm. A search for extrapulmonary small-cell carcinoma is warranted when chest studies are negative. These have been recorded in skin, tongue, larynx, cervix, prostate, breast, and ovary *(70*; S. Vernino and V.A. Lennon, unpublished observations). The clinical course of LES, with and without cancer, is generally progressive in the first year, with less fluctuation and a lower spontaneous remission rate than autoimmune myasthenia gravis. Many patients will improve with effective treatment of the underlying malignancy. It has been reported that SCLC in the context of LES may have a less aggressive natural history and a better response to therapy *(50)*. Whether this relates to early diagnosis because of the paraneoplastic syndrome or reflects a more effective immune response to the tumor is unclear. In the absence of cancer, LES may produce long-term disability on account of weakness and fatigue *(31)*. Most patients benefit from continued therapy with an oral cholinesterase inhibitor and 3-4-diaminopyridine, an agent that increases the release of ACh induced by nerve stimulus. Guanidine is also beneficial *(34)* in this regard, but its use is limited by renal and bone marrow toxicity. Immunosuppressive therapy also is beneficial *(31,79,80)*, but symptomatic response to immunosuppressive therapy tends to be less in LES than in myasthenia gravis.

## DIAGNOSIS

### Clinical Manifestations

LES should be suspected in a patient who complains of generalized fatigue or weakness that worsens with exertion and should be considered along with myasthenia gravis when a patient presents with prolonged apnea following a surgical procedure involving a neuromuscular blocking drug *(5,81)*. Factors that increase the likelihood of LES include early and prominent involvement of hip flexor muscles, xerostomia, impotence and other manifestations of autonomic dysfunction, reduced or absent reflexes (in lower limbs initially and more diffuse in the established disease), a history of smoking or lung cancer or autoimmunity, a family history of lung cancer or autoimmunity, and facilitation of tendon reflexes or strength on clinical examination.

The diagnosis of LES should also be suspected when a patient with another lung cancer-related paraneoplastic syndrome has prominent weakness or is seropositive for P/Q-type calcium channel antibody, or when a patient has respiratory failure of undetermined cause, or is referred with a diagnosis of seronegative myasthenia gravis.

### Electrodiagnostic Studies

For unambiguous electrodiagnosis of LES it is critically important that the patient be well rested and warm, that medications affecting the neuromuscular junction be withheld for several hours before testing, and that clinically weak muscles be tested. When weakness is moderate to severe, electrodiagnostic studies reveal a pathognomonic pattern *(44)* (**Table 2**). The baseline amplitude of the CMAP is reduced. A decrement is observed with slow rates of repetitive nerve stimulation, and facilitation of more than 200% (doubling of the baseline amplitude) is observed following brief exercise or high-frequency repetitive nerve stimulation. Needle examination shows low-amplitude varying MUP. Fibrillation potentials are usually absent but may occur in severe cases. Single-fiber EMG shows increased jitter and blocking that transiently improve at higher firing rates. The electrodiagnostic findings are usually demonstrated most readily in small intrinsic hand muscles.

**Table 2**
**Electrodiagnostic Characteristics of Lambert-Eaton Syndrome**[a]

| Severity of Weakness | Nerve Conduction Studies (CMAP Amplitude) | Needle Examination |
|---|---|---|
| Moderate-severe | 1. Baseline (initial stimulus): low<br>2. During RS at 2–3 Hz: decrement<br>3. After brief exercise or after RS at 20–50 Hz: facilitation > 200% | 1. Insertional activity: normal<br>2. Motor unit potentials: small with amplitude variation<br>3. Single-fiber EMG: increased jitter and blocking |
| Mild | 1. Baseline (initial stimulus): normal<br>2. During RS at 2–3 Hz: decrement<br>3. After brief exercise or after RS at 20–50 Hz: facilitation < 200% | 1. Insertional activity: normal<br>2. Motor unit potentials: normal to small with amplitude variation<br>3. Single-fiber EMG: increased jitter and blocking |

[a]CMAP = compound muscle action potential elicited by supramaximal stimulation of nerve in clinically weak muscle, with patient well rested and warm and with neuromuscular active medication withheld; RS = repetitive stimulation; EMG = electromyography.

When weakness is mild, as in the early course of LES, the CMAP amplitude may be reduced only slightly or may be in the lower range of normal. In this setting the CMAP decrement is usually modest, and facilitation is often less than 200%. Needle EMG is normal or shows only mild MUP amplitude variation. Mild cases of LES are difficult to differentiate from myasthenia gravis *(44)*. The distribution of clinical symptoms, the profile of serum autoantibodies, and the result of stimulated single-fiber EMG testing can help, but in some cases the correct diagnosis requires continued observation and retesting at a later date after the disease progresses.

### Serological Tests

P/Q-type ($Ca_v2.1$) channel antibodies are detectable in more than 90% of nonimmunosuppressed patients with LES with or without cancer of any type *(25)* (**Table 3**). N-type ($Ca_v2.2$) channel antibodies are detectable in 75% of LES patients with lung cancer, and in 40% without cancer risk *(25)*, but generally not in LES patients who have other types of cancer *(22)*. Eighteen percent of SCLC patients without clinical evidence of LES have P/Q-type calcium channel antibodies, and 22% have N-type calcium channel antibodies *(25)*. Nicotinic AChR antibodies, of muscle or ganglionic type, or striational antibodies are found additionally in approx 13% of patients with LES, with and without cancer *(26,82,83)*. Table 3 summarizes the frequency of neuronal,

Table 3

Serum Profiles of Organ-Specific Autoantibodies in Lambert-Eaton
Syndrome (LES) and Generalized Myasthenia Gravis (MG)[a]

| | Frequency (% Seropositive) | | | | |
|---|---|---|---|---|---|
| Antibody | LES Without Cancer | LES With Lung Cancer | MG Without Thymoma | MG With Thymoma | Nonautoimmune Neurologic Diseases |
| Calcium channel, P/Q | 91 | 99 | <5 | <5 | <5 |
| Calcium channel, N | 40 | 75 | <5 | <5 | <5 |
| Muscle AChR | 7 | 7 | 90 | >95 | <5 |
| Striational | 5 | 5 | 30 | 80 | <2 |
| Thyrogastric[b] | 55 | 20 | 50[c] | 30 | 20 |
| Ganglionic AChR | 10 | 10 | <2 | <2 | <2 |
| One or more of above | 96 | 100 | 95 | 100 | 20 |

[a]Nonimmunosuppressed adult patients. Based on refs. *14, 22, 26, 82,* and authors' unpublished data. AChR = acetylcholine receptor. These autoantibodies are significantly less frequent in LES patients who have lung cancer than in those without lung cancer risk factors *(82).*

[b]Thyroperoxidase, thyroglobulin, gastric parietal cell, intrinsic factor blocking, or glutamic acid decarboxylase (GAD65) antibody.

[c]Prevalence highest in ocular myasthenia.

muscle, and other organ-specific autoantibodies in adult patients with LES, myasthenia gravis, and nonautoimmune neurological disorders. Calcium channel antibodies of N-type and P/Q-type also serve as serologic markers of paraneoplastic neurologic disorders affecting the central and peripheral nervous system in the context of SCLC, ovarian carcinoma, and breast carcinoma *(25,84).* Calcium channel antibody values in those patients tend to be lower than in untreated LES patients. IgG autoantibody markers of SCLC that are specific for neuronal nuclear and cytoplasmic antigens [e.g., ANNA-1, CRMP-5, amphiphysin, PCA-2, ANNA-2, and ANNA-3 *(65,75,76)*] are rarely found in patients with paraneoplastic LES unless there is a coexisting encephalomyelopathy or neuropathy.

## Differential Diagnosis

The differential diagnosis of LES includes autoimmune myasthenia gravis and congenital myasthenic syndromes and defects of neuromuscular transmission induced by drugs or toxins. A congenital myasthenic syndrome that resembles LES has been reported *(85,86);* however, these patients were severely affected at birth. Autoimmune myasthenia gravis can usually be distinguished from LES by differences in clinical manifestations as well as electrodiagnostic tests and autoimmune serologic tests *(26)*. Cases of mild LES or severe myasthenia gravis can yield quite similar electrophysiologic findings with baseline CMAP amplitudes in the low normal range, a decrement at low rates of repetitive nerve stimulation, and facilitation of less than 200% following exercise or high rates of repetitive stimulation *(44)*. The distribution of weakness and the autoantibody profile *(26)* usually differentiate the disorders. Sometimes additional time for observation and retesting is needed, as LES typically progresses in severity if not treated. Although cases of an overlap or combination of LES and myasthenia gravis have been reported, no instance of a dual syndrome has been documented by in vitro microelectrode studies performed on biopsied intercostal or anconeus nerve-muscle preparations. These reports may reflect misinterpretation of autoantibody profiles *(87)*.

Botulism usually presents as an acute and severe weakness of cranial, axial, and limb muscles, requiring ventilatory support and emergent hospitalization. LES usually presents more gradually and rarely presents with respiratory failure. Electrodiagnostic studies in botulism reveal CMAPs of low amplitude with less prominent decrement and facilitation than LES. On needle EMG, fibrillation potentials are typically widespread in botulism but are rare in LES. The diagnosis of botulism is usually made on clinical grounds and confirmed by electrodiagnostic studies and demonstration of the toxin in the stool. Toxins delivered through the bite of venomous snakes and spiders may produce findings similar to botulism. These as well as acute intoxication with magnesium, neuromuscular blocking drugs, and organophosphates are unlikely to be mistaken for the diagnosis of LES.

## TREATMENT

### Symptomatic Treatment

#### Cholinesterase Inhibitors

This is the first line of treatment. However, because the quantal content is usually severely reduced in LES, the beneficial effect of acetylcholinesterase inhibition is usually modest unless it is combined with medications that simultaneously increase the release of ACh (e.g., 3,4-diaminopyridine or guanidine).

#### Guanidine

The beneficial effect of guanidine was initially described by Lambert and colleagues *(8,10)*. Guanidine increases intracellular calcium within the nerve terminal by inhibiting calcium uptake by organelles *(88)*. Its clinical utility is limited by significant hemopoietic and renal toxicity *(89,90)*, but guanidine is reported to be effective with less risk of toxicity when the dose is strictly limited and the drug is used in combination with pyridostigmine *(34,91)*.

## 3,4-Diaminopyridine

The effectiveness of 3,4-diaminopyridine (DAP) in LES has been documented in placebo-controlled prospective trials and in long-term follow-up studies *(30,92)*. This agent blocks $K_v$ channels in the nerve terminal, thus prolonging the action potential and enhancing $Ca^{2+}$ entry. Objective measures of strength are improved, including respiratory muscle function. Electromyographically there is an increase in amplitude of the CMAP and less CMAP decrement, and SFEMG reveals less jitter and block *(92–94)*. The peak beneficial effect of a single oral dose of 3,4-DAP occurs in about 1 h and lasts for 2–5 h *(93)*. The usual effective dose is 10–20 mg 4–5 times daily *(79,80,92)*. Adverse effects include perioral and acral paresthesiae, light-headedness, headache, insomnia, and seizures. Seizures are rare if the baseline electroencephalogram (EEG) is normal and the daily dose does not exceed 100 mg. Cardiac arrhythmia was described in a patient exposed to an intentional overdose of 3,4-DAP *(95)*. There is a theoretical risk of cardiac arrhythmia in patients with the prolonged QT syndrome, but 3,4-DAP toxicity has not been reported in that setting. Because 3,4-DAP is not approved for routine use in the United States, its use requires application as an investigational drug on a compassionate use basis. The drug is contraindicated if preliminary screening by electrocardiogram and EEG reveals a prolonged QT interval or epileptiform discharges. It is Mayo Clinic practice to monitor complete blood count, liver function, and serum creatinine three times a year, but the authors have not yet encountered bone marrow, liver, or kidney toxicity attributable to 3,4-DAP therapy.

## Treatment of the Associated Neoplasm

When cancer is found, its effective treatment may be followed by amelioration of LES manifestations, or even remission *(50)*. This has been documented particularly for SCLC treated by chemotherapy and radiation. Because neurologic improvement is not universal, patients should be cautioned that their neuromuscular disorder may need continued symptomatic treatment or immunotherapy even if their underlying cancer is cured.

## Immunotherapy

Immunotherapy for LES is generally approached as for myasthenia gravis and other autoimmune neurologic disorders. It is reserved for patients who fail to respond adequately to symptomatic therapy or, in the case of paraneoplastic LES, when tumor therapy is not accompanied by neurologic improvement. Alleviation of symptoms in LES is generally less dramatic than in myasthenia gravis *(31)*. Nevertheless, benefit has been documented with plasmapheresis *(96)*, intravenous immunoglobulin *(97–99)*, and corticosteroids *(31)*. In patients who are considered at high risk for cancer, immunotherapy is customarily reserved for those who are severely disabled by weakness and failing to respond to symptomatic therapy. Reluctance to treat stems from fear of compromising the patient's survival by promoting evasion of the suspected tumor from an effective immune response. Parenthetically, however, we do not recall having observed noteworthy emergence of metastatic cancer in two decades of using prednisone and azathioprine to treat numerous LES patients at risk for lung cancer. This anecdotal observation implies that an inherently effective cancer immune response is not impaired by the standard immunosuppressant protocols used to treat neurologic autoimmune disorders.

The type of immunotherapy chosen is tailored to the individual patient's need, depending on the magnitude and duration of benefit. Plasmapheresis is beneficial in LES, but because the duration of benefit is limited to several weeks, it is generally reserved for severely weak patients, particularly in the setting of respiratory insufficiency. Occasionally plasmapheresis is used as maintenance therapy at a frequency of 1–2 exchanges every 3–4 months. This usually requires placement of a central line or arteriovenous shunt, which increases the risk of complications from infection, coagulation disorders, and fluid/electrolyte imbalance.

Evidence for the benefit of intravenous immunoglobulin therapy is less convincing than for plasmapheresis. Its high cost and relatively short duration of action have limited its use as a maintenance therapy in LES. Treatment protocols have administered 400-500 mg/kg daily for 2–5 consecutive days or intermittent infusions at a frequency of 1–2 every 2–8 weeks.

Oral corticosteroid therapy benefits most LES patients, but improvement of strength is less dramatic than observed in myasthenia gravis. In one reported study, long-term treatment with prednisilone at 20–30 mg daily or on alternate days produced modest symptomatic benefit in most patients *(31)*. Azathioprine also is effective either as a steroid-sparing agent or as a stand-alone immunosuppressant *(31)*. Insufficient data are available concerning the efficacy of cyclosporine, cyclophosphamide, or mycophenolate as alternative immunosuppressants in LES. In principle, experimental treatment strategies that are being investigated for myasthenia gravis should be applicable to the treatment of LES, including the deletion of antigen-specific B-cells or T-cells and interference with costimulatory molecules that perpetuate the autoimmunization process.

## REFERENCES

1. Ertel EA, Campbell KP, Harpold MM, et al. Nomenclature of voltage-gated calcium channels [Letter to the Editor]. *Neuron* 2000;25:533–535.
2. Anderson HJ, Churchill-Davidson HC, Richardson AT. Bronchial neoplasm with myasthenia: prolonged apnoea after administration of succinylcholine. *Lancet* 1953; 2:1291–1293.
3. Sciamanna MA, Griesmann GE, Williams CL, Lennon VA. Nicotinic acetylcholine receptors of muscle and neuronal ($\alpha$7) types coexpressed in a small cell lung carcinoma. *J Neurochem* 1997;69:2302–2311.
4. Griesmann GE, Harper CM, Lennon VA. Paraneoplastic myasthenia gravis and lung carcinoma: distinction from Lambert-Eaton myasthenic syndrome and hypothesis of aberrant muscle acetylcholine receptor expression. *Muscle Nerve* 1998; (Suppl 7):S122.
5. Churchill-Davidson HC. Muscle relaxants. In: Langton Hewer C, ed. *Recent Advances in Anesthesia and Analgesia*, 9th ed. London, J and A Churchill, 1963, pp. 79–110.
6. Lambert EH, Rooke ED, Eaton LM, Hodgson CH. Myasthenic syndrome occasionally associated with bronchial neoplasm. In: Viets HR, ed. *Myasthenia Gravis*. Springfield, IL, Charles C. Thomas, 1961, pp. 362–410.
7. Lambert EH, Eaton LM, Rooke ED. Defect of neuromuscular transmission associated with malignant neoplasm. *Am J Physiol* 1956;187:612–621.
8. Eaton LM, Lambert EH. Electromyography and electrical stimulation of nerves in diseases of the motor unit: observations on myasthenic syndrome associated with malignant tumors. *JAMA* 1957;163:1117–1124.
9. Lambert EH, Rooke ED, Eaton LM, Hodgson CH. Myasthenic syndrome occasionally associated with bronchial neoplasm: neurophysiologic studies. In: Viets HR, ed. *Myasthenia Gravis*. Springfield, IL, Charles C. Thomas, 1961, pp. 362–410.
10. Lambert EH, Rooke ED. Myasthenic state and lung cancer. In: Brain WR, Norris FH, eds. *The Remote Effects of Cancer on the Nervous System (Contemporary Neurology Symposia)*, vol. 1. New York, Grune & Stratton, 1965, pp. 67–80.
11. Elmqvist D, Lambert EH. Detailed analysis of neuromuscular transmission in a patient with the myasthenic syndrome sometimes associated with bronchogenic carcinoma. *Mayo Clin Proc* 1968;43:689–713.
12. Lambert EH, Elmqvist D. Quantal components of end-plate potentials in the myasthenic syndrome. *Ann NY Acad Sci* 1971;183:183–199.
13. Gutmann L, Crosby TW, Takamori M, Martin JD. The Eaton-Lambert syndrome and autoimmune disorders. *Am J Med* 1972;53:354–356.
14. Lennon VA, Lambert EH, Whittingham S, Fairbanks V. Autoimmunity in the Lambert-Eaton myasthenic syndrome. *Muscle Nerve* 1982;5:S21–S25.
15. Fukunaga H, Engel AG, Osame M, Lambert EH. Paucity and disorganization of presynaptic membrane active zones in the Lambert-Eaton myasthenic syndrome. *Muscle Nerve* 1982;5:686–697.
16. Engel AG. Anatomy and molecular architecture of the neuromuscular junction. In: Engel AG, ed. *Myasthenia Gravis and Myasthenic Syndromes*. New York, Oxford University Press, 1999, pp. 3–40.
17. Lang B, Newsom-Davis J, Wray D, Vincent A, Murray N. Autoimmune etiology for myasthenic (Eaton-Lambert) syndrome. *Lancet* 1981;2:224–226.

18. Fukunaga H, Engel AG, Lang B, Newsom-Davis J, Vincent A. Passive transfer of Lambert-Eaton myasthenic syndrome with IgG from man to mouse depletes the presynaptic membrane active zones. *Proc Natl Acad Sci USA* 1983;80:7636–7640.
19. Kim YI. Passively transferred Lambert-Eaton syndrome in mice receiving purified IgG. *Muscle Nerve* 1986;9:523–530.
20. Lambert EH, Lennon VA. Selected IgG rapidly induces Lambert-Eaton myasthenic syndrome in mice: complement independence and EMG abnormalities. *Muscle Nerve* 1988;11:1133–1145.
21. Roberts A, Perera S, Lang B, Vincent A, Newsom-Davis J. Paraneoplastic myasthenic syndrome IgG inhibits $^{45}$Ca flux in human small cell carcinoma line. *Nature* 1985;317:737–739.
22. Lennon VA, Lambert EH. Autoantibodies bind solubilized calcium channel-omega-conotoxin complexes from small cell lung carcinoma: a diagnostic aid for Lambert-Eaton myasthenic syndrome. *Mayo Clin Proc* 1989;64:1498–1504.
23. Sher E, Canal N, Piccolo G, et al. Specificity of calcium channel autoantibodies in Lambert-Eaton myasthenic syndrome. *Lancet* 1989;ii:640–643.
24. Leys K, Lang B, Johnston L, Newsom-Davis J. Calcium channel autoantibodies in the Lambert-Eaton myasthenic syndrome. *Ann Neurol* 1991;29:307–314.
25. Lennon VA, Kryzer TJ, Griesmann GE, et al. Calcium-channel antibodies in the Lambert-Eaton syndrome and other paraneoplastic syndromes. *N Engl J Med* 1995; 332:1467–1471.
26. Lennon VA. Serologic profile of myasthenia gravis and distinction from Lambert-Eaton myasthenic syndrome. *Neurology* 1997;48(Suppl 5):S23–S27.
27. Chalk CH, Murray NM, Newsom-Davis J, O'Neill JH, Spiro SG. Response of the Lambert-Eaton myasthenic syndrome to treatment of associated small-cell lung carcinoma. *Neurology* 1990;40:1552–1556.
28. Streib EW, Rothner AD. Lambert-Eaton myasthenic syndrome: long-term treatment of three patients with prednisone. *Ann Neurol* 1981;10:448–453.
29. Newsom-Davis J, Murray NM. Plasma exchange and immunosuppressive drug treatment in the Lambert-Eaton myasthenic syndrome. *Neurology* 1984;34:480–485.
30. Lundh H, Nilsson O, Rosen I. Current therapy of the Lambert-Eaton myasthenic syndrome. *Prog Brain Res* 1990;84:163–170.
31. Maddison P, Lang B, Mills K, Newsom-Davis J. Long-term outcome in Lambert-Eaton myasthenic syndrome without lung cancer. *J Neurol Neurosurg Psychiatry* 2001;70:212–217.
32. Lundh H, Nilsson O, Rosen I. Treatment of Lambert-Eaton syndrome: 3,4-diamino-pyridine and pyridostigmine. *Neurology* 1984;34:1324–1330.
33. McEvoy KM, Windebank AJ, Daube JR, Low PA. 3,4-Diaminopyridine in the treatment of Lambert-Eaton myasthenic syndrome. *N Engl J Med* 1989;321:1567–1571.
34. Oh Sj, Kim DS, Head TC, Claussen GC. Low dose guanidine and pyridostigmine: relatively safe and effective long-term symptomatic therapy in Lambert-Eaton myasthenic syndrome. *Muscle Nerve* 1997;20:1146–1152.
35. Tim RW. Massey JM. Sanders DB. Lambert-Eaton myasthenic syndrome: electro-diagnostic findings and response to treatment. *Neurology* 2000;54:2176–2178.
36. Lambert EH, Okihiro M, Rooke ED. Clinical physiology of the neuromuscular junction. In: Paul WM, Daniel EE, Kay CM, Monckton G, eds. *Muscle.* Oxford, Pergamon, 1965, pp. 487–497.

37. Sudhof TC. The synaptic vesicle cycle revisited. *Neuron* 2000;28:317–320.
38. Boonyapisit K, Kaminski HJ, Ruff RL. The molecular basis of neuromuscular transmission disorders. *Am J Med* 1999;106:97–113.
39. Anderson CR, Stevens CF. Voltage clamp analysis of acetylcholine produced endplate current fluctuation at frog neuromuscular junction. *J Physiol (Lond)* 1973;235: 655–691.
40. Jablecki CK. Electrodiagnostic evaluation of patients with myasthenia gravis and related disorders. *Neurol Clin* 1985;3:557–572.
41. Jones SW. Overview of voltage-dependent calcium channels. *J Bioenerg Biomembr* 1998;30:299–312.
42. Black JL, Lennon VA. Identification and cloning of human neuronal high voltage-gated calcium channel 3-2 and 3-3 subunits: neurological implications. *Mayo Clin Proc* 1999;74:357–361.
43. Molenaar PC, Newsom-Davis J, Polak RL, Vincent A. Eaton-Lambert syndrome: acetylcholine and choline acetyltransferase in skeletal muscle. *Neurology* 1982;32: 1061–1065.
44. Harper CM. Electrodiagnosis of endplate disease. In: Engel AG, ed. *Myasthenia Gravis and Myasthenic Syndromes*. New York, Oxford University Press, 1999, pp. 65–86.
45. O'Neill JH, Murray NM, Newsom-Davis J. The Lambert-Eaton myasthenic syndrome. A review of 50 cases. *Brain* 1988;111:577–596.
46. O'Suilleabhain P, Low PA, Lennon VA. Autonomic dysfunction in the Lambert-Eaton myasthenic syndrome: serological and clinical correlates. *Neurology* 1998;50: 88–93.
47. Waterman SA, Lang B, Newsom-Davis J. Effect of Lambert-Eaton myasthenic syndrome antibodies on autonomic neurones in the mouse. *Ann Neurol* 1997;42:147–156.
48. Komai K, Jwasa K, Takamori M. Calcium channel peptide can cause an autoimmune-mediated model of Lambert-Eaton myasthenic syndrome in rats. *J Neurol Sci* 1999;166:126–130.
49. Oguro-Okano M, Griesmann GE, Wieben ED, et al. Molecular diversity of neuronal type calcium channels identified in small cell lung carcinoma. *Mayo Clin Proc* 1992;67:1150–1159.
50. Maddison P, Newsom-Davis J, Mills KR, Souhami RL. Favorable prognosis in Lambert-Eaton myasthenic syndrome and small-cell lung carcinoma. *Lancet* 1999; 353:117,118.
51. Prior C, Lang B, Wray D, Newsom-Davis J. Action of Lambert-Eaton myasthenic syndrome IgG at mouse motor nerve terminals. *Ann Neurol* 1985;17:587–592.
52. Fukuoka T, Engel AG, Lang B, et al. Lambert-Eaton myasthenic syndrome: I. Early morphological effects of IgG on the presynaptic membrane active zones. *Ann Neurol* 1987;22:193–199.
53. De Aizpurua HJ, Lambert EH, Griesmann GE, Olivera BM, Lennon VA. Antagonism of voltage-gated calcium channels in small cell carcinomas of patients with and without Lambert-Eaton myasthenic syndrome by autoantibodies, $\omega$-conotoxin and adenosine. *Cancer Res* 1988;48:4719–4724.
54. Lang B, Vincent A, Murray NM, Newsom-Davis J. Lambert-Eaton myasthenic syndrome: immunoglobulin G inhibition of $Ca^{2+}$ influx in tumor cells correlates with disease severity. *Ann Neurol* 1989;25:265–271.

55. Meriney SD, Hulsizer SC, Lennon VA, Grinnell AD. Lambert-Eaton myasthenic syndrome immunoglobulins react with multiple types of calcium channels in small cell lung carcinoma. *Ann Neurol* 1996;40:739–749.

56. Garcia KD, Beam KG. Reduction of calcium currents by Lambert-Eaton syndrome sera: motoneurons are preferentially affected, and L-type currents are spared. *J Neurosci* 1996;16:4903–4913.

57. Lang B, Newsom-Davis J, Peers C, Prior C, Wray DW. The effect of myasthenic syndrome antibody on presynaptic calcium channels in the mouse. *J Physiol (Lond)* 1987;390:257-270.

58. Yu Z, Lennon VA. Mechanism of intravenous immune globulin therapy in antibody-mediated autoimmune diseases. *N Engl J Med* 1999;340:227–228.

59. Willcox N, Demaine AG, Newsom-Davis J, et al. Increased frequency of IgG heavy chain marker Glm(2) and of HLA-B8 in Lambert-Eaton myasthenic syndrome with and without associated lung carcinoma. *Hum Immunol* 1985;14:29–36.

60. Parsons KT, Kwok WW, Gaur LK, Nepom GT. Increased frequency of HLA class II alleles DRB1*0301 and DQB1*0201 in Lambert-Eaton myasthenic syndrome without associated cancer. *Hum Immunol* 2000;61:828–833.

61. Elrington GM, Murray NME, Spiro SG, Newsom-Davis J. Neurological paraneoplastic syndromes in patients with small cell lung cancer: a prospective survey of 150 patients. *J Neurol Neurosurg Psychiatry* 1991;54:764–767.

62. Seltzer V. Cancer in women: prevention and early detection. *J Womens Health Gender Based Med* 2000;9:483–488.

63. Dalmau J, Graus F, Rosenblum MK, Posner JB. Anti-Hu-associated paraneoplastic encephalomyelitis/sensory neuronopathy: a clinical study of 71 patients. *Medicine* 1992;71:59–72.

64. Lucchinetti CF, Kimmel DW, Lennon VA. Paraneoplastic and oncological profiles of patients seropositive for type 1 anti-neuronal nuclear autoantibodies. *Neurology* 1998;50:652–657.

65. Yu Z, Kryzer TJ, Griesmann GE, et al. CRMP-5 neuronal autoantibody: marker of lung cancer and thymoma-related autoimmunity. *Ann Neurol* 2001;49:146–154.

66. Gutmann L, Phillips LH, Gutmann L. Trends in the association of Lambert-Eaton myasthenic syndrome with carcinoma. *Neurology* 1992;42:848–850.

67. Argov Z, Shapira Y, Averbuch-Heller L, Wirguin I. Lambert-Eaton myasthenic syndrome (LES) in association with lymphoproliferative disorders. *Muscle Nerve* 1995;18:715–719.

68. Burns TM, Juel VC, Sanders DB, Phillips LH. Neuroendocrine lung tumors and disorders of the neuromuscular junction. *Neurology* 1999;52:1490–1491.

69. Collins DR, Connolly S, Burns M, et al. Lambert-Eaton myasthenic syndrome in association with transitional cell carcinoma: a previously unrecognized association. *Urology* 1999;54:162.

70. Dalmau J, Gultekin HS, Posner JB. Paraneoplastic neurologic syndromes: pathogenesis and physiopathology. *Brain Pathol* 1999;9:275–284.

71. Oyaizu T, Okada Y, Sagawa M, et al. Lambert-Eaton myasthenic syndrome associated with an anterior mediastinal small cell carcinoma. *J Thorac Cardiovasc Surg* 2001;121:1005–1006.

72. Kennelly KD, Dodick DW, Pascuzzi RM, Albain KS, Lennon VA. Neuronal autoantibodies and paraneoplastic neurological syndromes associated with extrapulmonary small cell carcinoma. *Neurology* 1997;48(Suppl 2):A31.

73. Eggers SD, Salomao DR, Dinapoli RP, Vernino S. Paraneoplastic and metastatic neurologic complications of Merkel cell carcinoma. *Mayo Clin Proc* 2001;76: 327–330.
74. Barr CW, Claussen G, Thomas D, et al. Primary respiratory failure as the presenting symptom in Lambert-Eaton myasthenic syndrome. *Muscle Nerve* 1993;6:712–715.
75. Vernino S, Lennon VA. New Purkinje cell antibody (PCA-2): marker of lung cancer-related neurological autoimmunity. *Ann Neurol* 2000;47:297–305.
76. Chan KH, Vernino S, Lennon VA. ANNA-3 anti-neuronal nuclear antibody: marker of lung cancer-related autoimmunity. *Ann Neurol* 2001;50:301–311.
77. Lee H-R, Lennon VA, Camilleri M, Prather CM. Paraneoplastic gastrointestinal motor dysfunction: clinical and laboratory characteristics. *Am J Gastroenterol* 2001; 96:373–379.
78. Vernino S, Low PA, Fealey RD, et al. Autoantibodies to ganglionic acetylcholine receptors in autoimmune autonomic neuropathies. *N Engl J Med* 2000;343:847–855.
79. Lundh H, Nilsson O, Rosen I, Johansson S. Practical aspects of 3,4-diaminopyridine treatment of the Lambert-Eaton myasthenic syndrome. *Acta Neurol Scand* 1993;88: 136–140.
80. Sanders DB. 3,4-Diaminopyridine (DAP) in the treatment of Lambert-Eaton myasthenic syndrome (LES). *Ann NY Acad Sci* 1998;841:811–816.
81. Small S, Ali HH, Lennon VA, et al. Anesthesia for unsuspected Lambert-Eaton myasthenic syndrome with autoantibodies and occult small cell lung carcinoma. *Anesthesiology* 1992;76:142–145.
82. Lennon VA. Serological diagnosis of myasthenia gravis and the Lambert-Eaton myasthenic syndrome. In: Lisak R, ed. *Handbook of Myasthenia Gravis*. New York, Marcel Dekker, 1994, pp. 149–164.
83. Vernino S, Adamski J, Kryzer TJ. Lennon VA. Neuronal nicotinic AChR antibody in subacute autonomic neuropathy and cancer-related syndromes. *Neurology* 1998; 50:1806–1813.
84. Lennon VA, Kryzer TJ. Correspondence: neuronal calcium channel autoantibodies coexisting with type 1 Purkinje cell cytoplasmic autoantibodies (PCA-1 or "anti-Yo"). *Neurology* 1998;51:327–328.
85. Albers JW, Faulkner JA, Dorovini-Zis K. Abnormal neuromuscular transmission in an infantile myasthenic syndrome. *Ann Neurol* 1984;16:28–34.
86. Bady B, Chauplannaz G, Carrier H. Congenital Lambert-Eaton myasthenic syndrome. *J Neurol Neurosurg Psychiatr* 1987;50:476–478.
87. Katz JS, Wolfe GI, Bryan WW, Tintner R, Barohn RJ. Acetylcholine receptor antibodies in the Lambert-Eaton myasthenic syndrome. *Neurology* 1998;50:470–475.
88. Kamenskaya MA, Elmqvist D, Thesleff S. Guanidine and neuromuscular transmission. Effect on transmitter release in response to repetitive nerve stimulation. *Arch Neurol* 1975;32:510–518.
89. Cherington M. Guanidine and germine in Eaton-Lambert syndrome. *Neurology* 1976;26:944–946.
90. Blumhardt LD, Joekes AM, Marshall J, Philalithis PE. Guanidine treatment and impaired renal function in the Eaton-Lambert syndrome. *BMJ* 1977;1:946–947.
91. Silbert PL, Hankey GJ, Barr AL. Successful alternate day guanidine therapy following guanidine-induced neutropenia in the Lambert-Eaton myasthenic syndrome. *Muscle Nerve* 1990;13:360–361.

92. McEvoy KM, Windebank AJ, Daube JR, Low PA. 3,4-Diaminopyridine in the treatment of Lambert-Eaton myasthenic syndrome. *N Engl J Med* 1989;321:1567–1571.
93. Harper CM, McEvoy KM, Windebank AJ, Daube JR. Effect of 3,4-diaminopyridine on neuromuscular transmission in patients with Lambert-Eaton myasthenic syndrome. *Electroencephalogr Clin Neurophysiol* 1990;75:557.
94. Kim DS, Claussen GC, Oh SJ. Single-fiber electromyography improvement with 3,4-diaminopyridine in Lambert-Eaton myasthenic syndrome. *Muscle Nerve* 1998; 21:1107–1108.
95. Boerma CE, Rommes JH, van Leeuwen RB, Bakker J. Cardiac arrest following an iatrogenic 3,4-diaminopyridine intoxication in a patient with Lambert-Eaton myasthenic syndrome. *Clin Toxicol* 1995;33:249–251.
96. Dau PC, Denys EH. Plasmapheresis and immunosuppressive drug therapy in the Eaton-Lambert syndrome. *Ann Neurol* 1982;11:570–575.
97. Bird SJ. Clinical and electrophysiologic improvement in Lambert-Eaton syndrome with intravenous immunoglobulin therapy. *Neurology* 1992;42:1422–1423.
98. Motomura M, Tsujihata M, Takeo G, et al. The effect of high-dose gamma-globulin in Lambert-Eaton myasthenic syndrome. *Neurol Ther* 1994;11:377–383.
99. Takano H, Tanaka M, Koike R, et al. Effect of intravenous immunoglobulin in Lambert-Eaton myasthenic syndrome with small-cell lung cancer: correlation with the titer of anti-voltage-gated calcium channel antibody. *Muscle Nerve* 1994;17: 1074–1075.

# 13

# Acquired Neuromyotonia

## Ian Hart and Angela Vincent

### INTRODUCTION

Neuromyotonia (NMT; Isaacs' syndrome) is a syndrome of nerve hyperexcitability that is usually diagnosed by clinical and electrodiagnostic studies (EDX) showing continuous skeletal muscle overactivity. Although the syndrome can be caused by several different pathogenic mechanisms, here we concentrate on the acquired form that is predominately autoimmune. We review the clinical features, the immune and tumor associations, and the association with antibodies to voltage-gated ion channels.

### CLINICAL FEATURES
### OF NMT AND RELATED SYNDROMES

The typical presenting features are myokymia (muscle twitching) and cramps *(1–5)*, which can be associated with muscle stiffness, pseudomyotonia (delayed muscle relaxation after contraction), pseudotetany (for example, Chvostek's and Trousseau's signs), and weakness. The limb and trunk muscles are most commonly affected, although facial, bulbar, and respiratory muscles can also be involved. There is often increased sweating. Muscle contraction often provokes or exacerbates the symptoms. Reflexes are usually normal but can be reduced or absent when there is an accompanying neuropathy. Chronic cases may develop muscle hypertrophy.

Some patients with NMT have sensory symptoms such as paresthesia and numbness without evidence of peripheral neuropathy, suggesting that sensory as well as motor nerves may be hyperexcitable *(6)*. Perhaps more interestingly, in view of the antibody-mediated pathology, central nervous system (CNS) symptoms ranging from personality change and insomnia to a psychotic-like state with delusions and hallucinations can occur. This association is often called *chorée fibrillaire*, or Morvan's syndrome *(7,8)*, which can also include autonomic dysfunction *(9,10)*. Although full-blown Morvan's syndrome is

From: *Current Clinical Neurology: Myasthenia Gravis and Related Disorders*
Edited by: H. J. Kaminski © Humana Press Inc., Totowa, NJ

**Table 1**
**Similarities Between Neuromyotonia**
**and the Cramp-Fasciculation Syndrome**[a]

| Feature | Neuromyotonia (42 patients) (% positive) | Cramp-Fasciculation Syndrome (18 patients) (% positive) |
|---|---|---|
| Cramps | 88 | 100 |
| Muscle twitching | 100 | 94 |
| Pseudomyotonia | 36 | 22 |
| Sensory symptoms | 33 | 39 |
| CNS symptoms | 29 | 22 |
| Other autoimmune diseases | 59 | 28 |
| Thymoma | 19 | 11 |
| Lung tumor | 10 | 4 |
| Other autoantibodies | 50 | 17 |
| VGKC antibodies | 38 | 28 |

[a]Data from ref. *13*. VGKC = voltage-gated potassium channel.

apparently rare, cases with a CNS disorder and relatively mild peripheral features may be more common (see below).

Neuromyotonia can occur at any age and, since the severity of the clinical features ranges from the inconvenient to the incapacitating, it is not at all clear how common the disorder is. The course is variably progressive, although spontaneous remissions can occur. A relationship to preceding or established infections has been reported in two cases *(11)*. No HLA association has been detected in 12 patients examined (I. Hart, unpublished data).

A review of the clinical features of NMT showed that very similar features are found in patients with cramp-fasciculation syndrome (CFS) *(12)*, a proportion of whom also have voltage-gated potassium channel (VGKC) antibodies (**Table 1**) *(13)*. This, together with other evidence for autoimmunity in some CFS patients *(13)*, strongly indicates that CFS and NMT should be considered parts of a spectrum of autoimmune peripheral nerve hyperexcitability. This may also apply to the myokymia/cramp syndrome *(14)* and other conditions associated with muscle hyperexcitability and hyperhidrosis *(15, 16)*. Gutmann et al. *(17)* discussed the relationship between electrical neuromyotonic and myokymic discharges and the clinical disorder and came to a similar conclusion. Here we discuss NMT, because most of the experimental studies have been performed in patients who fulfill this diagnosis.

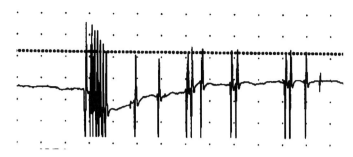

**Fig. 1.** Needle electromyography recording from the right extensor digitorum communis muscle of a neuromyotonia patient. There is a multiplet discharge with an intraburst frequency of 150 Hz followed at irregular intervals by several doublets and single discharges (fasciculations), all from a single motor unit.

## Electrophysiologic Features

The classical electrophysiologic feature of NMT is the spontaneous firing of single motor units as doublet, triplet, or multiplet discharges (**Fig. 1**). These neuromyotonic discharges occur at irregular intervals of 1–30 s and have an intraburst frequency of 40–400 Hz. They may be present in the absence of visible muscle twitching. In addition, voluntary or electrical activation may trigger prolonged afterdischarges at similar frequencies. Fasciculation and fibrillation potentials can also occur.

The spontaneous and repetitive muscle activity arises in the peripheral motor nerve, rather than in the muscle itself *(4,18)*. Isaacs showed that the discharges were abolished when curare was used to block neuromuscular transmission, but persisted after either proximal or distal nerve block. These observations, and recent studies using botulinum toxin, suggested that the activity was generated in the terminal arborization of the motor axons *(19)*. However, other studies indicate a more proximal initiation of the hyperactivity with reduction by proximal nerve block *(20–22)* or by epidural anesthesia *(23)*. The simplest explanation for these data is that the activity can originate at different sites including the lower motor neuron cell body in some cases.

Some patients with stiff person syndrome present with muscle hyperactivity and cramps. Sleep or general anesthesia abolishes muscle activity in stiff person syndrome but not in NMT, and this is a clinically important distinction between the two conditions.

Although it seems likely that NMT is usually a functional disorder of the motor nerve, rather than a secondary phenomenon caused by structural nerve or myelin damage, about 5–10% of patients have, in addition to NMT, electrical evidence of a subclinical idiopathic axonal or demyelinating polyneuropathy.

## Serum and Cerebrospinal Fluid Tests

Although most patients with NMT reported so far do not have marked CNS features, it is common to find a raised total IgG and oligoclonal bands in the cerebrospinal fluid (CSF) *(1)*. Curiously, VGKC antibodies (see below) are not usually found.

# PHYSIOLOGIC BASIS OF EXCITABILITY OF MOTOR AXONS IN NMT PATIENTS

It is possible to measure the response of subthreshold stimuli and the stimulus intensity (threshold) that is required to excite the motor nerve *(24, 25)*. One of these measures is the strength-duration time constant (SDTC), which is a property of the nodal membrane determined by the passive membrane time constant and the ion conductances acting at the nerve threshold. The SDTC was prolonged in the motor but not in the sensory axons in some NMT patients in one study *(26)*. However, a subsequent study, using more sensitive measures of both motor and sensory axonal excitability in the median nerve, found that all excitability indices were normal in all eight NMT patients examined *(27)*. Thus a general alteration of axonal membrane permeability is probably not present in these patients, as predicted by the previous studies, which indicated a distal pathology in most patients (see above).

# CLINICAL AND EXPERIMENTAL EVIDENCE FOR AN AUTOIMMUNE BASIS

## Associated Autoimmune Syndromes

As in disorders of the neuromuscular junction, one of the first indications that NMT had an autoimmune basis was the recognition of associated autoimmune diseases. These conditions include myasthenia gravis (MG) with or without thymoma, rheumatoid arthritis, systemic lupus erythematosus, and diabetes (**Table 1**). Individual patients with NMT and systemic sclerosis or idiopathic thrombocytopenia, or NMT occurring after bone marrow transplantation, are also reported *(28–36)*. Some patients may have an inflammatory neuropathy, although in these cases one might argue that the neuropathy is the primary event *(37)*.

The strongest tumor association is with thymoma. This occurs in patients with or without associated MG, and particularly in the former can precede the neuromyotonia by several years. Small cell lung cancers are also described in a few patients (**Table 1**) *(22)*, but in these cases the neuromyotonia usually precedes the cancer with latencies between onset of NMT and diagnosis of

SCLC of up to 4 years *(1)*. There are isolated reports of neuromyotonia with Hodgkin's lymphoma *(38)* or with a plasmacytoma and paraproteinemia *(39)*.

## Response to Immunotherapies

The first clinical experiment that suggested an autoimmune etiology for NMT was in a patient in whom plasma exchange resulted in marked reduction in the frequency of spontaneous motor unit potentials *(40)*. Although there have been no formal trials of immunotherapies, there are many anecdotal reports of improvement following plasma exchange, intravenous immunoglobulins, or corticosteroids *(1)*. In most patients, clinical improvement begins within 2–8 days of plasma exchange and lasts for about 1 month.

## PASSIVE TRANSFER OF IMMUNOGLOBULINS TO MICE

Passive transfer of NMT IgG to mice provides further evidence for the autoimmune basis of the disorder. After injection of purified IgG intraperitoneally for 10–12 days, there is an enhancement of neuromuscular transmission in mouse hemidiaphragm preparations, as demonstrated by a resistance to bath-applied curare *(41)*. Mice injected with NMT IgG release significantly more packets of acetylcholine from their motor nerve endings, consistent with the increased efficiency of neuromuscular transmission. However, there are no spontaneous motor unit potentials or double responses to single stimuli, as observed in the human disease *(40)*. Dorsal root ganglion cell cultures incubated with NMT IgG, however, show repetitive action potentials *(41)*. Together these studies suggest that an IgG autoantibody is responsible for at least some of the features of neuromyotonia. Moreover, the striking similarity between the changes seen in the mouse preparations and those found after small doses of the VGKC antagonists 3,4-diaminopyridine or 4-aminopyridine make it likely that the target of the antibodies is a VGKC *(40)*. The main function of neuronal VGKC is to restore the membrane potential after each action potential, thus closing the voltage-gated calcium channels and terminating neurotransmitter release. Thus, a reduction in VGKC numbers or function would lead to prolonged depolarization of the motor nerve with enhanced transmitter release.

Two other observations help to confirm that VGKCs are a major target in NMT. First, the snake toxin dendrotoxin from species of *Dendroaspis mambas (42)* blocks VGKC, increases the quantal content at the neuromuscular junction, and can produce repetitive or spontaneous activity in the motor nerve terminal *(41)*. In addition, and crucially, patch clamp studies with cultured PC-12 and NB-1 cell lines confirmed that NMT Ig suppresses voltage-dependent potassium currents *(43)*.

VGKCs function as delayed rectifiers or type A rapid inactivators and are involved in nerve repolarization *(44)*. A variety of studies suggests that they are mainly restricted to the paranodal and juxtanodal regions and nerve terminals of the peripheral motor nerves. In addition, they are also widely expressed in the CNS and peripheral sensory nerves. There are at least nine VGKC genes, termed $K_v1.1-1.9$. At the motor nerve terminal, the $K_v1.2$ appears to be the major type expressed, and since clinical neurophysiologic studies indicate that in most NMT patients the spontaneous activity originates from the terminal regions of the motor axons, this is likely to be a major antigenic target for the antibodies.

## ANTIBODIES TO VGKC

To look for antibodies to VGKCs, the same approach was used as in MG (see Chap. 8). VGKCs were extracted from human or mammalian brain and allowed to bind $[^{125}I]$ $\alpha$-dendrotoxin *(41,45)*. The labeled complex was then used in radioimmunoprecipitation assays. Dendrotoxin binds to $K_v1.1$, -1.2, and -1.6 VGKC proteins, and perhaps also $K_v1.3$ (unpublished observations). The results show significant levels of antibodies to VGKCs in around 40% of NMT patients (**Fig. 2**). A more sensitive, but more difficult technique is to measure antibody binding to cell lines or to *Xenopus* oocytes that have been made to express various VGKC genes. Using a sensitive molecular-immuno-histochemical assay, Hart et al. *(45)* showed antibody binding to VGKC proteins in 80–90% of patients (unpublished results). At present, however, it is not widely available (see below).

Functional VGKCs consist of four $\alpha$-subunits, each of which has six transmembrane regions (S1–6) *(44)*. Together, the $\alpha$-subunit S5 and S6 regions form the central ion pore. VGKC are expressed as gene products that need to combine as homomultimeric or heteromultimeric tetramers and to associate with intracellular $\beta$-subunits *(46)*. In the immunoprecipitation assay, only those VGKCs that include subtypes binding dendrotoxin are labeled. This means that antibodies to other subtypes associated with dendrotoxin-binding subunits in a heteromultimer will be detected, but antibodies to those that do not associate with dendrotoxin-binding subunits will not be found. In practice, the assay is also limited by the concentrations of the various channel subtypes in the brain extracts currently employed. For instance, in rabbit brain extracts, the $K_v1.2$ subtype seems to predominate, and many NMT autoantibodies appear to bind to it (Watanabe and Vincent, unpublished findings). However, there may be other subtypes or combinations of subtypes that are not present in the extract but that are potential targets for the antibodies. Attempts to improve the sensitivity of the assay by employing different neu-

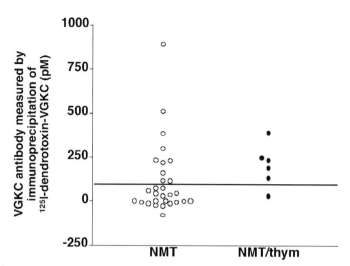

**Fig. 2.** Voltage-gated potassium channel (VGKC) antibodies in neuromyotonia patients without or with a thymoma. NMT = neuromyotonia; Thym = thymoma. (Data from Hart et al., submitted for publication.)

rotoxins (such as charybdotoxin, apamin, or margatoxin) have not been successful. In fact, margatoxin, which is thought to bind to the $K_v 1.3$ subtype as well as $K_v 1.2$, produced results that were essentially identical to those with dendrotoxin (Clover et al., in preparation).

Immunohistochemical assays show that different sera contain antibodies to different combinations of VGKC subunits, indicating heterogeneity of the antibody response *(45)* similar to that found for antibodies to acetylcholine receptors in MG. However, the studies need to be extended to all known VGKC subtypes in a more systematic manner. One way to do this would be to express each VGKC gene individually in a mammalian cell line, and to use fluorescence-activated cell sorting to measure binding of the antibodies to the expressed VGKCs. This method has the advantage that one would be measuring only antibodies to the extracellular determinants and could provide a precise and quantitative assay. However, it is technically difficult and time-consuming and will not be suitable for routine clinical testing.

In most NMT patients, the anti-VGKC antibodies are IgG. However, one patient with a plasmacytoma and IgM monoclonal gammopathy developed NMT *(39)*, and IgM purified from another NMT patient bound to an α-dendrotoxin-labeled protein by Western blotting and had immunoreactivity with both cultured PC-12 cells and human intramuscular nerve axons *(47)*. These findings suggest that in some patients NMT is IgM autoantibody-mediated. Recent studies of patients with Guillain-Barré syndrome (GBS) also indicate the presence of IgM antibodies to VGKC (Watanabe et al., in preparation).

The mechanism of action of NMT autoantibodies is probably to modulate the number of functional VGKCs, rather than to cause a complement-mediated attack on the motor nerve terminal or to block the ion channel directly. The lack of complement-mediated attack in both Lambert-Eaton syndrome (LES) and NMT is interesting, because previous studies in Miller-Fisher syndrome, in which there are IgG antibodies directed against the ganglioside GQ1b on the motor nerve terminal, indicate that complement can effectively damage the motor endplate *(48)*. One explanation could be that the antibodies in LES and NMT are of the IgG2 or IgG4 subclasses, which do not bind complement efficiently. Further studies on the subclasses of antibodies in LES and in NMT will need to be undertaken.

A direct block of function should be seen within 1 or 2 hours. When NMT IgG is applied to dorsal root ganglion cells, repetitive firing is observed after 24 h but not in the initial 2 h *(49)*. Similarly, in the patch clamp studies of PC-12 cells, application of the NMT IgG for short periods did not have any effect, and positive results were only found after 3 or more days *(47)*. Thus, autoantibodies appear to be able to reduce VGKC function by lowering the available numbers of channels rather than by directly affecting their activity.

### Other Possible Autoantibodies in NMT

A variety of neurotoxins, from species as diverse as dinoflagellates, scorpions, snails, and sea anemones, alter the closing of voltage-gated sodium channels to prolong sodium currents and produce repetitive firing of axons. Thus antibodies to sodium channels, if they also prolonged activations, could cause NMT. However, a patch clamp study of NB-1 cells did not detect any significant effect of NMT IgG on sodium currents *(49)*.

Other possible antigens targeted by the autoimmune process are the modulatory receptors that are present on the motor nerve terminal. These bind a variety of substances released by the motor nerve, such as acetylcholine, adenosine triphosphate, adenosine, and calcitonin gene-related peptide, or circulating substances such as epinephrine. These substances are thought to exist in order to regulate acetylcholine release and prevent overexcitation of the motor endplate by excessive acetylcholine. Therefore, any reduction in their expression could lead to muscle overactivity and manifestations of NMT.

A radioimmunoassay using $^{125}$I-labeled epibatidine (a specific agonist drug) identified autoantibodies to neuronal (rather than muscle) nicotinic acetylcholine receptors in sera from three of the six NMT patients studied *(50)*. However, it is not clear what effect these antibodies would have on the activity of the motor nerve terminal, as most studies in mammalian or amphibian muscles suggest that the functions of these presynaptic receptors are subtle and can only be demonstrated under relatively extreme conditions.

In some patients, autoantibodies may be directed against myelin antigens. The electromyographic features of NMT have been demonstrated in mice with targeted deletions in the genes for P0 or Pmp22 *(51,52)* and in the Trembler mouse which has a point mutation in Pmp22. The similarities with NMT are striking (discussed in ref. *53*) and suggest that manifestations of neuromyotonia may also be caused by antibodies to myelin proteins in humans.

## VGKC ANTIBODIES IN OTHER DISEASES

A study of 42 patients with NMT and 18 patients with CFS suggests considerable overlap between the two syndromes, as summarized in **Table 1**. Indeed, immunoglobulins from two CFS patients suppressed outward potassium currents of patch-clamped NB-1 cells in culture in a manner similar to NMT Ig *(49)*. In addition, VGKC antibodies were found in a patient with "neuromuscular hyperexcitabilty," very similar to a previous case of rippling muscle disease *(54)*. Both these patients had coexisting MG and are therefore assumed to have an autoimmune disease.

NMT can occur in patients with GBS *(37)*, an acute inflammatory demyelinating polyneuropathy, and at least one patient had VGKC antibodies (A. Selvan, G. Ebers, and A. Vincent, unpublished observations). Defects in myelination by themselves can induce nerve hyperexcitability, for example, in humans and mice with PMP22 gene mutations *(53)*, presumably by secondary effects on the regional expression of ion channels along the length of the axon *(51,52)*. In addition, however, purified Ig from two GBS patients reduced VGKC currents in NB-1 cells *(49)*. It will be interesting to see whether these sera immunoprecipitate VGKCs.

## CENTRAL NERVOUS SYSTEM ABNORMALITIES IN NMT

### Morvan's Syndrome

The clinical association of neuromyotonia with hallucinations, delusions, insomnia, and personality change was first recognized by Morvan, who called it *chorée fibrillare (7,8)*. Although he described the case fully, the central symptoms were only recorded in 1 of the 10 patients with symptoms and signs of NMT that he described. If they are sought specifically, the incidence of CNS manifestations in NMT is probably around 20% (**Table 1**) *(13)*.

The question arises as to whether autoantibodies enter the CNS by diffusion, or by leakage at sites where the blood-brain barrier is known to be weak,
or whether there is intrathecal synthesis of autoantibody. Oligoclonal bands
or an increase in CSF total IgG are commonly present in NMT patients, suggesting that there is intrathecal IgG synthesis (1). Preliminary immunohistochemical studies demonstrated binding of both CSF and serum IgG from
anti-VGKC antibody-positive NMT patients to neurons in the dentate nucleus
of the human cerebellum (55,56), and the pattern was similar to that of a polyclonal rabbit antiserum raised against a peptide of the $K_v1.1$ subtype. However, in general, the VGKC antibody levels in the CSF of patients are very
low, even when they have clear CNS manifestations (Vincent and Clover,
unpublished finding). Thus, the relationship between VGKC antibodies and
CNS abnormalities is not understood.

This is underscored by study of a patient with classical Morvan's syndrome
(**Fig. 3**; _10_). His onset was at 76 years of age, and no neoplasm was identified
_ante mortem_, although a small adenocarcinoma of the lung was found _post
mortem_. He developed severe insomnia, memory loss, confusion, and hallucinations over a few months, associated with extreme sweating, salivation,
and severe constipation. An electroencephalogram showed complete lack
of non-REM sleep, and a tendency to oscillate between a state of subwakeful-
ness and REM sleep. EDX studies showed florid neuromyotonic discharges,
and an electrocardiogram demonstrated cardiac arrhythmias. Strikingly, the
peripheral, autonomic and central features improved substantially after plasma
exchange. However, in addition to the VGKC antibodies, there were marked
changes in circadian rhythms of serum levels of various hormones under CNS
control, such as cortisol and melatonin. These changes could have been secondary to the effects of the autoantibodies on the CNS, or, conversely, the
effects of the autoantibodies on the periphery might have altered hormone
levels with secondary effects on CNS functions.

A rather similar case of "agrypnia excitata" was described, but VGKC antibodies were negative, and antibody binding to the CNS appeared to be to inhibitory synapses (57).

### Limbic Symptoms Without Overt Neuromyotonia

Two other patients were reported who contrast with Morvan's syndrome
(58). Both were diagnosed as having a limbic encephalitis on the basis of
memory loss, confusion, and anxiety with abnormalities of the hippocampus
on MRI. Neither was reported to have neuromyotonia or sleep disorders at the
time or subsequently, but both had excessive secretions—sweating in one
and salivation in the other. In a retrospective study, both patients had high

Morvan patient's serum       Control serum

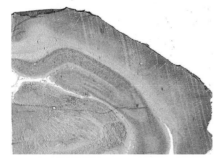 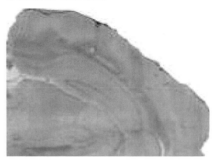

**Fig. 3.** Evidence for VGKC antibodies capable of binding CNS neurons in a patient with neuromyotonia, autonomic dysfunction, and CNS disorder (Morvan's syndrome; *10*). The patient's serum IgG antibodies (left) bind to thalamic neurons and to different layers of the hippocampus. In general, white matter is spared. The distribution is similar to that of antibodies to $K_v1.1$ and -1.2 subtypes. Control serum IgG (right) does not bind appreciably. (Courtesy of Ms. Linda Clover.)

levels of VGKC antibodies at the time of their limbic manifestations, and both improved when VGKC antibody levels fell—in one case after plasma exchange, and in the other spontaneously. Interestingly, one of these patients was a woman with a long history of MG with thymoma. The limbic manifestations arose following a recurrence of the thymoma, 13 years after the tumor had been removed. At the time, the MG was poorly controlled, but there was a striking dissociation between acetylcholine receptor autoantibody levels that fluctuated quite widely, and the single peak of VGKC antibodies that coincided with the limbic abnormalities. Plasma exchange was effective in reducing the CNS signs *(58)*.

These observations have stimulated us to look for antibodies to VGKC in a variety of patients with cognitive, psychiatric, or sleep disorders. Preliminary results suggest that VGKC antibodies are present in a proportion of these patients, that they are usually not present in those patients who have a neoplasm (except for thymomas, which are found with neuromyotonia), and that their presence may indicate a condition that will improve spontaneously, albeit slowly, or respond to immunosuppressive treatments.

## TREATMENT OF NMT

Antiepileptic drugs, such as carbamazepine and phenytoin, probably act by reducing sodium conductance and thus stabilize the nerve membrane, making it less excitable. Many patients require only these drugs, either separately or together. In general, baclofen, benzodiazepines, carbonic anhydrase inhibitors, and quinine are unhelpful.

Plasma exchange often produces short-term relief *(1)*, and, a trial of plasma exchange can help establish the diagnosis in the difficult situation of a patient with suspected autoimmune NMT but no VGKC antibodies. There is no evidence for a differential response to plasma exchange among patients with and without detectable VGKC antibodies. Nevertheless, a positive response to plasma exchange may be helpful in predicting those patients who are likely to benefit from long-term immunosuppression. Intravenous immunoglobulin has also been used, although reports suggest that some patients do not do well *(59)*, or do better with plasma exchange *(60)*. Combinations of prednisolone with azathioprine or methotrexate have helped some patients *(1)*. Randomized controlled trials are needed to evaluate these therapies more fully.

## REFERENCES

1. Newsom-Davis J, Mills KR. Immunological associations of acquired neuromyotonia (Isaacs' syndrome). Report of five cases and literature review. *Brain* 1993; 116:453–469.
2. Denny-Brown D, Foley DM. Myokymia and the benign fasciculation of muscular cramps. *Trans Assoc Am Physicians* 1948;61:88–96.
3. Gamstorp I, Wohlfart G. A syndrome characterized by myokymia, myotonia, muscular wasting and increased perspiration. *Acta Psychiatr Scand* 1959;34:181–194.
4. Isaacs H. A syndrome of continuous muscle-fibre activity. *J Neurol Neurosurg Psychiatry* 1961;24:319–325.
5. Mertens HG, Zschoke S. Neuromyotonie. *Klin Wochenschr* 1965;43:917–925.
6. Lance J W, Burke D, Pollard J. Hyperexcitability of motor and sensory neurons in neuromyotonia. *Ann Neurol* 1979;5:523–532.
7. Morvan A. De la chorée fibrillaire. *Gaz Hebdon Med Chir* 1890;27:173–200.
8. Serratrice G, Azulay JP. Que reste-t-il de la choreé fibrillaire de Morvan? *Rev Neurol* 1994;150:257–265.
9. Halbach M, Homberg V, Freund HJ. Neuromuscular, autonomic and central cholinergic hyperactivity associated with thymoma and acetylcholine receptor-binding antibody. *J Neurol (Berl)* 1987;234:433–436.
10. Liguori R, Vincent A, Clover L, et al. Morvan's syndrome: peripheral and central nervous system and cardiac involvement with antibodies to voltage-gated potassium channels. *Brain* 2001;124:2417–2426.
11. Maddison P, Lawn N, Mills KR, Vincent A, Donaghy M. Acquired neuromyotonia in a patient with spinal epidural abscess. *Muscle Nerve* 1998;21:672–674.
12. Tahmouch AJ, Alonso RJ, Tahmouch GP, et al. Cramp-fasciculation syndrome: a treatable hyperexcitable peripheral nerve disorder. *Neurology* 1991;41:1021–1024.
13. Hart IK, Maddison P, Vincent A, Newsom-Davis J, Vincent A, Mills KR. Phenotypic variants of autoimmune peripheral nerve hyperexcitability. *Brain*, in press.

14. Smith KKE, Claussen GY, Fesenmeier JT, Oh SJ. Myokymia-cramp syndrome: evidence of hyperexcitable peripheral nerve. *Muscle Nerve* 1994;17:1065–1067.
15. Wakayama Y, Ohbu S, Machida H. Myasthenia gravis, muscle twitch, hyperhidrosis, and limb pain associated with thymoma: proposal of a possible new myasthenic syndrome. *Tohoku J Exp Med* 1991:164:285–291.
16. Ho WKH, Wilson JD. Hypothermia, hyperhidrosis, myokymia and increased urinary excretion of catecholamines associated with a thymoma. *Med J Aust* 1993;158: 787–788.
17. Gutmann L, Libell D, Gutmann L. When is myokymia neuromyotonia? *Muscle Nerve* 2001;24:151–153.
18. Isaacs H. Continuous muscle fibre activity in an Indian male with additional evidence of terminal motor fibre abnormality. *J Neurol Neurosurg Psychiatry* 1967;30: 126–133.
19. Deymeer F, Oge AE, Serdaroglu P, et al. The use of botulinum toxin in localizing neuromyotonia to the terminal branches of the peripheral nerve. *Muscle Nerve* 1998; 21:643–646.
20. García-Merino A, Cabella A, Mora JS, Liaño H. Continuous muscle fiber activity, peripheral neuropathy, and thymoma. *Ann Neurol* 1991;29:215–218.
21. Irani PF, Purohit AV, Wadia HH. The syndrome of continuous muscle fiber activity. *Acta Neurol Scand* 1977;55:273–288.
22. Partanen VSJ, Soininen H, Saksa M, Riekkinen P. Electromyographic and nerve conduction findings in a patient with neuromyotonia, normocalcemic tetany and small-cell lung cancer. *Acta Neurol Scand* 1980;61:216–226.
23. Hosokawa S, Shinoda H, Sakai T, Kato M, Kuroiwa Y. Electrophysiological study on limb myokymia in three women. *J Neurol Neurosurg Psychiatry* 1987;50:877–881.
24. Bostock H, Cikurel K, Burke D. Threshold tracking techniques in the study of human peripheral nerve. *Muscle Nerve* 1998;21:137–158.
25. Burke D. Excitability of motor axons in neuromyotonia. *Muscle Nerve* 1999;22: 797–799.
26. Maddison P, Newsom-Davis J, Mills KR. Strength-duration properties of peripheral nerve in acquired neuromyotonia. *Muscle Nerve* 1999;22:823–830.
27. Kiernan MC, Hart IK, Bostock H. Excitability of motor axons in patients with spontaneous motor unit activity. *J Neurol Neurosurg Psychiatry* 2001;70:56–64.
28. Harman JB, Richardson AT. Generalized myokymia in thyrotoxicosis: report of a case. *Lancet* 1954;2:473–474.
29. Reeback J, Benton S, Swash M, Schwartz MS. Penicillamine-induced neuromyotonia. *BMJ* 1979;279:1464–1465.
30. Vilchez JJ, Cabello A, Benedito J, Villarroya T. Hyperkalaemic paralysis, neuropathy and persistent motor unit discharges at rest in Addison's disease. *J Neurol Neurosurg Psychiatry* 1980;43:818–822.
31. Benito-Leon J, Martin E, Vincent A, Fernandez-Lorente J, de Blas G. Neuromyotonia in association with essential thrombocythemia. *J Neurol Sci* 2000:173:78–79.
32. Gutmann L, Gutmann L, Schochet SS. Neuromyotonia and type 1 myofiber predominance in amyloidosis. *Muscle Nerve* 1996;19:1338–1341.
33. Hadjivassiliou M, Chattopadhyay AK, Davies-Jones GA, et al. Neuromuscular disorder as a presenting feature of coeliac disease. *J Neurol Neurosurg Psychiatry* 1997; 63:770–775.

34. Le Gars L, Clerc D, Cariou D, et al. Systemic juvenile rheumatoid arthritis and associated Isaacs' syndrome. *J Rheumatol* 1997;24:178–180.
35. Benito-Leon J, Miguelez R, Vincent A, et al. Neuromyotonia in association with systemic sclerosis. *J Neurol* 1999;246:976–977.
36. Liguori R, Vincent A, Avoni P, et al. Acquired neuromyotonia after bone marrow transplantation. *Neurology* 2000;54:1390–1931.
37. Vasilescu C, Alexianu M, Dan A. Muscle hypertrophy and a syndrome of continuous motor unit activity in prednisone-responsive Guillain-Barré polyneuropathy. *J Neurol (Berl)* 1984;231:276–279.
38. Caress JB, Abend WK, Preston DC, Logigian EL. A case of Hodgkin's lymphoma producing neuromyotonia. *Neurology* 1997;49:258–259.
39. Zifko U, Drlicek M, Machacek E, et al. Syndrome of continuous muscle fiber activity and plasmacytoma with IgM paraproteinemia. *Neurology* 1994;44:560–561.
40. Sinha S, Newsom-Davis J, Mills K, et al. Autoimmune aetiology for acquired neuromyotonia (Isaacs' syndrome). *Lancet* 1991;338:75–77.
41. Shillito P, Molenaar PC, Vincent A, et al. Acquired neuromyotonia: evidence for autoantibodies directed against K+ channels of peripheral nerves. *Ann Neurol* 1995;38:714–722.
42. Harvey AL, Rowan EG, Vatanpour H, Fatehi M, Castaneda O, Karlsson E. Potassium channel toxins and transmitter release. *Ann NY Acad Sci* 1994;710:1–10.
43. Sonoda Y, Arimura K, Kurono A, et al. Serum of Isaacs' syndrome suppresses potassium channels in PC-12 cell lines. *Muscle Nerve* 1996;19:1439–1446.
44. Ramaswami R, Gautam, M, Kamb A, et al. Human potassium channel genes: molecular cloning and functional expression. *Mol Cell Neurosci* 1990;1:214–223.
45. Hart IK, Waters C, Vincent A, et al. Autoantibodies detected to expressed K+ channels are implicated in neuromyotonia. *Ann Neurol* 1997;41:238–246.
46. Rettig J, Heinemann SH, Wunder F, et al. Inactivation properties of voltage-gated potassium channels altered by presence of β-subunit. *Nature* 1994;369:289–294.
47. Arimura K, Watanabe O, Kitajima I, et al. Antibodies to potassium channels of PC12 in serum of Isaacs' syndrome: western blot and immunohistochemical studies. *Muscle Nerve* 1997;20:299–305.
48. O'Hanlon GM, Plomp JJ, Chakrabarti M, et al. Anti-GQ1b ganglioside antibodies mediate complement-dependent destruction of the motor nerve terminal. *Brain* 2001;124:893–906.
49. Nagado T, Arimura K, Sonoda Y, et al. Potassium current suppression in patients with peripheral nerve hyperexcitability. *Brain* 1999;122:2057–2066.
50. Verino S, Adamski J, Kryzer TJ, et al. Neuronal nicotinic ACh receptor antibody in subacute autonomic neuropathy and cancer-related syndromes. *Neurology* 1998;50:1806–1813.
51. Toyka KV, Zielasek J, Ricker K, et al. Hereditary neuromyotonia: a mouse model associated with deficiency or increased gene dosage of the PMP22 gene. *J Neurol Neurosurg Psychiatry* 1997;63:812–813.
52. Zielasek J, Martini R, Suter U, Toyka KV. Neuromyotonia in mice with hereditary myelinopathies. *Muscle Nerve* 2000;23:696–701.
53. Vincent A. Understanding neuromyotonia. *Muscle Nerve* 2000;23:655–657.
54. Verino S, Auger RG, Emslie-Smith AM, et al. Myasthenia, thymoma, presynaptic antibodies, and a continuum of neuromuscular hyperexcitability. *Neurology* 1999;53:1233–1239.

55. Hart IK, Leys K, Vincent A, et al. Autoantibodies to voltage-gated potassium channels in acquired neuromyotonia. *Neuromuscul Disord* 1994;4:535.
56. Hart IK, Waters C, Newsom-Davis J. Cerebrospinal fluid and serum from acquired neuromyotonia patients seropositive for anti-potassium channel antibodies label dentate nucleus neurones. *Ann Neurol* 1996;40:554–555.
57. Batocchi AP, Marca GD, Mirabella, M, et al. Relapsing-remitting autoimmune agrypnia. *Ann Neurol* 2001;50:668–671.
58. Buckley C, Oger J, Clover L, et al. Potassium channel antibodies in two patients with reversible limbic encephalitis. *Ann Neurol* 2001;50:74–79.
59. Ishii A, Hayashi A, Ohkoshi N, et al. Clinical evaluation of plasma exchange and high dose intravenous immunoglobulin in a patient with Isaacs' syndrome. *J Neurol Neurosurg Psychiatry* 1994;57:840–842.
60. Van den Berg JS, van Engelen BG, Boerman RH, de Baets MH. Acquired neuromyotonia: superiority of plasma exchange over high-dose intravenous human immunoglobulin. *J Neurol* 1999;246:623–625.

# 14
# Congenital Myasthenic Syndromes

## Suraj A. Muley and Christopher M. Gomez

## INTRODUCTION

Congenital myasthenic syndromes (CMS) are a heterogeneous group of neuromuscular disorders that share clinical features with other neuromuscular transmission disorders but differ from acquired syndromes and among each other by their underlying molecular, genetic, and cellular pathogenesis. CMS may present in infancy or may not be recognized until childhood or later. Thus, a CMS may resemble neonatal or adult-onset myasthenia gravis (MG) or Lambert-Eaton syndrome (LES). Although impairment of neuromuscular transmission gives rise to similar clinical presentations, the sophisticated analysis of biopsied intact, muscle fibers from CMS patients using electrophysiologic, microscopic, and molecular techniques has identified several varieties of CMS in which impairment of neuromuscular transmission occurs through distinct molecular and cellular mechanisms. In many cases, recording of evoked or spontaneous miniature endplate potentials (MEPPs) or miniature endplate currents (MEPCs) or single channel currents has identified the presence and type of pre- or postsynaptic defect of neuromuscular transmission. Coupled with electron microscopic, biochemical, and genetic data, these studies have led to the identification of the affected protein, gene, and mutation in several patients. This detailed molecular information has provided insights into disease mechanisms that have begun to guide the development of therapeutic strategies.

## PREVALENCE AND CLASSIFICATION

The precise prevalence of CMS remains unknown. Underdiagnosis is likely because of incomplete characterization or misdiagnosis. The CMS are classified as presynaptic, synaptic, and postsynaptic (**Table 1**), based on the localization of the primary defect in neuromuscular transmission. In some cases

From: *Current Clinical Neurology: Myasthenia Gravis and Related Disorders*
Edited by: H. J. Kaminski © Humana Press Inc., Totowa, NJ

**Table 1**
**Classification of Congenital Myasthenic Syndromes (CMS)**

Presynaptic CMS
  CMS with episodic apnea (disorder of ACh resynthesis and packaging)
  CMS with deficiency of synaptic vesicles
  CMS resembling Lambert-Eaton syndrome
  CMS with nystagmus and ataxia (deficient action potential-dependent release
    of ACh)
Synaptic CMS
  Congenital endplate acetylcholinesterase deficiency
Postsynaptic CMS AChR deficiency (recessive AChR subunit mutations)
  Altered AChR channel kinetics
    Slow-channel CMS
    Low-affinity fast-channel CMS
    High-conductance fast-channel CMS
    CMS with AChR deficiency and short channel open time
  CMS with plectin deficiency
Poorly characterized CMS

[a]ACh = acetylcholine; AChR = acetylcholine receptor.

localization of the defect is difficult to establish. In 125 kinships studied at the Mayo Clinic, the defect was postsynaptic in 95, synaptic in 17, presynaptic in 9, and unclassified in 4 *(1)*. Genetic defects in most presynaptic disorders remain obscure, whereas those in the synaptic and in most postsynaptic disorders have been well established.

Presynaptic disorders result either from defects in acetylcholine (ACh) resynthesis and packaging or from reduction in the number of synaptic vesicles causing reduced quantal release of ACh. Acetylcholinesterase (AChE) deficiency is the only known synaptic disorder and is thought to be from impaired anchoring of the collagenic tail of AChE to the synaptic basal lamina. The postsynaptic disorders are from kinetic abnormalities and/or a deficiency of AChRs at the endplate, either of which may be predominant in a particular disorder.

## WORKUP AND DIAGNOSTIC STUDIES

CMS should be considered in any person presenting with fatigable ocular, bulbar, or limb weakness during infancy or early childhood, particularly (although not exclusively) with a positive family history. Decremental response in the compound muscle action potential (CMAP) elicited by repetitive nerve stimulation at low frequency (2 Hz) is strongly suggestive of impaired neuromuscular transmission, but may only be present in a few muscle groups. Single-fiber electromyography (SFEMG) will frequently reveal abnormal jitter and blocking. AChR antibody test is negative.

A tentative diagnosis of a particular CMS may be made based on the clinical features, electrophysiologic testing, and response to treatment. Prominent weakness of the cervical and wrist and finger extensor muscles and repetitive CMAPs in response to a single nerve stimulus are suggestive of either slow-channel CMS or endplate AChE deficiency. Lack of response to AChE inhibitors and a delayed pupillary light reflex suggests endplate AChE deficiency. Recurrent apneic episodes are common in patients with defective ACh resynthesis and packaging. A CMS with plectin deficiency has been described in patients with epidermolysis bullosa *(2)*. In tissue studies, AChE histochemistry in muscle biopsy may be used to establish the presence or absence of AChE at the endplate and electron microscopy to define the ultrastructure of the pre- and postsynaptic portions of the neuromuscular junction. Moreover, α-bunga-rotoxin (BGT) binding studies at the light and electron microscopic level can be used to quantitate AChRs. Biopsied, living muscle microelectrode studies (particularly recordings of endplate currents under voltage clamp conditions) are critical to characterize ACh release properties and the number and kinetic properties of the AChR channel. These tests may lead to a definitive diagnosis of a specific CMS. Moreover, in many cases these studies have identified the responsible gene and mutation.

## PRESYNAPTIC CONGENITAL MYASTHENIC SYNDROMES

### *Defect in Acetylcholine Resynthesis or Packaging*

#### *Clinical Features*

CMS with impaired resynthesis or packaging of ACh is an autosomal recessive disorder that was previously referred to as familial infantile myasthenia *(3–8)*. Clinical symptoms typically manifest at birth and consist of hypotonia, bulbar and respiratory weakness, ptosis, and extraocular muscle weakness, although ophthalmoparesis tends to be mild. Respiratory insufficiency with recurrent apnea is a hallmark of this disease and can result in death during infancy. Symptoms tend to improve with age in most patients, but in some they persist into adulthood and may cause respiratory failure precipitated by infections, fever, excitement, vomiting, or overexertion. Treatment with anticholinesterase drugs leads to improvement in muscle weakness and can be used prophylactically in anticipation of a crisis.

*Electrophysiologic and Morphologic Studies*

Routine nerve conduction studies and EMG are normal. In rested muscle the CMAP elicited by repetitive nerve stimulation at 2 Hz and the SFEMG may be normal. However, after exercise or after conditioning stimulus at 10 Hz, a decremental CMAP response with repetitive nerve stimulation and abnormal jitter are seen *(5,8,9)*. In vitro studies have shown that the EPP and MEPP amplitudes are normal in rested muscle preparations but decrease after a conditioning 10-Hz stimulus *(5,8,9)*. The endplate appears normal by electron microscopy, and the density and distribution of AChR on the junctional folds are normal *(5,8)*. These findings are similar to those found with muscle fibers poisoned by hemicholinium *(10–12)*, which depletes the nerve of choline by impairing its reuptake.

*Pathogenesis and Genetics*

Failed neuromuscular transmission and weakness result because the safety margin of neuromuscular transmission is compromised during sustained activity by the decreasing quantal size. Activity-dependent reduction in MEPP size suggests a defect in ACh synthesis and packaging. Expression of several genes may be responsible for the synthesis and packaging of neurotransmitter. Choline acetyltransferase, which catalyzes the reversible synthesis of ACh from acetyl coenzyme A (CoA) and choline at the synapse, has recently been found to be abnormal in some individuals with this disorder. Ten recessive mutations in five patients with this syndrome have thus far been identified *(13)*. Defects in other presynaptic proteins such as the choline transporter, vesicular ACh transporter, or vesicular proton pump may cause a similar phenotype, but no mutations in these proteins have thus far been identified.

## Paucity of Synaptic Vesicles and Reduced Quantal Release

*Clinical Features*

This rare CMS has been described in only a small number of patients. Clinical symptoms manifested during infancy with poor feeding, a weak cry, and delayed motor development. Fatigable weakness affecting the limb, bulbar, and periorbital muscles developed subsequently. Treatment with anticholinesterase drugs was partially effective *(14–16)*.

*Electrophysiologic and Morphologic Studies*

In this group of patients, as in most CMS, repetitive nerve stimulation at 2 Hz results in a decremental response in the CMAP. Interestingly, unlike with LES, there is no facilitation with high-frequency stimulation. Microelectrode studies reveal normal MEPP and MEPC amplitude and frequency. The time courses of decay of MEPC, single-channel conductance, and mean channel open time are normal. These studies indicate that the quantal size and the elementary properties of the AChR channel are normal in this syndrome. However, in one study the mean number of transmitter quanta released with 1-Hz stimulation was reduced by 20% *(15)*. This could be attributed to a reduction in the number of quanta immediately available for release. Moreover, quantitative electron microscopy revealed reduction in the number of synaptic vesicles to 20% of normal *(15)*.

## Pathogenesis and Genetics

Failed neuromuscular transmission and weakness in this disorder appear to result because the safety margin of neuromuscular transmission is compromised during sustained activity by the decreasing number of quanta released rather than by decreasing quantal size. The genetic basis of this disorder remains unknown. As in LES, there is a reduction in the quantal content of the EPP. Unlike in LES, in which there is reduction in the probability of quantal release, in this disorder there is reduction in the number of quanta immediately available for release. Accordingly, increment with stimulation at higher frequencies is not seen. The reduction in synaptic vesicular density may be a result of defective vesicle formation in the anterior horn cell, defective transport, impaired assembly, or impaired recycling.

## Other Presynaptic Congenital Myasthenic Syndromes

Two patients with CMS more closely resembling LES have been described *(17,18)*. One of these patients was mentally retarded with delayed motor milestones, and the other had severe bulbar and limb weakness along with respiratory insufficiency. Both patients were areflexic and hypotonic. CMAP amplitudes were reduced and facilitated with high-frequency stimulation, as with LES. The pre- and postsynaptic regions were structurally intact, and the synaptic vesicular density was normal *(18)*. The defect is thought to reside either in the presynaptic voltage-gated P/Q-type calcium channel or in a component of the synaptic vesicle release complex.

A new presynaptic CMS characterized by deficiency of the action potential-dependent release without reduction in the spontaneous release of neurotransmitter from the nerve terminal has recently been described *(19)*. In addition to myasthenic symptoms, these patients had nystagmus and ataxia. Deficiency of the quantal release of the neurotransmitter is thought to be the basis of this disorder, but the genetic defect remains unknown.

## SYNAPTIC DEFECT

### *Congenital Endplate AChE Deficiency*

#### *Clinical Features*

Congenital endplate acetylcholinesterase deficiency (CEAD) is an autosomal recessive disorder that begins at birth or early childhood and is characterized by fatigability and severe weakness affecting facial, cervical, axial, and limb muscles *(20,21)*. Involvement of axial muscles leads to lordosis and kyphoscoliosis. There is difficulty with feeding, crying, and respiratory distress along with delayed motor milestones. Extraocular muscle involvement is common. Tendon reflexes are hypoactive. Pupillary light reactions are reduced and in the appropriate clinical context are pathognomonic of CEAD *(20–24)*. Symptoms are refractory to treatment with anticholinesterase drugs. Treatment with quinidine worsens weakness, ephedrine is ineffective, and pseudoephedrine and prednisone result in variable response *(18)*. Atracurium, which causes intermittent AChR blockade, caused improvement in a respiratory-dependent patient with severe weakness *(25)*.

#### *Electrophysiologic and Morphologic Studies*

Single nerve stimuli elicit a repetitive CMAP response, a hallmark of this disease shared only by the congenital and acquired slow-channel syndromes. A decremental response in the CMAP is seen on repetitive nerve stimulation at multiple frequencies, reflecting impaired neuromuscular transmission. Microelectrode studies reveal normal to moderately reduced MEPP and MEPC amplitudes. Also, there is prolongation of the decay times of MEPPs, EPPs, and MEPCs *(18,20,21)*, indicating that the AChR activation events are prolonged. In biopsied muscle endplate, AChE is virtually undetectable using histochemical, electron cytochemical, and immunohistochemical approaches *(20,21)*. Quantitative electron microscopy reveals decrease in the nerve terminal size and presynaptic membrane length with extension of Schwann cell processes into the primary synaptic cleft *(18)*. AChR is lost from the endplates with degeneration of junctional folds *(20,26)*.

#### *Pathogenesis and Genetics*

Asymmetric AChE is concentrated at the endplate by means of a collagenic tail (ColQ) that anchors its catalytic subunit to the basal lamina at the neuromuscular junction. The genetic alteration underlying EAD consists of loss-of-function mutations of the gene encoding ColQ *(23,27)*. Eighteen mutations in ColQ have been identified to date *(28)*. These include missense mutations in the proline-rich attachment domain (which impair attachment of catalytic subunits), truncation mutations in the collagen domain (leading to a truncated ColQ protein), hydrophobic missense residues in the C-terminal domain (preventing triple helical assembly of the collagen domain), and mutations in the C-terminal region (producing insertion-incompetent AChE) *(29)*.

As revealed by comparable studies using AChE inhibitors, disappearance of released ACh from the synaptic cleft is delayed without the enzyme and depends on passive diffusion. The persistence of ACh in the cleft greatly prolongs the AChR activation events owing to the multiple rebinding of ACh, resulting in prolonged AChR opening and endplate currents. Prolonged AChR opening leads to overload of the subsynaptic region with sodium and calcium, which initiates autolytic biochemical processes that are responsible for the degenerating junctional folds. Reduced nerve terminal size appears to result from a retrograde feedback mechanism. Fatigability and weakness result from the reduced safety margin of neuromuscular transmission, which is caused by 1) decreased number of readily releasable quanta; 2) AChR deficiency secondary to degenerating junctional folds; 3) increased ACh at the synapse causing desensitization of AChRs *(30,31)*; and 4) failure to generate muscle fiber action potential because prolonged postsynaptic depolarization leads to inactivation of the perijunctional sodium channels *(18)*.

## GENETIC DISORDERS OF THE AChR

The AChR is a 250-kDa glycoprotein comprised of five homologous subunits that span the postsynaptic membrane and form a ligand-gated ion channel. Binding of ACh to two binding sites on the surface of each molecule causes opening of a cation channel through which sodium and calcium ions enter and give rise to synaptic currents in the neuromuscular junction. The subunits, two $\alpha$, and one each $\beta$, $\delta$, and $\varepsilon$ are each encoded by a separate gene. Genetic disorders of the AChR result in weakness and impaired neuromuscular transmission through a variety of mechanisms. Some mutations lead to AChR deficiency or reduced function and are recessively inherited. Others that affect the kinetics of channel gating are dominantly inherited.

In some of the diseases described below, only a few cases have been reported to date, and clinical data are sparse.

### *AChR Deficiency Caused by Recessive Mutations in the AChR Subunits*

#### *Clinical Features*

Hereditary AChR deficiency is an autosomal recessive CMS resulting from mutations causing a primary deficiency in endplate AChRs. The clinical phenotype can vary from mild to severe. In severe cases symptoms begin in infancy with delayed motor milestones, respiratory insufficiency, and feeding difficulties. Facial, limb, and extraocular muscle weakness with wasting begins in the first few years of life. Patients can lose their ability to walk in the first decade. Paraspinal muscle weakness leading to progressive kyphoscoliosis is common *(32)*. In milder cases motor milestones may be normal, and there is only mild ptosis and limitation of ocular movements. Symptoms may be overlooked until exposure to a muscle relaxant causes ventilatory failure and brings the disease to light *(33)*. Intermediate phenotypes also exist. Patients with a remitting-relapsing clinical course have also been observed *(34)*. In general, treatment with pyridostigmine and 3,4-diaminopyridine (3,4-DAP) is partially effective *(35)*.

*Electrophysiologic and Morphologic Studies*

Repetitive nerve stimulation at 2 Hz elicits decremental CMAPs, indicating that there is a reduced safety factor of neuromuscular transmission. Microelectrode studies show that the MEPP and MEPC amplitudes are decreased to 8–26% and 20–42%, respectively *(36)*. In some cases, single-channel studies of dissociated patient fibers have shown that the duration of channel opening episodes is prolonged and channel conductance is reduced *(33,36,37)*. As with other forms of CMS, there is an increased number of small EP regions distributed over an increased span of the muscle fiber. The endplate is structurally intact, although the junctional folds are simplified and somewhat reduced in size. The AChR index (ratio of the postsynaptic membrane reacting for AChR to the length of the primary synaptic cleft) is reduced, and the reaction for AChR on the junctional folds is patchy and reduced in intensity.

*Pathogenesis and Genetics*

Weakness and reduced safety factor are a result of the decreased MEPP and MEPC amplitudes. Synaptic responses are reduced because of a primary deficiency of AChRs that reduces the number of molecules available to generate synaptic currents. In some cases immunostaining confirms that there is deficiency of one of the subunits. In the case of the ε-subunit mutations, there is a compensatory expression of the fetal γ AChR subunit, a fact that accounts for the prolonged duration of channel opening and reduced channel conductance, properties of embryonic AChRs. Several genetic studies have demonstrated that this syndrome is caused by a group of mutations that severely reduce or eliminate the function of one entire subunit. Most cases arise from mutations in the gene encoding the AChR ε-subunit, although mutations in the α-, β-, and δ-subunits have also been described. Typically, affected patients bear two distinct mutations, one in each of their parental subunit alleles of the same subunit, i.e., they are compound heterozygotes. Rarely they are homozygotes. The ε- and δ-subunit mutations have been identified that cause premature termination of the translational chain *(33,36,38–41)*, alter the signal peptide or promoter *(42,43)*, interfere with assembly of the pentameric AChR *(36,37,42)* or disturb both AChR expression and kinetics *(36,41)*. β-subunit mutations have been identified that cause premature termination of the translational chain or impair AChR assembly by disrupting a specific interaction between the β- and δ-subunits *(44)*. Mutations affecting the α-, β-, or δ-subunits appear to cause a more severe phenotype, presumably because in those cases the fetal γ-subunit cannot substitute for the mutated subunit, as in the ε mutations.

## KINETIC ABNORMALITIES OF THE AChR

In these disorders impaired neuromuscular transmission results from impaired AChR ion channel gating. In some cases impaired gating leads directly to reduced synaptic currents, because of intrinsic dysfunction of the AChRs. In others, particularly in most cases of the slow-channel syndrome, impaired gating results in damage to the postsynaptic membrane, leading to loss of AChR and remodeling of the synaptic cleft.

### *Low-Affinity Fast-Channel Syndromes*

#### *ε-Subunit Mutations*

##### CLINICAL FEATURES

This CMS has been described in two unrelated patients who presented with myasthenic symptoms at birth *(42,45)*. Symptoms began in the neonatal period with stridor, ptosis, feeble cry, and difficulty feeding and continued during childhood with fatigable weakness, fluctuating ptosis, ocular palsies, difficulty chewing, and swallowing. Severe global weakness with inability to abduct arms against gravity developed during adulthood.

##### ELECTROPHYSIOLOGIC AND MORPHOLOGIC STUDIES

Routine EMG studies revealed short-duration motor unit potentials with moment-to-moment fluctuation of amplitude. Repetitive nerve stimulation showed 40, 24, and 7% decrements of evoked CMAP in the biceps, facial, and hypothenar muscles, respectively. MEPPs and MEPCs were small, but the number of AChRs per endplate was normal. Analysis of the ACh-induced current noise revealed that the mean single-channel conductance was normal but the noise power spectrum was abnormal, containing two components of different time-course. These abnormalities were thought to be from abnormal interaction of ACh with its receptor. Electron microscopy revealed that the synaptic vesicles were of normal size, the junctional folds were intact, and the density and distribution of the AChR on the folds were normal.

PATHOGENESIS AND GENETICS

Endplate noise analysis pointed to the presence of a kinetic abnormality of the AChR. Mutational analysis of two unrelated patients revealed that both patients were compound heterozygotes, each bearing mutations in both parental ε-subunit genes. Of the heteroallelic AChR ε-subunit gene mutations, both shared a common εP121L mutation also and had a unique mutation, one a signal peptide mutation (εG-8R) and the other a glycosylation consensus site mutation (εS143L). AChR expression studies in vitro demonstrated that the εG-8R and εS143L mutations resulted in severe reduction in surface AChR expression, but that the εP121L mutation gave normal expression. Normal endplate AChR number implies that the pathogenesis of the neuromuscular deficit is solely determined by the kinetic properties of the εP121L mutation. Studies of engineered εP121L AChR revealed markedly reduced rate of channel opening and reduced affinity of the open channel and desensitized states but little change in the affinity of the resting state for ACh *(41)*. The pathophysiology is related to abnormally infrequent and brief episodes of AChR channel opening because of alteration in ACh interaction with the AChR.

*α- and δ-Subunit Mutations*

Mutations affecting the M3 transmembrane domain of the α-subunit have recently been described *(46)*. In a few patients mild myasthenic symptoms were present at birth, and repetitive nerve stimulation revealed a decremental response. Each patient had two heterozygous missense mutations in the α-subunit of the AChR: αF233V in the M1 domain and αV285I in the M3 domain. Patch clamp studies revealed that the αV285I-AChR channels had normal conductance and burst durations that were 2.4-fold shorter and showed increased resistance to desensitization *(46)*. A partially characterized fast-channel syndrome causing severe congenital weakness has also been described with a δ-subunit mutation, δE59K *(43)*.

**High-Conductance Fast-Channel Syndrome**

*Clinical Features*

This autosomal recessive CMS has been described among two sisters who had myasthenic symptoms that manifested in the neonatal period with poor feeding, weak cry, and nocturnal respiratory insufficiency in infancy *(14,47)*.

Ptosis and extraocular muscle weakness developed at 3 years of age. Leg weakness leading to walking difficulties was also seen in both patients.

## Electrophysiologic and Morphologic Studies

Routine EMG studies revealed myopathic motor unit potentials (MUPs) in limb muscles. A 6–8% decrement on femoral nerve stimulation was seen only 3 min after exercise. Single-fiber EMG of the frontalis muscle revealed a neuromuscular transmission defect. Microelectrode studies revealed that MEPCs were abnormally large and their decay constant abnormally short. Analysis of ACh-induced current noise revealed that the mean single-channel conductance was increased 1.7-fold and the mean channel open time was 30% shorter than normal. On electron microscopy, the number of AChRs per endplate was normal, and only a few endplates were simplified or degenerating.

## Pathogenesis and Genetics

The pathophysiology is thought to be related to increased conductance and reduced open time of the AChR channel and possibly a structural abnormality at the endplate. The genetic basis has not been established, but a mutation affecting the pore of the AChR channel is thought to alter channel kinetics and cause this syndrome.

## AChR Deficiency and Short-Channel Open Time

A single patient with this CMS has been described. The patient had myasthenic symptoms at birth *(48)*. She was unable to suck and was fed with a nasogastric tube for 6 months. She also developed respiratory failure requiring mechanical ventilation. In the first year of life she had diffuse weakness, stridor, difficulty closing her mouth, difficulty chewing, and slurred and hypernasal speech. Motor milestones were delayed. She had a high arched palate with malocclusion. Symptoms progressed through childhood with facial, bulbar, and limb weakness. Treatments with pyridostigmine and prednisone were partially effective. A decremental response on repetitive nerve stimulation was seen and varied with age, implying impairment of neuromuscular transmission. Postsynaptic regions appeared normal on electron microscopy but the density of AChR on the junctional folds was reduced. The number of transmitter quanta released per nerve impulse were normal, but the amplitude of the MEPPs and MEPCs was low. The mean channel open time was reduced, but the mean channel conductance was normal. Thus, the neuromuscular transmission defect in this patient can be explained on the basis of reduced AChR density on junctional folds and their shorter open time, which gives rise to reduced amplitude of MEPCs. A genetic defect in an AChR subunit is the most likely cause of this syndrome, although genetic studies have yet to demonstrate such a defect.

## Slow-Channel Syndrome

### Clinical Features

The slow-channel congenital myasthenic syndrome (49,50) is an autosomal dominant, or occasionally sporadic, disorder presenting any time from infancy to middle age. Clinical features of the disease vary between different families depending on the mutation and between different members of the same family. The severe form of the disease presents in infancy and progresses through childhood, often causing respiratory insufficiency and loss of ambulation. There is weakness, fatigability, and atrophy of muscles with selective involvement of the cervical, scapular, finger extensor, and sometimes masticatory muscles. Ptosis and extraocular muscle involvement tend to be milder. Milder forms of the disease present in childhood or adult life and progress slowly or intermittently. Diagnosis is suggested by the presence of selective severe involvement of cervical and finger extensor muscles. AChE inhibitors either have no effect or worsen symptoms.

### Electrophysiologic Features and Microscopy

Routine nerve conduction studies and EMG are normal. As with CEAD, single-nerve stimuli elicit repetitive CMAPs in many muscles. Decremental response to repetitive stimulation at 2–3 Hz is seen mainly in clinically affected muscles. In vitro microelectrode studies indicate marked prolongation of endplate potentials and currents, which sometimes have biexponential decay phases. MEPP and MEPC amplitudes are reduced in some muscle fibers. Patch clamp of the motor endplate in acutely dissociated muscle fibers reveals the presence of AChRs with both normal and abnormally prolonged open times, accounting for the decays (51–56). Light microscopy reveals type 1 fiber predominance, atrophic fibers, tubular aggregates, and vacuoles in fiber regions near endplates (49,56). Electron microscopy reveals a variety of changes that comprise what has been termed the endplate myopathy. At the postsynaptic membrane and at the junctional folds, there are occasionally networks of labyrinthine membranous structures and pinocytotic vesicles, areas of degeneration of postsynaptic folds, and others with apparent hypertrophy of postsynaptic folds. The synaptic cleft may be widened focally or globally and may contain accumulations of electron-dense or granular debris or reduplicated basement membrane. The junctional sarcoplasm may contain membrane-bound structures resembling autophagic vacuoles or dilated mitochondria. There may be degenerating mitochondria and nuclei with con-

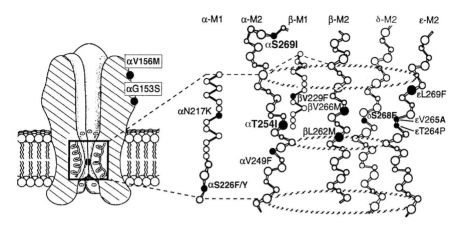

**Fig. 1.** Schematic illustration showing locations of AChR mutations (solid circles) causing slow-channel congenital myasthenic syndrome.

densed chromatin resembling apoptotic nuclei. Morphometric studies reveal decrease in nerve terminal size, increase in synaptic vesicle density, and reduction in the postsynaptic membrane length and density owing to degeneration of junctional folds *(18,49,50,56)*. BGT binding studies have sometimes shown a loss of AChRs from junctional folds, but at times the AChR number is normal or increased *(49,50,56)*.

*Pathogenesis and Genetics*

Weakness and fatigability are the result of impaired safety factor of neuromuscular transmission, which arises from reduced MEPC amplitudes. The abnormal MEPC decay phases, in the face of intact AChE imply the presence of a kinetic abnormality of the endplate AChRs that results in prolonged activation events. In all, 15 distinct missense mutations in AChR subunit genes (eight in the α-subunit, three in the ε-subunit, three in the β-subunit, and one in the δ-subunit) have been reported to date (**Fig. 1**) *(52–61)*. The mutations involve different functional domains (M1, M2, ACh binding site) encoded by these genes.

When studied in vitro, the AChRs containing the mutant subunits manifest several properties predicted to result in prolonged activation events in vivo. Most mutations cause a slowing of channel closing rate, and some cause increased affinity for ACh or spontaneous channel openings even in the absence of ACh. Some mutations alter channel kinetics by disturbing the equilibrium between different allosteric states of the AChR *(55)*. Mutations in the M2 domain tend to be more disabling than those in the M1 or extracellular domain

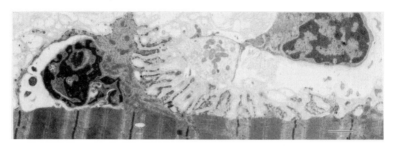

**Fig. 2.** Neuromuscular junction from deltoid muscle demonstrating the focal degeneration of postsynaptic folds, overabundant endocytotic vesicles in the postsynaptic membrane, autophagic vacuoles, and degenerating subsynaptic nucleus typically observed among patients with congenital myasthenic syndromes. (*See* Chapter 1.)

(ACh binding site). Prolonged opening of the AChR channel causes sodium and calcium overload, which may activate a variety of intracellular enzymatic pathways, such as proteases, phospholipases, and DNAses that could be responsible for the degenerative changes seen in the postsynaptic region *(49, 62–64)*. These changes directly damage postsynaptic folds as well as the underlying subsynaptic nuclei responsible for expression of the AChR genes, resulting in reduced AChR density. They may also impair the efficiency of AChR activation by causing a widened, debris-filled synaptic space (**Fig. 2**) *(49,57, 61)*. Weakness may result from other mechanisms as well, such as abnormal desensitization (even at low concentrations of ACh), depolarization blockade of perijunctional sodium channels, and slowed channel opening.

Quinidine, a long-acting open-channel blocker of wild-type AChR, shortens the duration of channel-open intervals in a concentration-dependent manner *(65)* and has been shown to improve symptoms *(66)*. Fluoxetine, another long-acting, open-channel blocker of AChR, may also be useful in symptomatic treatment *(18)*.

## CMS with Plectin Deficiency

This CMS has been described in a patient with epidermolysis bullosa simplex *(2)*. Myasthenic symptoms started at 9 years of age with progressive fatigable weakness in ocular, facial, limb, and truncal muscles. EMG revealed myopathic motor units, and on repetitive nerve stimulation a decremental CMAP response was seen. Microscopy revealed necrotic muscle fibers and degenerating junctional folds. Plectin, which is normally present in the sarcolemma, nuclear membrane, and intermyofibrillar network of muscle fibers, was absent. The presence of a myopathy and a myasthenic syndrome in this disorder suggests that plectin may be important in maintaining the structural integrity of the muscle and also in neuromuscular transmission.

## REFERENCES

1. Engel AE. 73rd ENMC International Workshop: congenital myasthenic syndromes. 22–23 October, 1999, Naarden, The Netherlands. *Neuromuscul Disord* 2001;11: 315–321.
2. Banwell BL, Russel J, Fukudome T, et al. Myopathy, myasthenic syndrome, and epidermolysis bullosa simplex due to plectin deficiency. *J Neuropathol Exp Neurol* 1999;58:832–846.
3. Greer M, Schotland M. Myasthenia gravis in the newborn. *Pediatrics* 1960;26:101–108.
4. Conomy JP, Levinsohn M, Fanaroff A. Familial infantile myasthenia gravis: a cause of sudden death in young children. *J Pediatr* 1975;87:428–430.
5. Hart Z, Sahashi K, Lambert EH, Engel AG, Lindstrom J. A congenital, familial, myasthenic syndrome caused by a presynaptic defect of transmitter resynthesis or mobilization. *Neurology* 1979;29:559.
6. Robertson WC, Chun RW, Kornguth SE. Familial infantile myasthenia. *Arch Neurol* 1980;37:117–119.
7. Gieron MA, Korthals JK. Familial infantile myasthenia gravis. Report of three cases with follow-up until adult life. *Arch Neurol* 1985;42:143–144.
8. Mora M, Lambert EH, Engel AG. Synaptic vesicle abnormality in familial infantile myasthenia. *Neurology* 1987;37:206–214.
9. Engel AG, Lambert EH. Congenital myasthenic syndromes. *Electroencephalogr Clin Neurophysiol Suppl* 1987;39:91–102.
10. Wolters C, Leeuwin RS, Van Wijngaarden KV. The effect of prednisolone on the rat phrenic nerve-diaphragm preparation treated with hemicholinium. *Eur J Pharmacol* 1974;29:165–167.
11. Jones S, Kwanbunbumpen, S. Some effects of nerve stimulation and hemicholinium on quantal transmitter release at the mammalian neuromuscular junction. *J Physiol (Lond)* 1970;207:51–61.
12. Jones S, Kwanbunbumpen S. The effects of nerve stimulation and hemicholinium on synaptic vesicles at the mammalian neuromuscular junction. *J Physiol (Lond)* 1970;207:31–50.
13. Ohno K, Tsujino A, Brengman JM, et al. Choline acetyltransferase mutations cause myasthenic syndrome associated with episodic apnea in humans. *Proc Natl Acad Sci USA* 2001;98:2017–2022.
14. Engel AG, Walls TJ, Nagel A, Uchitel O. Newly recognized congenital myasthenic syndromes: I. Congenital paucity of synaptic vesicles and reduced quantal release. II. High-conductance fast-channel syndrome. III. Abnormal acetylcholine receptor (AChR) interaction with acetylcholine. IV. AChR deficiency and short channel-open time. *Prog Brain Res* 1990;84:125–137.
15. Walls TJ, Engel AG, Nagel AS, Harper CM, Trastek VF. Congenital myasthenic syndrome associated with paucity of synaptic vesicles and reduced quantal release. *Ann NY Acad Sci* 1993;681:461–468.

16. Patrosso M, Maselli R, Gospe SM, et al. Synapsin I gene analysis in a boy affected by an unusual congenital myasthenic syndrome. *Muscle Nerve* 1994:(Suppl 1): S187.

17. Bady B, Chauplannaz G, Carrier H. Congenital Lambert-Eaton myasthenic syndrome. *J Neurol Neurosurg Psychiatry* 1987;50:476–478.

18. Engel A, Ohno K, Sine S. Congenital myasthenic syndromes. In: Engel A, ed. *Myasthenia Gravis and Myasthenic Disorders.* New York, Oxford University Press, 1999, pp. 251–297.

19. Maselli RA, Kong DZ, Bowe CM, et al. Presynaptic congenital myasthenic syndrome due to quantal release deficiency. *Neurology* 2001;57:279–289.

20. Engel AG, Lambert EH, Gomez MR. A new myasthenic syndrome with end-plate acetylcholinesterase deficiency, small nerve terminals, and reduced acetylcholine release. *Ann Neurol* 1977;1:315–330.

21. Hutchinson DO, Walls TJ, Nakano S, et al. Congenital endplate acetylcholinesterase deficiency. *Brain* 1993;116:633–653.

22. Hutchinson DO, Engel AG, Walls TJ, et al. The spectrum of congenital end-plate acetylcholinesterase deficiency. *Ann NY Acad Sci* 1993;681:469–486.

23. Ohno K, Brengman J, Tsujino A, Engel AG. Human endplate acetylcholinesterase deficiency caused by mutations in the collagen-like tail subunit (ColQ) of the asymmetric enzyme. *Proc Natl Acad Sci USA* 1998;95:9654–9659.

24. Ohno K, Brengman JM, Milone M, et al. Congenital end-plate acetylcholinesterase deficiency: novel missense and null mutations in the collagen-like tail subunit of the asymmetric enzyme. *Am J Hum Genet* 1998;63:A377.

25. Breningstall GN, Kurachek SC, Fugate JH, Engel AG. Treatment of congenital endplate acetylcholinesterase deficiency by neuromuscular blockade. *J Child Neurol* 1996;11:345–346.

26. Salpeter M, Kasprzak H, Feng H, Fertuck H. End-plates after esterase inactivation in vivo: correlation between esterase concentration, functional response and fine structure. *J Neurocytol* 1979;8:95–115.

27. Donger C, Krejci E, Serradell AP, et al. Mutation in the human acetylcholinesterase-associated collagen gene, COLQ, is responsible for congenital myasthenic syndrome with end-plate acetylcholinesterase deficiency (Type Ic). *Am J Hum Genet* 1998;63:967–975.

28. Ohno K, Engel AG. Congenital myasthenic syndromes: gene mutations. *Neuromuscul Disord* 2000;10:534–536.

29. Ohno K, Engel AG, Brengman JM, et al. The spectrum of mutations causing endplate acetylcholinesterase deficiency. *Ann Neurol* 2000;47:162–170.

30. Magleby KL, Pallotta BS. A study of desensitization of acetylcholine receptors using nerve-released transmitter in the frog. *J Physiol* 1981;316:225–250.

31. Katz B, Thesleff, S. A study of the 'desensitization' produced by acetylcholine at the motor end-plate. *J Physiol (Lond)* 1957;138:63–80.

32. Sieb JP, Kraner S, Schrank B, et al. Severe congenital myasthenic syndrome due to homozygosity of the 1293insG epsilon-acetylcholine receptor subunit mutation. *Ann Neurol* 2000;48:379–383.

33. Engel AG, Ohno K, Bouzat C, Sine SM, Griggs RC. End-plate acetylcholine receptor deficiency due to nonsense mutations in the epsilon subunit. *Ann Neurol* 1996; 40:810–817.

34. Milone M, Shen X-M, Ohno K, et al. Unusual congenital myasthenic syndrome caused by alpha subunit mutations and a relapsing-remitting clinical course. *Neurology* 1999;52:A185.
35. Palace J, Wiles CM, Newsom-Davis J. 3,4-Diaminopyridine in the treatment of congenital (hereditary) myasthenia. *J Neurol Neurosurg Psychiatry* 1991;54:1069–1072.
36. Ohno K, Quiram PA, Milone M, et al. Congenital myasthenic syndromes due to heteroallelic nonsense/missense mutations in the acetylcholine receptor epsilon subunit gene: identification and functional characterization of six new mutations. *Hum Mol Genet* 1997;6:753–766.
37. Milone M, Wang HL, Ohno K, et al. Mode switching kinetics produced by a naturally occurring mutation in the cytoplasmic loop of the human acetylcholine receptor epsilon subunit. *Neuron* 1998;20:575–588.
38. Middleton L, Ohno K, Christodoulou K, et al. Chromosome 17p-linked myasthenias stem from defects in the acetylcholine receptor epsilon-subunit gene. *Neurology* 1999; 53:1076–1082.
39. Ohno K, Anlar B, Ozdirim E, et al. Myasthenic syndromes in Turkish kinships due to mutations in the acetylcholine receptor. *Ann Neurol* 1998;44:234–241.
40. Ohno K, Fukudome T, Nakano S, et al. Mutational analysis in a congenital myasthenic syndrome reveals a novel acetylcholine receptor epsilon subunit mutation. *Soc Neurosci Abstr* 1996;22:234.
41. Brownlow S, Webster R, Croxen R, et al. Acetylcholine receptor delta subunit mutations underlie a fast-channel myasthenic syndrome and arthrogryposis multiplex congenita. *Clin Invest* 2001;108:125–130.
42. Ohno K, Wang HL, Milone M, et al. Congenital myasthenic syndrome caused by decreased agonist binding affinity due to a mutation in the acetylcholine receptor epsilon subunit. *Neuron* 1996;17:157–170.
43. Nichols P, Croxen R, Vincent A, et al. Mutation of the acetylcholine receptor epsilon-subunit promoter in congenital myasthenic syndrome. *Ann Neurol* 1999;45:439–443
44. Quiram PA, Ohno K, Milone M, et al. Mutation causing congenital myasthenia reveals acetylcholine receptor beta/delta subunit interaction essential for assembly. *J Clin Invest* 1999;104:1403–1410.
45. Uchitel O, Engel AG, Walls TJ, et al. Congenital myasthenic syndromes: II. Syndrome attributed to abnormal interaction of acetylcholine with its receptor. *Muscle Nerve* 1993;16:1293–1301.
46. Milone M, Ohno K, Brengman JM, et al. Low-affinity fast-channel congenital myasthenic syndrome caused by new missense mutations in the acetylcholine receptor alpha subunit. *Neurology* 1998;50:A432–A433.
47. Engel AG, Uchitel OD, Walls TJ, et al. Newly recognized congenital myasthenic syndrome associated with high conductance and fast closure of the acetylcholine receptor channel. *Ann Neurol* 1993;34:38–47.
48. Engel AG, Nagel A, Walls TJ, Harper CM, Waisburg HA. Congenital myasthenic syndromes: I. Deficiency and short open-time of the acetylcholine receptor. *Muscle Nerve* 1993;16:1284–1292.
49. Engel AG, Lambert EH, Mulder DM, et al. A newly recognized congenital myasthenic syndrome attributed to a prolonged open time of the acetylcholine-induced ion channel. *Ann Neurol* 1982;11:553–569.

50. Oosterhuis HJ, Newsom-Davis J, Wokke JH, et al. The slow channel syndrome. Two new cases. *Brain* 1987;110:1061–1079.
51. Ohno K, Hutchinson DO, Milone M, et al. Congenital myasthenic syndrome caused by prolonged acetylcholine receptor channel openings due to a mutation in the M2 domain of the epsilon subunit. *Proc Natl Acad Sci USA* 1995;92:758–762.
52. Engel AG, Ohno K, Milone M, et al. New mutations in acetylcholine receptor subunit genes reveal heterogeneity in the slow-channel congenital myasthenic syndrome. *Hum Mol Genet* 1996;5:1217–1227.
53. Milone M, Wang HL, Ohno K, et al. Slow-channel myasthenic syndrome caused by enhanced activation, desensitization, and agonist binding affinity attributable to mutation in the M2 domain of the acetylcholine receptor alpha subunit. *J Neurosci* 1997;17:5651–5665.
54. Sine SM, Ohno K, Bouzat C, et al. Mutation of the acetylcholine receptor alpha subunit causes a slow-channel myasthenic syndrome by enhancing agonist binding affinity. *Neuron* 1995;15:229–239.
55. Wang HL, Auerbach A, Bren N, et al. Mutation in the M1 domain of the acetylcholine receptor alpha subunit decreases the rate of agonist dissociation. *J Gen Physiol* 1997;109:757–766.
56. Gomez CM, Maselli R, Gammack J, et al. A beta-subunit mutation in the acetylcholine receptor channel gate causes severe slow-channel syndrome. *Ann Neurol* 1996; 39:712–723.
57. Gomez CM, Gammack JT. A leucine-to-phenylalanine substitution in the acetylcholine receptor ion channel in a family with the slow-channel syndrome. *Neurology* 1995;45:982–985.
58. Croxen R, Newland C, Beeson D, et al. Mutations in different functional domains of the human muscle acetylcholine receptor alpha subunit in patients with the slow-channel congenital myasthenic syndrome. *Hum Mol Genet* 1997;6:767–774.
59. Gomez CM, Maselli R, Staub J, et al. Novel δ and β subunit acetylcholine receptor mutations in the slow-channel syndrome demonstrate phenotypic variability. *Soc Neurosci Abstr* 1998;24:A573.
60. Ohno K, Wang H-L, Shen X-M, et al. Slow-channel mutations in the center of the M1 transmembrane domain of acetylcholine receptor alpha subunit. *Neurology* 2000; 54(Suppl 3):A183.
61. Gomez CM, Maselli RA, Vohra BP, et al. Novel delta subunit mutation in slow-channel syndrome causes severe weakness by novel mechanisms. *Ann Neurol* 2002; 51:102–112.
62. Evans RH. The entry of labelled calcium into the innervated region of the mouse diaphragm muscle. *J Physiol* 1974;240:517–533.
63. Takeuchi N. Effects of calcium on the conductance change of the end-plate membrane during the action of the transmitter. *J Physiol (Lond)* 1963;167:141–155.
64. Jackson MJ, Jones DA, Edwards RH. Experimental skeletal muscle damage: the nature of the calcium-activated degenerative processes. *Eur J Clin Invest* 1984;14: 369–374.
65. Sieb JP, Milone M, Engel AG. Effects of the quinoline derivatives quinine, quinidine, and chloroquine on neuromuscular transmission. *Brain Res* 1996;712:179–189.
66. Harper CM, Engel AG. Quinidine sulfate therapy for the slow-channel congenital myasthenic syndrome. *Ann Neurol* 1998;43:480–484.

# 15

# Toxic Neuromuscular Transmission Disorders

## James F. Howard, Jr.

## INTRODUCTION

The neuromuscular junction (NMJ) is uniquely sensitive to the effects of neurotoxins. Unlike the blood-brain barrier, which protects the brain and spinal cord, and the blood-nerve barrier, which protects peripheral nerve, there are no barriers to protect the NMJ from the deleterious effects of these agents. Several forms of neurotoxins are directed against the NMJ. Many occur as natural substances of plants or animals, other result from the actions of widely prescribed pharmaceutical compounds, and still others are environmental hazards. In nearly all instances of NMJ neurotoxicity, there is a reduction in the safety factor of neuromuscular transmission by one of several mechanisms. These neurotoxins may affect either the presynaptic or the postsynaptic elements of the NMJ. The clinical features of these neurotoxins are quite varied; many have associated toxicity of other parts of the central, peripheral, or autonomic nervous systems. Many will have other systemic effects as well. While feared as the purveyor of morbidity and mortality, many of these neurotoxins have led to significant advances in our understanding of the molecular mechanisms of pharmacology and physiology and their associated diseases. For example, the recognition that $\alpha$-bungarotoxin binds to the acetylcholine receptor (AChR) advanced our knowledge of the diagnosis and treatment of myasthenia gravis (MG) (1). Worldwide, the most common neurotoxicity of the NMJ results from envenomation. Of more concern to the clinical neurologist are those situations that result from the direct effects of various pharmacologic agents routinely used in the practice of medicine that produce significant aberrations of neuromuscular transmission in susceptible individuals. The potential for environmental intoxication has been limited by the stringent regulation of federal and international regulatory agencies.

The neurotoxins of interest may be broadly classified into three major categories: biologic, environmental, and pharmacologic. This chapter focuses on the direct effects of neurotoxins affecting neuromuscular transmission of

From: *Current Clinical Neurology: Myasthenia Gravis and Related Disorders*
Edited by: H. J. Kaminski © Humana Press Inc., Totowa, NJ

humans but is not meant to be a treatise on the broad topic of neuromuscular neurotoxicology. It is not possible to elaborate on all the pharmacologic and physiologic effects of particular toxins beyond the scope of the NMJ nor to discuss in detail the neuromuscular blocking effects of these neurotoxins in animals or experimental preparations.

All forms of NMJ neurotoxicity are characterized by progressive, typically symmetric, muscle weakness. Muscles of eye movement or the eyelid are most often involved, as well as the muscles of neck flexion and the pectoral and pelvic girdles. There may be involvement of bulbar and respiratory musculature depending on the toxin involved, the dose acquired, and the duration of toxin exposure. Cognition and sensation are spared, unless other elements of the central nervous system are simultaneously involved. Muscle stretch reflexes are often preserved or only minimally diminished, particularly during the early phases of the illness, but they may be lost if the weakness is severe.

## PHARMACOLOGIC NEUROTOXICITY

The adverse effects of drugs on synaptic transmission may be classified as acting 1) *presynaptically*, with a reduction in acetylcholine (ACh) release secondary to local anesthetic-like activity on the nerve terminal, alteration or impairment of calcium flux into the nerve terminal, or a hemicholinium effect; 2) *postsynaptically*, with antibody blockade of ACh receptors, curare-like effects, or potentiation of depolarizing or nondepolarizing neuromuscular blocking agents; or 3) in varying degrees, *both*. Each of these pharmacologic interactions may result in any of the clinical situations described above. Since the publication of the summaries of Barrons, Howard, and Kaeser, describing disorders of neuromuscular transmission occurring as the result of adverse drug reactions many more reports have surfaced adding to the list of potentially dangerous drugs *(2–6)*. An up-to-date list of these potential drug-disorder interactions is maintained on the web site of the Myasthenia Gravis Foundation of America (http://www.myasthenia.org/drugs/reference.htm). Unfortunately, much of the literature is anecdotal, and there are only a few comprehensive in vitro studies of drug effects on neuromuscular transmission in animal or human nerve-muscle preparations. The potential adverse effects of these medications must be taken into consideration when deciding which drugs to use in treating patients who have disorders of synaptic transmission.

With the possible exceptions of D-penicillamine, interferon-α, and botulinum toxin, no drugs are absolutely contraindicated in patients with MG and Lambert-Eaton syndrome (LES). There are, however, numerous drugs that interfere with neuromuscular transmission and will make the weakness of these patients worse or prolong the duration of neuromuscular block in patients receiving muscle relaxants. Drug-induced disturbances of synaptic transmission resemble MG, with varying degrees of ptosis, ocular, facial, bulbar, respiratory, and generalized muscle weakness. Treatment includes discontinuation of the offending drug and (when necessary) reversing the neuromuscular block with intravenous infusions of calcium, potassium, or cholinesterase inhibitors. In rare instances, these drugs may induce an autoimmune form of MG (D-penicillamine and interferon-α). In these situations, the treating physician must utilize therapies that are typically used for other forms of autoimmune MG.

Although it is most desirable to avoid drugs that may adversely affect neuromuscular transmission, in certain instances they must be used for the management of other illness. In such situations a thorough knowledge of the deleterious side effects can minimize their potential danger. If at all possible, it is wise to use the drug within a class of drugs that has been shown to have the least effect on neuromuscular transmission. Unfortunately, studies of such comparisons are few.

The most frequently encountered problems are the effects of antibiotics (aminoglycosides and macrolides) and β-adrenergic blocking agents, which acutely worsen the strength of patients with MG. Less commonly encountered are prolonged muscle weakness and respiratory embarrassment postoperatively in patients with disorders of neuromuscular transmission.

### Antibiotics

The aminoglycoside antibiotics may produce neuromuscular weakness irrespective of their route of administration *(7)*. The weakness is related to serum levels of the drug and is reversible in part by cholinesterase inhibitors, calcium infusion, and the aminopyridines *(8)*. These drugs have pre- and postsynaptic actions; many have elements of both. Neuromuscular toxicity data exist for several of the antibiotics including amikacin, gentamicin, kanamycin, neomycin, netilmicin, streptomycin, and tobramycin *(9)*. Of the group, neomycin is the most toxic and tobramycin the least. Clinically, gentamicin, kanamycin, neomycin, tobramycin, and streptomycin have been implicated in producing muscle weakness in nonmyasthenic patients *(4)*. Neuromuscular blockade is not limited to the aminoglycoside antibiotics. Myasthenic patients given erythromycin or azithromycin will report a mild exacerbation of their weakness *(10,11)*. The polypeptide and monobasic amino acid antibiotics, penicillins, sulfonamides, tetracyclines, and fluroquinolones cause transient worsening of myasthenic weakness, potentiate the weakness of neuromuscular blocking agents, or block synaptic transmission for other reasons *(12)*. Lincomycin and clindamycin can cause neuromuscular blocking, which is not readily reversible with cholinesterase inhibitors *(13,14)*. Polymyxin B, colistimethate, and colistin are also reported to produce neuromuscular weakness, particularly in patients with renal disease or when used in combination with other antibiotics or neuromuscular blocking agents *(7,15)*. These drugs, ampicillin, the tetracycline analogs oxytetracycline and rolitetracycline, and (more recently) ciprofloxacin *(16)* all exacerbate MG, although the mechanisms for each medication are not fully understood *(17,18)*.

## Cardiovascular Drugs

Many cardiovascular drugs are implicated in adversely affecting the strength of patients with MG and LES, and they (along with the antibiotics) account for the majority of adverse drug reactions in patients with neuromuscular disorders. β-adrenergic blockers may cause exacerbation of MG, or their use may coincide with the onset of myasthenic manifestations *(19,20)* . Even drugs instilled topically on the cornea are capable of producing such weakness *(21, 22)*. Atenolol, labetolol, metoprolol, nadolol, propranolol, and timolol cause a dose-dependent reduction in the efficacy of neuromuscular transmission in normal rat skeletal muscle and human myasthenic intercostal muscle biopsies *(20)*. Different β-blockers have reproducibly different pre- and postsynaptic effects on neuromuscular transmission. Of the group, propranolol is most effective in blocking neuromuscular transmission and atenolol the least.

The effects of calcium channel blockers on skeletal muscle are not understood, and studies have provided conflicting information. Some demonstrated neuromuscular blockade with postsynaptic curare-like effects, presynaptic inhibition of ACh release, and both pre- and postsynaptic effects *(23–25)*. The oral administration of calcium channel blockers to cardiac patients without neuromuscular disease does not produce altered neuromuscular transmission by single-fiber electromyography (SFEMG) measures *(26)*. Acute respiratory failure was temporally associated with administration of an oral dose of verapamil in a patient with LES and small cell carcinoma of the lung *(27)*. One patient with moderately severe, generalized MG developed acute respiratory failure following verapamil initiation (author's observations). Low doses of verapamil and its timed-release preparation have been used successfully for the treatment of hypertension in patients with MG receiving cyclosporine (author's observations).

Procainamide may produce acute worsening of strength in patients with MG *(28)*. The rapid onset of neuromuscular block and the rapid resolution of symptoms following discontinuation of the drug suggest the drug has a direct toxic effect on synaptic transmission, rather than inducting an autoimmune response against the neuromuscular junction. The postulated mechanism of action is primarily at the presynaptic membrane, with impaired formation of ACh or its release, although it is known to have postsynaptic blocking effects as well.

The earliest report of quinidine (the steroisomer of quinine) administration aggravating MG was by Weisman *(29)*. There are several reports of the unmasking of previously unrecognized MG following treatment with quinidine *(30, 31)*. The neuromuscular block is both presynaptic; impairing either the formation or release of ACh or, in larger doses, postsynaptic, with a curare-like action *(32)*. It has been claimed that the ingestion of small amounts of quinine, for example in a gin and tonic, may acutely worsen weakness in a myasthenic patient, although this cannot be substantiated with objective reports.

## Rheumatologic Drugs

D-penicillamine (D-P) is used in the treatment of rheumatoid arthritis (RA), Wilson's disease, and cystinuria. A number of autoimmune diseases occur in patients receiving D-P, of which MG is the most frequent *(33–35)*. The MG induced by D-P is usually mild and may be restricted to the ocular muscles. In many patients the symptoms are not recognized, and it may be difficult to demonstrate mild weakness of the limbs in the presence of severe arthritis. It is unlikely that D-P has a direct effect on neuromuscular transmission, as MG begins after prolonged D-P therapy in most patients and has a relatively low incidence in patients receiving D-P for Wilson's disease compared with those receiving it for RA *(36)*. It is more likely that D-P induces MG by stimulating or enhancing an immunological reaction against the neuromuscular junction. When MG begins while the patient is receiving D-P, it remits in 70% of patients within 1 year after discontinuation of the drug *(37)*. In a few patients, the MG persists after D-P is discontinued, implying that a subclinical myasthenic state existed prior to the initiation of the D-P (author's observations).

Chloroquine is used primarily as an antimalarial drug, but in higher doses it is also used in the treatment of several collagen vascular disorders including RA, discoid lupus erythematosus, and porphyria cutanea. It may produce a number of neurologic side effects, among which are disorders of neuromuscular transmission. Reported mechanisms of action for this have been both pre- and postsynaptic, but chloroquine may also alter immune regulation, producing a clinical syndrome of MG similar to that reported with D-P. One patient with RA and another with systemic lupus erythematosus developed the typical clinical, physiologic, and pharmacologic picture of MG following prolonged treatment with chloroquine. Antibodies to the AChR were identified and subsequently slowly disappeared, as did the clinical and electrophysiologic abnormalities, with discontinuation of the drug *(38,39)*. A patient is described with a transient postsynaptic disorder of neuromuscular transmission following 1 week of chloroquine therapy that was thought to be caused by a direct toxic effect on the neuromuscular junction rather than a derangement of immune function *(40)*.

## Other Drugs

### Interferon-α

Generalized MG may occur after starting interferon-α therapy for leukemia, during interferon-α2b treatment for malignancy, and during treatment for chronic active hepatitis C *(41–45)*. Myasthenic crisis may even develop with interferon alpha therapy *(46)*. The mechanism of interferon-induced MG is not known. Expression of interferon-γ at motor endplates of transgenic mice results in generalized weakness and abnormal NMJ function, which improves with cholinesterase inhibitors. Immunoprecipitation studies identified an 87-kDa target antigen recognized by sera from these transgenic mice and from human MG patients. Such studies suggest that the expression of interferon-γ at the motor endplates provoked an autoimmune humoral response, similar to that occurring in human MG *(47)*.

Numerous other drugs may interfere with neuromuscular transmission. Many local anesthetics, certain anticonvulsants, magnesium, iodinated contrast dyes, and of course the neuromuscular blocking agents used by anesthesiologists during surgery are included in this list. Adverse drug-disorder interactions are reported frequently. It is beyond the scope of this chapter to discuss them all in detail, and the reader is referred to a more comprehensive review of the topic *(19)* or to the web address of the MG Foundation of America given above.

## BIOLOGIC NEUROTOXINS

### Botulism

Botulism is caused by a clostridial neurotoxin that blocks the release of ACh from the motor nerve terminal* *(48)*. The result is a long-lasting, severe muscle paralysis. Botulism may be classified clinically according to presentation, as noted in **Table 1**. Of eight different types of botulinum toxins, types A and B cause most cases of botulism in the United States. Type E is trans-

---

*Although tetanus toxin also binds to the neuromuscular junction, its mechanism of action is distinctly different. This toxin is translocated into the nerve terminal and then moves in a retroaxonal fashion to the synaptic space between the α-motoneuron and inhibitory neurons. There it inhibits exocytosis, resulting in paresis. Because it does not directly involve the motor nerve terminal, it will not be discussed further.

**Table 1**
**Clinical Classification of Botulism**

Classic form
Infantile form
Wound botulism
Traumatic or surgical
Drug abuse
Intranasal
Intravenous
Hidden form

mitted in seafood, and type A is thought to produce the most severe manifestations. The classic form of the disease usually follows ingestion of foods that were contaminated by inadequate sterilization. Not all persons ingesting contaminated food become symptomatic. Nausea and vomiting are the first symptoms, and the neuromuscular features begin 12–36 h after exposure. The clinical findings are stereotypical. Ptosis, blurred vision, dysphagia, and dysarthria are the presenting features. The pupils may be dilated and poorly reactive to light. Descending weakness progresses for 4–5 days and then plateaus. Respiratory paralysis may occur rapidly. Most patients have autonomic dysfunction, such as dry mouth, constipation, urinary retention, and cardiovascular instability.

Infantile botulism is caused by the chronic absorption of toxin from *Clostridium botulinum* growing in the infant gastrointestinal tract *(49)*. Honey is a common source of contamination. The onset of symptoms (constipation, lethargy, and poor suck) usually occurs between 6 weeks and 6 months of age. A descending pattern of weakness occurs and may produce widespread cranial nerve and limb muscle involvement. The pupils are poorly reactive, and the tendon reflexes are hypoactive. Most babies will require ventilatory support.

Wound botulism occurs owing to the contamination of a wound with *Clostridium botulinum*. Its rarity may be related to the difficulty of spore germination in a wound environment. The clinical presentation of wound botulism is similar to the classical form of the disease, as noted above. It may occur as a complication of intranasal and parenteral use of cocaine *(50)*.

The term hidden botulism is used when no source of botulism or exposure can be identified. Some argue that these cases represent adult forms of infantile botulism *(51)*. This is suggested by the high prevalence of colonic diverting procedures among these patients.

Response to antitoxin treatment is generally poor, probably because once toxin binds to the nerve terminal it is no longer accessible to the antitoxin. Antibiotic therapy is not effective unless the botulism is the infantile or hidden form of the disease. Otherwise, treatment is supportive, with respiratory assistance when necessary. Cholinesterase inhibitors are not usually beneficial; guanidine or 3,4-diaminopyridine (3,4-DAP) may improve strength but not respiratory function. Recovery takes many months but is usually complete.

EMG abnormalities evolve as the disease progresses and may not be present at onset of symptoms. CMAP amplitude is decreased in affected muscles, but motor and sensory nerve conduction is normal. Some patients demonstrate a decremental pattern, and at some time most have posttetanic facilitation in some muscles of 30–100% to low-frequency stimulation. These findings are similar to those of LES but have a more restricted distribution. SFEMG shows markedly increased jitter and blocking. The organism can be recovered from the stool of infected infants or in the hidden form of the disease.

### Envenomation

Most biologic toxins of animal origin affect the cholinergic system and either facilitate the release of neurotransmitter from the presynaptic nerve terminal or block the AChR. In general, bites from snakes, scorpions, and ticks are more common during summer months when they are inadvertently encountered. In contrast, exposure to marine toxins may occur at any time, as they are acquired through ingestion and less rarely by injection or penetration. Specific geographic loci can be demonstrated for each of these vectors. For example, tic envenomation predominates in states west of the Rocky Mountains, the western provinces of Canada, and Australia. The geography of snake envenomation is species-specific. The cobras are found in Asia and Africa, the kraits in Southeast Asia, the mambas in Africa, the coral snake in North America, and the sea snakes in the waters of the Pacific near Australia and New Guinea.

### Arthropods

The venoms of the phylum Arthropod are used to incapacitate prey for feeding or as a defense against predators *(52)*, an observation made in antiquity. Few of the arthropods, however, produce toxicity at the NMJ; when it is produced, it is by three mechanisms (**Table 2**). In the first there is an initial augmentation of ACh release followed by presynaptic depletion of neurotransmitter. The second leads to a facilitation of ACh release without a subsequent presynaptic depletion of neurotransmitter. The third mechanism causes a depletion of ACh release with a subsequent presynaptic depletion of neurotransmitter.

**Table 2**
**Mechanisms of Arthropod Blockade of Synaptic Transmission**[a]

| |
|---|
| Facilitation of ACh release with subsequent exhaustion of neurotransmitter |
| Facilitation of ACh release without subsequent exhaustion of neurotransmitter |
| Depletion of ACh release with subsequent exhaustion of neurotransmitter |

[a]ACh = acetylcholine.

SPIDER BITES

Only a few spider venoms affect the neuromuscular junction. The funnel web spider and the redback spider of Australia are the most dangerous spiders in this group. In North America, only the bite of the black widow spider is of concern. The usual victim of a black widow spider bite is a small boy, perhaps the result of inquisitiveness into nooks and crannies.

Lathrotoxins found in the venoms from the spider genus *Latrodectus* (black widow spider) cause systemic lathrodectism. These toxins produce a marked facilitation in neurotransmitter release by depolarization of the presynaptic nerve terminal and increasing $Ca^{2+}$ influx into the nerve terminal at all neurosecretory synapses including the NMJ *(53–55)*. There is subsequent depletion of neurotransmitter from the nerve terminal, resulting in a blockade of synaptic transmission. This toxin exerts its effects on the presynaptic nerve terminal by several mechanisms. The toxin binds to neurexin and thereby activates the presynaptic protein complex of neurexin, syntaxin, synaptotagmin, and the N-type calcium channel to facilitate massive ACh release *(56)*. Neurotransmitter release in nerve-muscle preparations, as measured by MEPP frequency, increases several hundred-fold within a few minutes *(57)*. There is a subsequent depletion of synaptic vesicles and disruption of the highly organized active zone region of the presynaptic nerve terminal, thus inhibiting the docking of synaptic vesicles to the terminal membrane and effective recycling of vesicular membrane *(58–63)*.

Signs of a black widow spider bite begin within minutes of the bite and reflect the massive release of neurotransmitter from peripheral, autonomic, and central synapses *(64)*. Severe muscle rigidity and cramps precede generalized muscle weakness owing to the depolarizing neuromuscular blockade. The black widow spider bite is rarely fatal, but cardiovascular collapse may occur in the elderly or in young children. Treatment is primarily supportive. The administration of calcium gluconate may be helpful in alleviating muscle cramps and rigidity *(65)*. Magnesium salts may be beneficial by reducing neurotransmitter release *(64)*. The administration of horse serum antivenom is effective and rapidly reverses the neurotoxic effects *(66)*.

**Table 3**
**Comparative Features of Ascending Paralysis**[a]

| Clinical and Laboratory Features | Tick Paralysis | Landry-Guillain-Barré Syndrome |
|---|---|---|
| Rate of progression | Hours to days | Days to 1–2 weeks |
| Sensory loss | Absent | Mild |
| Muscle stretch reflexes | Diminished or absent | Diminished or absent |
| Time to recovery | <24 h after tick removal | Weeks to months |
| CSF WBC count | <10/mm$^2$ | <10/mm$^2$ |
| CSF protein | Normal | Elevated |

[a]CSF = cerebrospinal fluid.

TICK PARALYSIS

Tick paralysis, a worldwide disorder, was first described at the turn of the 20th century in North America and Australia, although there is a vague reference to an earlier case in the early 1800s *(67–70)*. It is one of several kinds of neuromuscular disorders that result from tick venom exposure. Tick paralysis results from the introduction of a neurotoxin from one of more than 60 tick species *(71,72)*. In North America, the *Dermacentor andersoni, D. variabilis, D. occidentalis, Amblyomma americanum,* and *A. maculatum* species are toxic. The vectors in Europe and the Pacific are *Ixodes ricinus* and *I. cornuatus*, and that in Australia is *I. holocyclus*. Geographically, tick paralysis is more common in States west of the Rocky Mountains and in British Columbia and Alberta *(73)*.

The symptoms are stereotypical. Within 5–6 days of attachment, there is a prodrome of paresthesia, headache, malaise, nausea, and vomiting. The prodromal period parallels the feeding pattern of the tick. Over the next 24–48 h, an ascending paralysis occurs. It begins symmetrically in the lower extremities and progresses to involve the trunk and arms. In most instances when a tick is found, it is fully engorged. In contrast to the vectors found most commonly in North America (*Dermacentor* and *Amblyomma* species*)*, the weakness of the Australian tick is more severe and much slower to resolve. In these patients there is often a worsening of clinical signs 24–48 h after he removal of the tick *(74)*. Sensation is preserved, but muscle stretch reflexes are often diminished or not present, suggesting the Landry-Guillain-Barré syndrome (**Table 3**), a common misdiagnosis *(75)*. There is no demonstrable response to cholinesterase inhibitors *(76,77)*. There is some indication of an association between the proximity of the site of attachment to the brain and the severity of the disease. Antitoxin may be of benefit in some situations, but the high frequency of acute allergic reactions makes its widespread use less useful *(78)*. Resolution of manifestations is dependent in part on how quickly the tick is removed, suggesting that the amount of muscle weakness is a dose-dependent process. Often improvement begins within hours of removing the tick. Paralyses caused by the *Dermacentor* species may continue over several days. However, prolonged weakness is reported *(79)*. Death may occur owing to respiratory failure from severe bulbar and respiratory muscle weakness, and the clinical picture may be clouded by the presences of central nervous system manifestations *(73,80)*.

Whereas once these envenomations carried a 12–25% mortality, they are now rarely fatal, owing to improvements in critical care over the latter half of the 20th century *(67,81)*. Children are more prone to the disorder than adults, possibly because of their play habits and their lower body mass relative to the amount of toxin acquired. The head and neck is the most common site for tick attachment, although any part of the body may be bitten. Some studies suggest that girls are more often affected because their (on average) longer hair allows the tick to remain hidden for longer periods and therefore allows prolonged feeding *(75,82)*. The identification of a tick bite is often delayed, resulting in misdiagnosis. Tick paralysis may be confused with Landry-Guillain-Barré syndrome, myasthenia gravis, spinal cord disease, periodic paralysis, diphtheria, heavy metal intoxication, insecticide poisoning, porphyria, and hysteria *(75,83)*. In many instances the tick is located by the nurse, the house officer, the mortician, or autopsy personnel *(75,81,84)*. Careful, systematic inspection of the scalp, neck, and perineum, often with a fine-toothed comb, is necessary to locate the tick.

The mechanisms of paralysis following tick envenomation remain controversial. The most potent toxin is from the Australian tick, *I. holocyclus*. Holocyclotoxin, isolated from the salivary glands of female ticks, causes a temperature-dependent blockade of neuronally evoked release of ACh *(85)*. Others have suggested a postsynaptic block of neuromuscular transmission *(86)*. The tick paralysis of the *Dermacentor* species is understood less clearly, and no direct abnormality of synaptic transmission may occur, rather, the abnormality may be caused by impaired depolarization of the nerve terminal with the consequence of decreased ACh release *(87,88)*. Prolonged distal motor latencies, slowed nerve conduction velocities, and reduced compound muscle action potential (CMAP) amplitudes are described *(72,89–92)*.

### Scorpion Bites

The peptides contained in scorpion neurotoxins may cause a variety of neurologic effects, the most significant of which are those that modulate $Na^+$ and $K^+$ channel function. Some, however, affect the NMJ and produce an enhanced presynaptic depolarization resulting in neurotransmitter release *(93)*. Increased excretion of catecholamines is demonstrated after scorpion sting and may relate to the primary effect of the venom or to a secondary sympathetic adrenergic surge. Treatment is nonspecific and focuses on maintaining respiratory, cardiac, and coagulation function. Antivenom appears not to be efficacious *(94,95)*.

*Snake Bites*

Four major groups are responsible for envenomation by snake bite: *Viperidae* (true vipers) *Crotalidae* (rattlesnakes and pit vipers) *Elapidae* (American coral snake, cobras, kraits, mambas), and *Hydrophidae* (sea snakes). Neuromuscular blockade occurs primarily from the *Elapidae* and *Hydrophidae* species *(96–98)*. One *Crotalidae* species, *Croatulus durissus terrificus*, a South American rattlesnake, has a very potent neuromuscular blocking venom. Other rattlesnakes and pit vipers act through hematologic and cardiovascular mechanisms. Venom is produced and stored in salivary glands, and inoculation occurs through fangs or modified premaxillary teeth *(96)*.

Snake toxins may act by presynaptic or postsynaptic mechanisms. Presynaptic toxins, the β-neurotoxins (β-bungarotoxin, notexin, and taipoxin) act to inhibit the normal release of ACh from the presynaptic terminal of the neuromuscular junction. Often, there is an initial augmentation of ACh release followed by presynaptic depletion of neurotransmitter. They tend to be more potent than postsynaptic toxins. Postsynaptic neurotoxins, the α-neurotoxins, produce a curare-mimetic, nondepolarizing neuromuscular block and vary in the degree of the reversibility of the block in experimental preparations.

Most venoms are a mixture of the two types of neurotoxin, although one type may predominate in a given venom. For example, the venom of the Thai cobra is composed primarily of a single postsynaptic neurotoxin *(99)*. In contrast, the venom of *Bungarus multicintus* contains β-bungarotoxin, four other presynaptic toxins, α-bungarotoxin, and two other postsynaptic toxins *(100)*. The venoms of *Hydrophidae* species are more toxic than those of land snakes, although the amount of toxin injected by sea snakes is smaller than that of land-based snakes *(101,102)*. The α-neurotoxins (postsynaptic) like curare bind to the muscle nicotinic AChR. They have a slower onset of action and a longer duration of effect and are 15–40 times more potent than D-tubocurarine *(103)*. There are numerous subforms of β-neurotoxins (presynaptic). Most have a phospholipase component that is essential for the presynaptic effects of the toxin. All suppress the release of ACh from the nerve terminal, although there is some variability in the precise mechanism by which this occurs. In experimental preparations, toxins from different species potentiate each other, suggesting different binding sites at the neuromuscular junction *(104)*. Taipoxin from the Australian and Papua New Guinean taipan snake is unique. In addition to its potent presynaptic blockade of synaptic transmission, it also has a direct myotoxic component. This produces rapid muscle necrosis and degeneration. There is species variation in the susceptibility to toxin exposure. The venom of the Australian mulga snake is fatal in humans, produces ptosis in monkeys, and does not produce a neuromuscular block in the rabbit *(105,106)*.

The clinical course of snake envenomation follows a specific pattern. After the bite of a pit viper or cobra, there is local pain, which is often absent following the bite of other *Elapidae (*mambas, kraits, coral snakes) and *Hydrophidae*. Swelling typically follows within an hour of the bites from *Viperidae, Crotalidae*, or the cobra but is not seen following bites from other *Elapidae* and *Hydrophidae*. A preparalytic stage develops with headache, vomiting, loss of consciousness, paresthesias, hematuria, or hemoptysis *(107)*. These manifestations are not common after envenomation by cobras or mambas. The time between snake bite and paralysis may vary from 0.5 to 19 h *(108)*. The first signs of neuromuscular toxicity are usually ptosis and ophthalmoparesis, although these are absent following the bite of the South American rattlesnake. Facial and bulbar weakness develops over hours following the ocular signs *(109)*. For 2–3 days, limb, diaphragmatic, and intercostal weakness may continue to evolve *(96,110)*, and, without appropriate treatment, cardiovascular collapse, seizures, and coma ensue. There is no sensory abnormality other than that from the bite itself. Other systemic effects of neurologic importance relate to coagulation deficits. Cerebral and subarachnoid hemorrhage may occur after bites from many species and is the leading cause of death following viper bites in several regions of the world *(111,112)*.

Treatment consists of antivenom, which is most effective in bites that do not contain significant amounts of phospholipase, a component of presynaptic neurotoxins *(109,113,114)*. If the type of snake is known, a high-titer monovalent type is administered, but more often the snake variety is not known, necessitating the use of polyvalent antivenom. The goal of antivenom is to shorten the duration of weakness, and frequently the addition of respiratory, cardiovascular, and hematologic support is required. Supportive measures are the mainstay of care for most victims of coral snake bite. Intensive care treatment and airway maintenance is similar to that used for patients with MG. Some authors recommend treatment with cholinesterase inhibitors in cases that are predominantly caused by a postsynaptic abnormality and suggest that electrodiagnostic testing may be useful in determining their effectiveness *(115,116)*.

*Marine Toxins*

The rapid rise in marine pollution has spurred a renewed interest in marine toxins. Previously they were only of interest to the physiologist and pharmacologist, who use them in the investigation of biologic systems. Examples of marine neurotoxicology are scattered throughout the literature dating to biblical times (*Exodus* 7:20–21). The reader is referred to Southcott's paper for an excellent review of the subject *(117)*. Marine neurotoxins affecting the NMJ are rare and occur primarily from poisonous fish, a few mollusks, and perhaps dinoflagellates. Unlike the poisoning from arthropods and snakes, most marine intoxications occur as the result of ingestion. Unique to some marine toxins is the increase in concentration of toxin through successive predatory transvection up the food chain.

Dinoflagellates are single-celled, biflagellated, algae-like organisms. Diatoms, similar to dinoflagellates, are not flagellated and are encased by a silica shell. The toxins produced by these organisms cause a variety of systemic and neurologic effects, but NMJ effects are rare and indirect. Paralytic shellfish poisoning results from neurotoxins produced by less than 1% of the 2000–3000 species of known dinoflagellates and diatoms *(118)*. The toxin is rapidly absorbed through the gastrointestinal tract, and symptoms begin within 30 min of ingestion. Characteristically, there is an initial burning or paresthesias of the face and mouth, spreading quickly to involve the neck and limbs. Slowly, the sensations abate and are replaced with numbness, some ataxia, and (in severe cases) progressive generalized weakness and respiratory failure. Overall, the mortality approaches 10%. Most neurotoxins from dinoflagellates and diatoms are sodium channel blockers (e.g., saxitoxin and tetrodotoxin). Brevetoxin, a milder neurotoxin that causes the nonlethal neurotoxic shellfish poisoning, depolarizes cholinergic systems, by opening sodium channels and resulting in neuromuscular transmission alterations indirectly. Ciguatoxin, from *Gambierdiscus toxicus*, is commonly found in the Caribbean and South Pacific regions. This heat-stable lipid enhances the release of ACh from the NMJ by prolonged sodium channel opening. Onset of symptoms is within hours of ingestion, and respiratory muscle paralysis may occur quickly. Recovery usually occurs within a few weeks.

Conontoxins are a diverse group of toxins from predatory cone snails that inject their venom through a small harpoon-like dart *(119)*. It is only the fish predatory species (*Conus geographus, C. textile, C. marmoreus*, and *C. omaria*) of this mollusk that appears to be dangerous to humans *(120–122)*. The effects of these toxins are variable among species and within a single species, and several have direct effects on the NMJ. α-Conotoxins block the binding of

ACh to the ligand binding site *(123–125)*. These venoms function similarly to the snake α-neurotoxins described earlier. The ω-Conotoxins block the voltage-gated calcium channel of the presynaptic nerve terminal *(126)*. The latter toxin has played an important role in understanding of LES and serves as the basis for the currently used antibody assay *(127,128)*. Following the injection of toxin, there is intense local pain quickly followed by malaise, headache, and (within 30 min) progressive generalized weakness. Respiratory failure often occurs within 1–2 h. Most cone shell bites are preventable. These shells should be handled carefully with forceps and thick gloves. The proboscis protrudes from the small end of the shell, but it is flexible and long enough to sting the holder at the other end. The live shells should never be placed in a pocket, as the dart may penetrate cloth *(117)*. Treatment is directed toward respiratory and cardiovascular support. There is no available antivenom. There is no literature discussing the potential efficacy of cholinesterase inhibitors. More than 60% of stings are fatal *(122,129)*.

The most venomous fish is the stonefish, *Synanceja horrida, S. traachynis,* and *S. verrucosa* found in the Indo-Pacific oceans and Red Sea as well as the genus *Inimicus* found off the coast of Japan *(130)*. The toxin, stonustoxin, is inflicted by injection through the 13 dorsal spines when the victim steps on the small fish that is buried in the sand. Neuromuscular blockade results from induced neurotransmitter release with depletion of ACh stores, similar to that of other presynaptic toxins *(131,132)*. Envenomation results in immediate, excruciating pain that may last for 1–2 days. Severe edema occurs owing to the actions of hyaluronidase, which promotes the rapid spread of venom through the tissue; tissue necrosis may occur *(117)*. In addition to gastrointestinal, autonomic, and cognitive effects, the victim may experience generalized muscle weakness owing to the mechanism noted above. Death occurs from cardiotoxicity. Treatment is supportive, and in some patients a specific antitoxin may be administered.

*Plant Toxins*

Rarely, plant neurotoxins affect the human NMJ, but more toxic effects are observed in animals. Neurotoxicity is dependent on the potency, concentration, and interaction with other toxins or substrates in the victim. Many are alkaloids. Coniine, the neurotoxin from the herb *Conium maculatum* (poison hemlock), produces a rapidly ascending paralysis, often resulting in death. Sensory abnormalities are common and prominent *(133)*. The death of Socrates is attributed to hemlock *(134)*. The mechanisms of action of this piperidine alkaloid neurotoxin are not completely understood. There is evidence that the toxin acts as a curare mimetic *(135)*.

## OCCUPATIONAL NEUROTOXINS

### Heavy Metals

Numerous polyvalent cations affect neuromuscular transmission and are often used to study basic mechanisms of synaptic transmission. These include barium, erbium, cadmium, cobalt, gadolinium, lanthanum, manganese, nickel, praseodymium, triethyltin, and zinc (136–148). Nearly all these intoxicants have multiple effects on synaptic transmission, but they predominantly block the release of ACh as well as facilitate spontaneous quantal release of neurotransmitter. They exert their effects by block of the flux of $Ca^{2+}$ through voltage-gated calcium channels, and they disrupt intracellular stores of $Ca^{2+}$ (149).

Heavy metal intoxication is a rare cause of clinical NMJ toxicity. Interest in this topic arose from the 1971 contamination of grain in Iraq with a methylmercury fungicide. Despite appropriate warnings, the grain was fed to animals, ground for flour, and used for making bread (150). Symptoms began within 1 month of consumption, ultimately affecting more than 6500 people and killing nearly 8% (151). Patients experienced ataxia, fatigue, generalized muscle weakness, and occasionally optic atrophy. Although one of the expected abnormalities following mercurial poisoning is a peripheral neuropathy (based on the Minamata experience), extensive electrodiagnostic examinations of the affected population did not demonstrate this (152,153). Repetitive nerve stimulation studies demonstrated a decremental response that was partially reversible with cholinesterase inhibitors (154). Similar abnormalities were demonstrated in experimental animals (155).

### Organophosphate and Carbamate Poisoning

The earliest use of a cholinesterase inhibitor as a neurotoxin is attributed to tribesman in Africa, who used the Calabar bean as a right of passage or an "ordeal poison" (116). Organophosphates (OPs) are a class of more than 20,000 compounds that irreversibly inhibit cholinesterases including acetylcholinesterase (AChE) (156). They are widely used in the agricultural, manufacturing, and pharmaceutical industries as well as for weapons of mass destruction (157,158). Exposure to OP compounds occurs in the workplace, in food, in drinking water, and in the environment. OP intoxication is infrequent in the United States because OP-containing insecticides are not readily available. However, these are used commonly in many other countries, where intoxication most commonly results from attempted suicide by ingestion of insecticides, indiscriminate handling, and storage by poorly informed workers (159–162).

**Table 4**
**Neuromuscular Syndromes**
**of Organophosphate Poisoning**

Acute cholinergic crisis
Intermediate syndrome
Myopathy
Delayed toxin-induced neuropathy

The physiochemical properties of these compounds vary. They may be solid, liquid, or gaseous and soluble in various media. Some are highly corrosive, and others are not; some are highly volatile, and others not. Dermal contact, respiratory inhalation, and gastrointestinal absorption may lead to OP absorption. These various physiochemical properties lend themselves to the wide range of applications noted above as well as to the inherent danger of their use *(163)*.

Four neuromuscular toxicologic syndromes occur from OP poisoning: an acute cholinergic crisis (type 1 and 2), an intermediate syndrome, a myopathy, and a delayed induced neuropathy (**Table 4**) *(164)*. Only the type 2 cholinergic crisis and the intermediate syndrome are the result of NMJ toxicity. OP compounds exert their NMJ toxicity by the irreversible inhibition of AChE. This results in the excessive accumulation of ACh at the NMJ as well as other cholinergic synapses of the central, peripheral, and autonomic nervous systems *(165)*. The excessive accumulation of ACh produces a depolarizing neuromuscular block at the NMJ that is followed by desensitization of the AChR *(166–168)*. Electrodiagnostic studies demonstrate normal nerve conduction studies, reduced CMAP amplitudes, a decremental response to repetitive nerve stimulation, and CMAP afterdischarges to a single nerve stimulus *(161,169)*.

Carbamate salts and esters, which are primarily used as pesticides, are synthetic analogs of the alkaloid physostigmine (eserine). They may directly or indirectly affect the NMJ. Like the OP compounds, carbamates also inhibit the action of AChE at cholinergic synapses. They are easily absorbed into the central nervous system because of their lipid solubility characteristics. Unlike OP compounds, the effects of carbamate agents are reversible. However, the manifestations of carbamate poisoning are indistinguishable from those of OP poisoning. Neurotoxicity occurs rapidly following significant exposure to both classes of compounds. Mortality rates are high, with death usually occurring from respiratory paralysis, which develops in 40% of poison victims *(170)*.

*Pesticides*

OP chemistry had its origin around 1820, when Lassainge synthesized triethyl phosphate, but not until the turn of the century did they become commonly used for their insecticidal properties. The OP insecticides are all derivatives of phosphoric acid. There are many subclasses within this group of compounds, and their various moieties (e.g., sulfur, amides) confer variation in overall toxicity. Despite recognition of their toxicity, their use continues to rise, particularly in developing countries where demand was predicted to more than double in the 1990s *(171)*. Most fatal intoxications result from suicidal ingestion *(159–162,172–175)*. Reports of carbamate NMJ toxicity are few *(176)*. The largest episode of carbamate poisoning occurred in 1985 when aldicarb was illegally used as an insecticide on watermelons *(177)*. Seventy-seven percent of 1376 exposed individuals were poisoned, each exhibiting a dose-related spectrum of nicotinic and muscarinic cholinergic receptor toxicity. Fatalities are rare and only occur at high exposure levels *(178–181)*. Symptoms appear rapidly, often within an hour, peaking in 2–3 h, with full recovery within 72 h *(182)*.

*Agents of War and Terrorism*

The highly dangerous toxicity of OP compounds was recognized in 1932, leading to the development of GB (sarin) and GA (tabun) in 1937, GD (soman) in 1944, and VX (venom X) in 1952 *(183)*. Little is known about a Russian agent, coded VR-55 *(184)*. Great Britain ceased nerve gas weapons research in 1959, and the United States transiently discontinued its efforts between 1969 and 1981 *(185)*. Other countries continue to develop their weapons programs. It is speculated that GA was used in the 1980s during the Iraq-Iran conflict, causing innumerable deaths *(184)*. Local effects (sweating, mucosal irritation) occur within seconds, and paralysis and apnea may occur after even 1–2 min of exposure. Comparative inhalation toxicities are summarized in **Table 5**. Absorption may be through inhalation, ingestion, or cutaneous contact. VX is the most potent and GA the least. Terrorist attacks in Japan resulted in the exposure of civilians to GB and VX *(186–190)*.

*Treatment*

Treatment is directed toward the prevention of chemical exposure by appropriate clothing and the decontamination of exposed victims *(191)*. Aggressive cardiopulmonary support is necessary. Atropine is an effective antidote to block excessive cholinergic activity at muscarinic receptors in both organophosphate and carbamate intoxications. AChE reactivators (oximes, e.g., 2-PAM) and anticholinergics are often helpful for acute OP intoxications, but they appear to have little effect in reversing weakness caused by the inter-

**Table 5**
**Comparative Human LCt$_{50}$ and LD$_{50}$ to Nerve Agents$^a$**

| Nerve Agent | Aerosolized (LCt$_{50}$) | Percutaneous (LD$_{50}$) |
|---|---|---|
| VX vapor | 10 mg/min/m$^3$ | 6–10 mg |
| Soman vapor | 50 mg/min/m$^3$ | 350 mg |
| Sarin vapor | 100 mg/min/m$^3$ | 1700 mg |
| Tabun vapor | 400 mg/min/m$^3$ | 1000 mg |

LCt$_{50}$ = the dose of vapor necessary to cause death in 50% of the exposed population where $C$ is concentration and $t$ is time; LD$_{50}$ = the dose of cutaneous exposure necessary to cause death in 50% of the exposed population.

mediate syndrome. Oximes dissociate the toxic phosphate moiety from the esteratic site on AChE, thus reactivating esterase and restoring normal neuromuscular transmission *(192)*. Soman is the least responsive of the nerve agents to oxime therapy because the agent-enzyme complex rapidly undergoes "aging," a time-dependent conformational change that is no longer responsive to reactivators *(193)*. In contrast to OP intoxications, oxime reactivators are contraindicated in carbamate poisoning as these compounds enhance the effects of the carbamate and promote further junctional toxicity *(194)*. When the offending compound is not known, it is possible to assay the reactivation of AChE activity in vivo and possibly differentiate between OP and carbamate poisoning *(195)*. Neuromuscular blockade with curariform drugs blocks repetitive discharges, although it is not clear whether there is any clinical benefit to their use *(196)*. The carbamate pyridostigmine was used as a "pretreatment" for organophosphorous poisoning during the Gulf War, but such use is controversial. Although studies showed that a 40% inhibition in AChE activity by physostigmine protected experimental animals from acute cholinergic toxicity following exposure to soman, such findings have not been conclusively demonstrated for pyridostigmine *(197)*.

## REFERENCES

1. Fambrough DM, Drachman DB, Satymurti S. Neuromuscular function in myasthenia gravis: decreased acetycholine receptors. *Science* 1973;182:293–295.
2. Barrons RW. Drug-induced neuromuscular blockade and myasthenia gravis. *Pharmacotherapy* 1977;17:1220–1232.
3. Howard JF. Adverse drug effects on neuromuscular transmission. *Semin Neurol* 1990;10:89–102.
4. Kaeser HE. Drug-induced myasthenic syndromes. *Acta Neurol Scand* 1984;70: 39–37.

5. Swift TR. Disorders of neuromuscular transmission other than myasthenia gravis. *Muscle Nerve* 1981;4:334–353.
6. Argov Z, Mastaglia FL. Disorders of neuromuscular transmission caused by drugs. *N Engl J Med* 1979;301:409–413.
7. Pittinger C, Adamson R. Antibiotic blockade of neuromuscular function. *Annu Rev Pharmacol* 1972;12:109–184.
8. Singh YN, Marshall IG, Harvey AL. Reversal of antibiotic-induced muscle paralysis by 3,4-diaminopyridine. *J Pharm Pharmacol* 1978;30:249–250.
9. Caputy AJ, Kim YI, Sanders DB. The neuromuscular blocking effects of therapeutic concentrations of various antibiotics on normal rat skeletal muscle: a quantitative comparison. *J Pharmacol Exp Ther* 1981;217:369–378.
10. Snavely SR, Hodges GR. The neurotoxicity of antibacterial agents [Review] [293 refs]. *Ann Intern Med* 1984;101:92–104.
11. Cadisch R, Streit E, Hartmann K. [Exacerbation of pseudoparalytic myasthenia gravis following azithromycin (Zithromax)] [German]. *Schw Med Wochenschr J Suisse Med* 1996;126:308–310.
12. Roquer J, Cano A, Seoane JL, Pou SA. Myasthenia gravis and ciprofloxacin [Letter]. *Acta Neurol Scand* 1996;94:419–420.
13. Samuelson RJ, Giesecke AH Jr, Kallus FT, Stanley VF. Lincomycin-curare interaction. *Anesth Analg* 1975;54:103–105.
14. Fogdall RP, Miller RD. Prolongation of a pancuronium-induced neuromuscular blockade by clindamycin. *Anesthesiology* 1974;41:407–408.
15. McQuillen MP, Engbaek L. Mechanism of colistin-induced neuromuscular depression. *Arch Neurol* 1975;32:235–238.
16. Moore B, Safani M, Keesey J. Possible exacerbation of myasthenia gravis by ciprofloxacin [Letter]. *Lancet* 1988;1:882.
17. Decker DA, Fincham RW. Respiratory arrest in myasthenia gravis with colistimethate therapy. *Arch Neurol* 1971;25:141–144.
18. Argov Z, Brenner T, Abramsky O. Ampicillin may aggravate clinical and experimental myasthenia gravis. *Arch Neurol* 1986;43:255–256.
19. Howard JF Jr. Adverse drug interactions in disorders of neuromuscular transmission. *J Neurol Orthop Med Surg* 1991;12:26–34.
20. Howard JF, Johnson BR, Quint SR. The effects of beta-adrenergic antagonists on neuromuscular transmission in rat skeletal muscle. *Society for Neuroscience Abstracts* 1987;13:147.
21. Coppeto JR. Timolol-associated myasthenia gravis. *Am J Ophthalmol* 1984;98:244–245.
22. Verkijk A. Worsening of myasthenia gravis with timolol maleate eyedrops. *Ann Neurol* 1985;17:211–212.
23. Bikhazi GB, Leung I, Foldes FF. Interaction of neuromuscular blocking agents with calcium channel blockers. *Anesthesiology* 1982;57:A268.
24. Van der Kloot W, Kita H. The effects of verapamil on muscle action potentials in the frog and crayfish and on neuromuscular transmission in the crayfish. *Comp Biochem Physiol* 1975;50C:121–125.
25. Ribera AB, Nastuk WL. The actions of verapamil at the neuromuscular junction. *Comp Biochem Physiol C: Comp Pharm Toxicol* 1989;93C:137–141.
26. Adams RJ, Rivner MH, Salazar J, Swift TR. Effects of oral calcium antagonists on neuromuscular transmission. *Neurology* 1984;34(Suppl 1):132–133.

27. Krendel DA, Hopkins LC. Adverse effect of verapamil in a patient with the Lambert-Eaton syndrome. *Muscle Nerve* 1986;9:519–522.
28. Kornfeld P, Horowitz SH, Genkins G, Papatestas AE. Myasthenia gravis unmasked by antiarrhythmic agents. *Mt Sinai J Med* 1976;43:10–14.
29. Weisman SJ. Masked myasthenia gravis. *JAMA* 1949;141:917–918.
30. Shy ME, Lange DJ, Howard JF, et al. Quinidine exacerbating myasthenia gravis: a case report and intracellular recordings. *Ann Neurol* 1985;18:120.
31. Stoffer SS, Chandler JH. Quinidine-induced exacerbation of myasthenia gravis in patient with myasthenia gravis. *Arch Intern Med* 1980;140:283–284.
32. Miller RD, Way WL, Katzung BG. The neuromuscular effects of quinidine. *Proc Soc Exp Biol Med* 1968;129:215–218.
33. Balint G, Szobor A, Temesvari P, Zahumenszky Z, Bozsoky S. Myasthenia gravis developed under D-penicillamine treatment. *Scand J Rheumatol* 1975;(Suppl 8): 12–21.
34. Bucknall RC, Balint G, Dawkins RL. Myasthenia gravis associated with penicillamine treatment for rheumatoid arthritis. *BMJ* 1975;1:600–602.
35. Czlonskowska A. Myasthenia syndrome during penicillamine treatment. *BMJ* 1975; 2:726–727.
36. Masters CL, Dawkins RL, Zilko PJ, Simpson JA, Leedman RJ. Penicillamine-associated myasthenia gravis, antiacetylcholine receptor and antistriational antibodies. *Am J Med* 1977;63:689–694.
37. Albers JW, Beals CA, Levine SP. Neuromuscular transmission in rheumatoid arthritis, with and without penicillamine treatment. *Neurology* 1981;31:1562–1564.
38. Sghirlanzoni A, Mantegazza R, Mora M, Pareyson D, Cornelio F. Chloroquine myopathy and myasthenia-like syndrome. *Muscle Nerve* 1988;11:114–119.
39. Schumm F, Wietholter H, Fateh-Moghadam A. Myasthenie-syndrom unter chloroquin-therapie. *Deutsc Med Wochenschr* 1981;25:1745–1747.
40. Robberecht W, Bednarik J, Bourgeois P, Van Hees J, Carton H. Myasthenic syndrome caused by direct effect of chloroquine on neuromuscular junction. *Arch Neurol* 1989;46:464–468.
41. Perez A, Perella M, Pastor E, Cano M, Escudero J. Myasthenia gravis induced by alpha-interferon therapy. *Am J Hematol* 1995;49:365–366.
42. Batocchi AP, Evoli A, Servidei S, et al. Myasthenia gravis during interferon alpha therapy. *Neurology* 1995;45:382–383.
43. Lensch E, Faust J, Nix WA, Wandel E. Myasthenia gravis after interferon alpha treatment. *Muscle Nerve* 1996;19:927–928.
44. Piccolo G, Franciotta D, Versino M, et al. Myasthenia gravis in a patient with chronic active hepatitis C during interferon-alpha treatment [Letter]. *J Neurol Neurosurg Psychiatry* 1996;60:348.
45. Mase G, Zorzon M, Biasutti E, et al. Development of myasthenia gravis during interferon-alpha treatment for anti-HCV positive chronic hepatitis [Letter]. *J Neurol Neurosurg Psychiatry* 1996;60:348–349.
46. Konishi T. [A case of myasthenia gravis which developed myasthenic crisis after alpha-interferon therapy for chronic hepatitis C] [Review] [14 refs] [Japanese]. *Rinsho Shinkeigaku Clin Neurol* 1996;36:980–985.
47. Gu D, Wogensen L, Calcutt N, et al. Myasthenia gravis-like syndrome induced by expression of interferon in the neuromuscular junction. *J Exp Med* 1995;18:547–557.

48. Cherington M. Clinical spectrum of botulism. *Muscle Nerve* 1998;21:701–710.
49. Pickett J, Berg B, Chaplin E, Brunstetter-Shafer M. Syndrome of botulism in infancy: clinical and electrophysiologic study. *N Engl J Med* 1976;295:770–792.
50. MacDonald KL, Rutherford SM, Friedman SM, et al. Botulism and botulism-like illness in chronic drug users. *Ann Intern Med* 1985;102:616–618.
51. McCroskey LM, Hatheway CL, Woodruff BA, Greenberg JA, Jurgenson P. Type F botulism due to neurotoxigenic *Clostridium baratii* from an unknown source in an adult. *J Clin Microbiol* 1991;29:2618–2620.
52. Maretic Z. Epidemiology of envenomation. In: Bettini S, ed. *Arthropod Venoms*. Berlin, Springer-Verlag, 1978, pp. 185–212.
53. Rosenthal L. Alpha-lathrotoxin and related toxins. *Pharmacol Ther* 1989;42:115–134.
54. Hurlbut WP, Iezzi N, Fesce R, Ceccarelli B. Correlation between quantal secretion and vesicle loss at the frog neuromuscular junction. *J Physiol (Lond)* 1990;424:501–526.
55. Henkel AW, Sankaranarayanan S. Mechanisms of α-lathrotoxin action. *Cell Tissue Res* 1999;296:229–233.
56. Ushkaryov YA, Petrenko AG, Geppert M, Sudhof TC. Neurexins: synaptic cell surface proteins related to the α-lathrotoxin receptor and laminin. *Science* 1992;257:50–56.
57. Longenecker HE, Hurlbut WP, Mauro A, Clark AW. Effects of black widow spider venom on the frog neuromuscular junction. Effects on end-plate potential, miniature end-plate potential and nerve terminal spike. *Nature* 1970;225:701–703.
58. Clark AW, Hurlbut WP, Mauro A. Changes in the fine structure of the neuromuscular junction of the frog caused by black widow spider venom. *J Cell Biol* 1972;52:1–14.
59. Clark AW, Mauro A, Longenecker HE, Hurlbut WP. Effects of black widow spider venom on the frog neuromuscular junction. Effects on the fine structure of the frog neuromuscular junction. *Nature* 1970;225:703–705.
60. Ceccarelli B, Grohovaz F, Hurlbut WP. Freeze-fracture studies of frog neuromuscular junctions during intense release of neurotransmitter. I. Effects of black widow spider venom and Ca$^{2+}$-free solutions on the structure of the active zone. *J Cell Biol* 1979;81:163–177.
61. Pumplin DW, Reese TS. Action of brown widow spider venom and botulinum toxin on the frog neuromuscular junction examined with the freeze-fracture technique. *J Physiol* 1977;273:443–457.
62. Gorio A, Rubin LL, Mauro A. Double mode of action of black widow spider venom on frog neuromuscular junction. *J Neurocytol* 1978;7:193–202.
63. Howard BD. Effects and mechanisms of polypeptide neurotoxins that act presynaptically. *Annu Rev Pharmacol Toxicol* 1980;20:307–336.
64. Gilbert WW, Stewart CM. Effective treatment of arachiodism by calcium salts. *Am J Med Sci* 1935;189:532–536.
65. Miller TA. Bite of the black widow spider. *Am Fam Physician* 1992;45:181–187.
66. D'Amour EF, Becker FE, Van Riper W. The black widow spider. *Q Rev Biol* 1936;11:123–160.
67. Temple IU. Acute ascending paralysis, or tick paralysis. *Med Sentinel* 1912;20:507–514.
68. Todd JL. Tick bite in British Columbia. *Can Med Assoc J* 1912;2:1118–1119.

69. Cleland JB. Injuries and diseases of man in Australia attributable to animals (except insects). *Australas Med Gaz* 1912;32:295–299.
70. Gregson JD. *Tick Paralysis—An Appraisal of Natural and Experimental Data.* Report 6-23. Ottawa, Canada Department of Agriculture, 1973, pp. 1–109.
71. Anonymous. Tick paralysis—Washington, 1995. From the Centers for Disease Control and Prevention. *JAMA* 1996;275:1470.
72. Gothe R, Kunze K, Hoogstraal H. The mechanisms of pathogenicity in the tick paralyses. *J Med Entomol* 1979;16:357–369.
73. Weingart JL. Tick paralysis. *Minn Med* 1967;50:383–386.
74. Brown AF, Hamilton DL. Tick bite anaphylaxis in Australia. *J Assoc Emerg Med* 1998;15:111–113.
75. Felz MW, Smith CD, Swift TR. A six-year-old girl with tick paralysis [see comments]. *N Engl J Med* 2000;342:90–94.
76. Cherington M, Synder RD. Tick paralysis. Neurophysiologic studies. *N Engl J Med* 1968;278:95–97.
77. Swift TR, Ignacio OJ. Tick paralysis: electrophysiologic studies. *Neurology* 1975; 25:1130–1133.
78. Grattan-Smith PJ, Morris JG, Johnston HM, et al. Clinical and neurophysiological features of tick paralysis. *Brain* 1997;120:1975–1987.
79. Donat JR, Donat JF. Tick paralysis with persistent weakness and electromyographic abnormalities. *Arch Neurol* 1981;38:59–61.
80. Lagos JC, Thies RE. Tick paralysis without muscle weakness. *Arch Neurol* 1969; 21:471–474.
81. Rose I. A review of tick paralysis. *Can Med Assoc J* 1954;70:175–176.
82. Dworkin MS, Shoemaker PC, Anderson DE. Tick paralysis: 33 human cases in Washington State, 1946–1996. *Clin Infect Dis* 1999;29:1435–1439.
83. Jones HR Jr. Guillain-Barré syndrome in children. *Current Opin Pediatr* 1995;7: 663–668.
84. Stanbury JB, Huyck JH. Tick paralysis: critical review. *Medicine* 1945;24:219–242.
85. Stone BF, Aylward JH. Holocyclotoxin—the paralysing toxin of the Australian paralysis tick *Ixodus holocyclus*; chemical and immunological characterization. *Toxicon* 1992;30:552–553.
86. Rose I, Gregson JD. Evidence of neuromuscular block in tick paralysis. *Nature* 1959;178:95–96.
87. Gothe R, Neitz AWH. Tick paralyses: pathogenesis and etiology. In: Harris KF, ed. *Adv Dis Vector Res* 1991;8:177–204.
88. Stone BF. Tick paralysis, particularly involving *Ixodes holocyclus* and other *Ixodes* species. *Adv Dis Vector Res* 1988;5:61–85.
89. Esplin DW, Phillip CB, Hughes LE. Impairment of muscle stretch reflexes in tick paralysis. *Science* 1960;132:958–959.
90. Cherington M, Snyder RD. Tick paralysis: neurophysiological studies. *N Engl J Med* 1968;278:95–97.
91. DeBusk FL, O'Connor S. Tick toxicosis. *Pediatrics* 1972;50:328–329.
92. Haller JS, Fabara JA. Tick paralysis. Case report with emphasis on neurological toxicity. *Am J Dis Child* 1972;124:915–917.
93. Warnick JE, Albuquerque EX, Diniz CR. Electrophysiological observations on the action of the purified scorpion venom, *tityustoxin*, on nerve and skeletal muscle of the rat. *J Pharmacol Exp Ther* 1976;198:155–167.

94. Belghith M, Boussarsar M, Haguiga H, et al. Efficacy of serotherapy in scorpion sting: a matched-pair study. *J Toxicol Clin Toxicol* 1999;37:51–57.

95. Sofer S, Shahak E, Gueron M. Scorpion envenomation and antivenom therapy. *Pediatrics* 1994;124:973–978.

96. Campbell CH. The effects of snake venoms and their neurotoxins on the nervous system of man and animals. *Contemp Neurol Ser* 1975;12:259–293.

97. Vital-Brazil O. Venoms: their inhibitory action on neuromuscular transmission. In: Cheymol J, ed. *Neuromuscular Blocking and Stimulating Agents*. New York, Pergamon, 1972, pp. 145–167.

98. Lee CY. Elapid neurotoxins and their mode of action. *Clin Toxicol* 1970;3:457–472.

99. Karlsson E, Arnberg H, Eaker D. Isolation of the principal neurotoxin of two *Naja naja* subspecies. *Eur J Biochem* 1971;21:1–16.

100. Lee CY, Chang SL, Kau ST, Luh SH. Chromatographic separation of the venon of *Bungarus multicinctus* and characteristics of its components. *J Chromatogr* 1972; 72:71–82.

101. Tu AT, Tu T. Sea snakes from southeast Asia and Far East and their venoms. In: Halstead BW, ed. *Poisonous and Venomous Marine Animals of the World*. Washington, DC, US Government Printing Office, 1970, pp. 885–903.

102. Barme M. Venomous sea snakes of Vietnam and their venoms. In: Keegan HL, MacFarlane W, eds. *Venomous and Poisonous Animals and Noxious Plants of the Pacific Region*. Oxford, Oxford University Press, 1963, pp. 373–378.

103. Karlsson E. Chemistry of protein toxins in snake venoms. In: Lee CY, ed. *Snake Venoms*. New York, Springer-Verlag, 1979, pp. 159–212.

104. Chang CC, Su MJ. Mutual potentiation at nerve terminals, between toxins from snake venoms that contain phospholipase A activity: β bungarotoxin, crotoxin, taipoxin. *Toxicon* 1980;18:641–648.

105. Rowlands JB, Mastaglia FL, Kakulas BA, Hainsworth D. Clinical and pathological aspects of a fatal case of mulga (*Pseudechis australis*) snakebite. *Med J Aust* 1969;1:226–230.

106. Kellaway CH. The peripheral action of the Australian snake venoms. 2. The curarilike action in mammals. *Aust J Exp Biol Med Sci* 1932;10:181–194.

107. Bouquier JJ, Guibert J, Dupont C, Umdenstock R. Les piqures de vipère chez l'enfant. *Arch Fr Pediatr* 1974;31:285–296.

108. Mitrakul C, Dhamkrong-At A, Futrakul P, et al. Clinical features of neurotoxic snake bite and response to antivenom in 47 children. *Am J Trop Med Hyg* 1984;33: 1258–1266.

109. Reid HA. Cobra-bites. *BMJ* 1964;2:540–545.

110. Warrell DA, Barnes HJ, Piburn MF. Neurotoxic effects of bites by the Egyptian cobra (*Naja haje*) in Nigeria. *Trans R Soc Trop Med Hyg* 1976;70:78,79.

111. Kerrigan KR. Venomous snake bites in Eastern Ecuador. *Am J Trop Med Hyg* 1991;44:93–99.

112. Ouyang C, Teng C-M, Huang T-F. Characterization of snake venom components acting on blood coagulation and platelet function. *Toxicon* 1992;30:945–966.

113. Reid HA. Antivenom in sea-snake bite poisoning. *Lancet* 1975;i:622–623.

114. Theakston RDG, Phillips RE, Warrell DA, et al. Envenoming by the common krait (*Bungarus caeruleus*) and Sri Lankan cobra (*Naja naja naja*): efficacy and complications with Haffkine antivenom. *Trans R Soc Trop Med Hyg* 1990;84:301–308.

115. Kumar S, Usgaonkar RS. Myasthenia gravis like picture resulting from snake bite. *J Ind Med Assoc* 1968;50:428–429.
116. Pettigrew LC, Glass JP. Neurologic complications of coral snake bite. *Neurology* 1985;35:589–592.
117. Southcott RV. The neurologic effects of noxious marine creatures. In: Hornabrook RW, ed. *Topics on Tropical Neurology*. Philadelphia, FA Davis, 1975, pp. 165–258.
118. Steidinger KA, Steinfield HJ. Toxic marine dinoflagellates. In: Spector DL, ed. *Dinoflagellates*. New York, Academic, 1984, pp. 201–206.
119. Olivera BM, Gray WR, Zeikus R, et al. Peptide neruotoxins from fish-hunting cone snails. *Science* 1985;230:1338–1343.
120. Kohn AJ. Venomous marine snails of the genus *Conus*. In: Keegan HC, McFarlane WV, eds. *Venomous and Poisonous Animals and Noxious Plants of the Pacific Region*. Oxford, Pergamon, 1963, p. 83.
121. Kohn AJ. Recent cases of human injury due to venomous marine snails of the genus *Conus*. *Hawaii Med J* 1958;17:528–532.
122. Cruz LJ, White J. Clinical toxicology of *Conus* snail stings. In: Meier J, White J, eds. *CRC Handbook on Clinical Toxicology of Animal Venoms and Poisons*. Boca Raton, FL, CRC, 1995, pp. 177–128.
123. Gray WR, Luque A, Olivera BM, Barrett J, Cruz LJ. Peptide toxins from *Conus geographus* venom. *J Biol Chem* 1981;256:4734–4740.
124. Hopkins C, Grilley M, Miller C, et al. A new family of Conus peptides targeted to the nicotinic acetylcholine receptor. *J Biol Chem* 1995;270:22,361–22,367.
125. McIntosh M, Cruz LJ, Hunkapiller MW, Gray WR, Olivera BM. Isolation and structure of a peptide toxin from the marine snail *Conus magnus*. *Arch Bioch Biophys* 1982;218:329–334.
126. McCleskey EW, Fox AP, Feldman D, et al. Calcium channel blockade by a peptide from *Conus*: specificity and mechanism. *Proc Nat Acad Sci USA* 1987;84:4327–4331.
127. Adams DJ, Alewood PF, Craik DJ, Drinkwater RD, Lewis RJ. Conotoxins and their potential pharmaceutical applications. *Drug Dev Res* 1999;46:219–234.
128. De Aizpurua HJ, Lambert EH, Griesmann GE, Olivera M, Lennon VA. Antagonism of voltage-gated calcium channels in small cell carcinomas of patients with and without Lambert-Eaton myasthenic syndrome by autoantibodies omega-conotoxin and adenosine. *Cancer Res* 1988;48:4719–4724.
129. Yoshiba S. [An estimation of the most dangerous species of cone shell, *Conus (Gastridium) geographus* Linne, 1758, venom's lethal dose in humans]. *Jpn J Hyg* 1984; 39:565–572.
130. Halstead BW. *Poisonous and Venomous Marine Animals of the World*. Washington, DC, US Government Printing Office, 1970, pp. 1–1006.
131. Gwee MC, Gopalakrishnakone P, Yuen R, Khoo HE, Low KS. A review of stonefish venoms and toxins. *Pharmacol Ther* 1994;64:509–528.
132. Kreger AS, Molgo J, Comella JX, Hansson B, Thesleff S. Effects of stonefish (*Synanceia trachynis*) venom on murine and frog neuromuscular junctions. *Toxicon* 1993;31:307–317.
133. Hardin JW, Arena JW. *Human Poisoning from Native and Cultivated Plants*, 1st ed. Durham, NC, Duke University Press, 1974, pp. 1–174.
134. Davies Ml, Davies TA. Hemlock: murder before the Lord. *Med Sci Law* 1994;34: 331–333.

135. Panter KE, Keeler RF. Piperidine alkaloids of poison hemlock (*Conium maculatum*). In: Cheeke P, ed. *Toxicants of Plant Origin*, vol 1. Alkaloids. Boca Raton, FL, CRC, 1989, pp. 109–130.
136. Silinsky EM. On the role of barium in supporting the asynchronous release of acetylcholine quanta by moter nerve impulses. *J Physiol (Lond)* 1978;274:157–171.
137. Silinsky EM. Can barium support the release of acetylcholine by nerve impulses? *Br J Pharmacol* 1977;59:215–217.
138. Metral S, Bonneton C, Hort-Legrand C, Reynes J. Dual action of erbium on transmitter release at the neuromuscular synapse. *Nature* 1978;271:773–775.
139. Cooper GP, Manalis RS. Cadmium: effects on transmitter release at the frog neuromuscular junction. *Eur J Pharmacol* 1984;99:251–256.
140. Forshaw PJ. The inhibitory effect of cadmium on neuromuscular transmission in the rat. *Eur J Pharmacol* 1977;42:371–377.
141. Weakly JN. The action of cobalt ions on neuromuscular transmission in the frog. *J Physiol (Lond)* 1973;234:597–612.
142. Molgo J, del Pozo E, Banos JE, Angaut-Petit D. Changes in quantal transmitter release caused by gadolinium ions at the frog neuromuscular junction. *Br J Pharmacol* 1991;104:133–138.
143. Kajimoto N, Kirpekar SM. Effects of manganese and lanthanum on spontaneous release of acetylcholine at frog motor nerve terminals. *Nature* 1972;235:29–30.
144. Balnave RJ, Gage PW. The inhibitory effect of manganese on transmitter release at the neuromuscular junction of the toad. *Br J Pharmacol* 1973;47:339–352.
145. Kita H, Van der Kloot W. Action of Co and Ni at the frog neuromuscular junction. *Nature* 1973;245:52–53.
146. Alnaes E, Rahaminoff R. Dual action of praseodymium ($Pr^{3+}$) on transmitter release at the frog neuromuscular synapse. *Nature* 1975;247:478–479.
147. Allen JE, Gage PW, Leaver DD, Leow ACT. Triethyltin decreases evoked transmitter release at the mouse neuromuscular junction. *Chem Biol Interact* 1980;31:227–231.
148. Benoit PR, Mambrini J. Modification of transmitter release by ions which prolong the presynaptic action potential. *J Physiol (Lond)* 1970;210:681–695.
149. Cooper GP, Manalis RS. Influence of heavy metals on synaptic transmission. *Neurotoxicology* 2001;4:69–84.
150. Rustam H, Hamdi T. Methylmercury poisoning in Iraq; a neurological study. *Brain* 1974;97:499–510.
151. Bakir F, Damluji SF, Amin-Saki L, et al. Methylmercury poisoning in Iraq. *Science* 1973;181:230–241.
152. Igata A. Neurological aspects of methlmercury poisoning in Minamata. In: Tsubaki T, Takahashi H, eds. *Recent Advances in Minamata Disease Studies*. Tokyo, Kodansha, 1986, pp. 41–57.
153. LeQuense P, Damluji SF, Berlin M. Electrophysiological studies of peripheral nerves in patients with organic mercury poisoning. *J Neurol Neurosurg Psychiatry* 1974;37:333–339.
154. Rustam H, von Burg R, Amin-Saki L, Elhassani S. Evidence of a neuromuscular disorder in methymercury poisoning. *Arch Environ Health* 1975;30:190–195.
155. Atchinson WD, Narahashi T. Methylmercury induced depression of neuromuscular transmission in the rat. *Neurotoxicology* 1982;3:37–50.

156. Taylor P. Anticholinesterase agents. In: Gilman AG, Goodman LS, Rall TW, Murad F, eds. *The Pharmacological Basis of Therapeutics.* New York, MacMillan, 1985, pp. 110–129.
157. Edmundson RS. *Dictionary of Organophosphorous Compounds.* London, Chapman and Hall, 1988 (electronic resource).
158. Gunderson CH, Lehmann CR, Sidell FR, Jabari B. Nerve agents: a review. *Neurology* 1992;42:946–950.
159. Fernando R. *Pesticides in Sri Lanka.* Colombo, Friedrich-Ebert-Stiftung, 1989, pp. 1–255.
160. Besser R, Gutmann L, Dilimann U, Weilemann LS, Hopf HC. End plate dysfunction in acute organophosphate intoxication. *Neurology* 1989;39:561–567.
161. Gutmann L, Besser R. Organophosphate intoxication: pharmacologic, neurophysiologic, clinical, and therapeutic considerations. *Semin Neurol* 1990;10:46–51.
162. Jeyaratnam J. Acute pesticide poisoning: a major health problem. *World Health Stat Q* 1990;43:139–145.
163. Aldridge WN, Reiner E. *Enzyme Inhibitors as Substrates.* Amsterdam, North-Holland, 1972, pp. 1–328.
164. Marrs TC. Organophosphate poisoning. *Pharmacol Ther* 1993;58:51–66.
165. Namba T, Nolte CT, Jackrel J, Grob D. Poisoning due to organophosphorous insecticides. *Am J Med* 2001;50:475–492.
166. Karalliedde L, Senanayake N. Organophosphorous insecticide poisoning. *Br J Anaesth* 1989;63:736–750.
167. De Wilde V, Vogblaers D, Colarddyn F, et al. Postsynaptic neuromuscular dysfunction in organophosphate induced intermediate syndrome. *Klin Wochenschr* 1991; 69:177–183.
168. Good JL, Khurana RK, Mayer RF, Cintra WM, Albuquerque EX. Pathophysiological studies of neuromuscular function in subacute organophosphate poisoning induced by phosmet. *J Neurol Neurosurg Psychiatry* 1993;56:290–294.
169. Maselli RA, Soliven BC. Analysis of the organophosphate-induced electromyographic response to repetitive nerve stimulation: paradoxical response to edrophonium and D-tubocurarine. *Muscle Nerve* 1991;14:1182–1188.
170. Tsao TC, Juang Y, Lan R, Shieh W, Lee C. Respiratory failure of acute organophosphate and carbamate poisoning. *Chest* 1990;98:631–636.
171. WHO/UNEP. *Public Health Impact of Pesticides Used in Agriculture.* Geneva, World Heath Organization, 1990, pp. 1–128.
172. Haddad LM. Organophosphate poisoning—intermediate syndrome. *J Toxicol Clin Toxicol* 1992;30:331–332.
173. De Bleecker J, Willems J, Van Den Neucker K, De Reuck J, Vogelaers D. Prolonged toxicity with intermediate syndrome after combined parathion and methyl parathion poisoning. *Clin Toxicol* 1992;30:333–345.
174. Güler K, Tascioglu C, Özbey N. Organophosphate poisoning. *Isr J Med Sci* 1996; 32:791–792.
175. Chaudhry R, Lall SB, Mishra B, Dhawan B. Lesson of the week—a foodborne outbreak of organophosphate poisoning. *BMJ* 1998;317:268–269.
176. Cranmer MF. Carbaryl. A toxicological review and risk analysis. *Neurotoxicology* 1986;7:247–328.

177. Goldman LR, Smith DF, Neutra RR, et al. Pesticide food poisoning from contaminated watermelons in California. *Arch Environ Health* 1990;45:229–236.
178. Freslew KE, Hagardorn AN, McCormick WF. Poisoning from oral ingestion of carbofuran (Furandan 4F), a cholinesterase-inhibiting carbamate insecticide, and its effects on cholinesterase activity in various biological fluids. *J Forens Sci* 1992; 37:337–344.
179. Jenis EH, Payne RJ, Goldbaum LR. Acute meprobamate poisoning: a fatal case following a lucid interval. *JAMA* 1969;207:361–362.
180. Klys M, Kosún J, Pach J, Kamenczak A. Carbofuran poisoning of pregnant women and fetus per ingestion. *J Forens Sci* 1989;34:1413–1416.
181. Maddock RK, Bloomer HA. Meprobamate overdosage. Evaluation of its severity and methods of treatment. *JAMA* 1967;201:123–127.
182. Ecobichon DJ. Carbamates. In: Spencer PS, Schaumburg HH, eds. *Experimental Clinical Neurotoxicology*. New York, Oxford University Press, 2000, pp. 289–298.
183. Maynard RL. Toxicology of chemical warfare agents. In: Ballantyne B, Marrs T, Turner T, ed. *General and Applied Toxicology*. New York, Stockton Press, 1993, p. 1253.
184. Spencer PS, Wilson BW, Albuquerque EX. Sarin, other "nerve agents" and their antidotes. In: Spencer PS, Schaumburg HH, eds. *Experimental Clinical Neurotoxicology*. New York, Oxford University Press, 2000, pp. 1073–1093.
185. Meselson M, Perry Robinson J. Chemical warfare and disarmament. *Sci Am* 1980; 242(4):34.
186. Nozaki H, Aikawa N, Fujishima S, et al. A case of VX poisoning and the difference from sarin. *Lancet* 1995;346:698–699.
187. Nozaki H, Aikawa N, Shinozawa Y, et al. Sarin poisoning in Tokyo subway. *Lancet* 1995;345:980–981.
188. Morita H, Yanagisawa N, Nakajima T, et al. Sarin poisoning in Matsumoto, Japan. *Lancet* 1995;346:290–293.
189. Nakajima T, Saro S, Morita H, Yanagisawa N. Sarin poisoning of a rescue team in the Matsumoto sarin incident in Japan. *Occup Environ Med* 1997;54:697–701.
190. Woodall J. Tokyo subway gas attack. *Lancet* 1997;350:296.
191. Holstege CP, Kirk M, Sidell FR. Chemical warfare. Nerve agent poisoning. *Crit Care Med* 1997;13:923–942.
192. Dawson RM. Review of oximes available for treatment of nerve agent poisoning. *J Appl Toxicol* 1994;14:317–331.
193. Becker G, Kawan A, Szinicz L. Direct reaction of oximes with sarin, soman or tabun *in vitro*. *Arch Toxicol* 1997;71:714–718.
194. Ecobichon DJ. Carbamic acid ester insecticids. In: Ecobichon DJ, Joy RM, eds. *Pesticides and Neurological Disease*. Boca Raton, FL, CRC, 1994, pp. 251–289.
195. Rotenberg M, Shefi M, Dany S, et al. Differentiation between organophosphate and carbamate poisoning. *Clin Chim Acta* 1995;234:11–21.
196. Besser R, Vogt T, Gutmann L. High pancuronium sensitivity of axonal nicotinic-acetylcholine receptors in humans during organophosphate intoxication. *Muscle Nerve* 1991;14:1197–1201.
197. Miller SA, Blick DW, Kerenyi SZ, Murphy MR. Efficacy of physostigmine as a pretreatment for organophosphate poisoning. *Pharmacol Biochem Behav* 1993;44: 343–347.

# 16
# Psychological and Social Consequences of Myasthenia Gravis

## Robert H. Paul and James M. Gilchrist

## INTRODUCTION

Clinical and basic science research in the field of myasthenia gravis (MG) has largely focused on understanding the etiology, clinical sequelae, and treatment of the disease. This emphasis has produced invaluable contributions to the conceptualization of MG and the implementation of effective treatments. However, in the absence of a cure, patients are required to manage a chronic disease, and this burden renders some individuals vulnerable to psychological distress. Previous textbooks have not reviewed the psychological aspects of MG, yet the issue is critical to optimize patient care. Mental health is ultimately associated with functional outcome because the manner in which individuals identify themselves with their illness, experience their symptoms, and interpret the impact of their disease influences adjustment to the condition. For this reason it is important to understand the factors that both challenge and support the psychological well-being of patients.

Broadly, the psychological aspects of MG can be categorized into two areas: 1) the effect of a patient's psychological health on the expression of their disease; and 2) the effect of disease on the psychological health of the patient. In the present chapter we examine the research in each of these areas. We then discuss the controversial issue of cognitive abnormalities caused by MG and the relationship between perceived fatigue and memory function. Finally, we review factors that support psychological health in chronic disease, with a particular emphasis on MG.

## THE EFFECTS OF PSYCHOLOGICAL HEALTH ON DISEASE

Concern that psychological health may directly affect disease expression is predicated on the theoretical perspective that psychological distress can lead to immune dysregulation. This interaction between psychological and

From: *Current Clinical Neurology: Myasthenia Gravis and Related Disorders*
Edited by: H. J. Kaminski © Humana Press Inc., Totowa, NJ

immunologic systems begins with the activation of the sympathetic nervous system during emotional arousal. During a stress response, the hypothalamus secretes a series of hormones that eventually initiate the release of cortisol from the adrenal cortex. The primary physiologic role of cortisol is stimulation of glucogenesis, protein degradation, and lipolysis, all of which generate energy supplies to support resistance to the perceived stressor *(1)*. A secondary effect of cortisol release is temporary immune dysregulation. This results from the binding of cortisol to receptors located on immune cells *(2,3)*. The interdependent circuits of the central nervous and immune systems provide a biologic basis for the notion that psychological factors directly impact disease states. However, at present there is no empirical support for the hypothesis that psychological factors affect the onset or the course of MG.

A few early case reports and case series described a relationship between psychological illness and the precipitation of MG *(4–7)*, but no controlled studies have confirmed this association. Furthermore, studies that have examined premorbid personality characteristics of MG patients have not identified meaningful relationships between personality and onset of MG. MacKenzie et al. *(8)* reported that 8/25 MG patients "came from markedly abnormal family backgrounds," although at least some of the examples (e.g., single-parent households) would not be considered abnormal today. Nine of 20 patients exhibited "abnormal" profiles on the Minnesota Multiphasic Personality Inventory (MMPI), a standard clinical measure designed to identify individuals with psychiatric illness. Scores were not reported, but elevations were noted on three subscales that measure depression, concerns about disease and illness, and specific somatic symptoms of physical disease. Obviously, these scales are sensitive to symptoms of *bona fide* medical illnesses *(9)*, and therefore it is not surprising that MG patients obtained higher scores on these scales. Unfortunately, the fact that actual scores were not provided makes it impossible to determine whether the elevated scores were clinically meaningful. Furthermore, the fact that elevations were not observed on scales more sensitive to premorbid personality characteristics (e.g., obsessive-compulsive behaviors or psychotic symptoms) argues against the notion of a pre-morbid or reactive "myasthenic personality."

Nearly identical results were reported in a second study conducted by Schwartz and Cahill *(10)*. In this study, 17 MG patients who volunteered for a psychotherapeutic intervention study were administered the MMPI, and elevations were found on the same three scales. The authors interpreted these results as a reflection of general reactive distress typical of patients with chronic disease. An elevated score was also obtained on a scale that measures psychotic behavioral characteristics, which was interpreted to reflect the tendency of MG patients to experience embarrassment and social isolation, rather than reflecting "overt psychosis." Although there may be some validity to this, it is important to recognize the selection bias present in this study. The participants were volunteers in a psychological intervention study, and MG patients seeking mental health treatment reportedly initiated the investigation. The fact that the participants in the study were self-selected for psychological treatment raises the possibility that this group does not adequately represent the larger population of MG patients.

A few reports suggest that psychological health can affect the clinical course of MG by inducing exacerbations. These effects are based on very dated and descriptive studies *(4,8,11)*. No controlled studies have demonstrated that psychological distress influences acetylcholine receptor antibody levels or alters receptor properties in the presence of antibodies. In the only prospective study, Magni et al. *(12)* found no association between the type or the number of significant life events and disease severity in a year of observation. In this study, 51 patients with a range of disease severity reported positive (e.g., marriage, promotion, birth of child) and negative (death of loved one, loss of job, and so on) life events during the 12 months immediately preceding entry into the study. Disease status and the number and type of life events were examined again after 12 months. At the follow-up assessment, individuals who exhibited improvement in their symptoms reported no difference in the number or type of life events during the study period compared with individuals who exhibited either no change or more severe disease symptoms. These results do not address the possibility of acute changes in disease status associated with stressful experiences, but the findings do indicate that overall clinical status is not affected by psychological events.

Although there is limited evidence that disease is directly affected by psychological health in MG, it is important to recognize that a patient may experience greater symptom severity during times of emotional distress, despite no change in disease activity. This point represents the critical distinction between a biomedical condition and how patients interpret and experience symptoms of the condition. Previous researchers have referred to the former as the "disease," and the latter as the "illness" *(13)*. These two dimensions of health co-vary, but they do not perfectly correlate. A full range of illness severity is possible at a given level of disease, and psychological health is an important factor determining the point on the continuum at which illness severity is expressed. This effect emanates from a patient's cognitive framework (i.e., schemata), which works to interpret life events and assign psychological valence to the experiences. During times of stress or depressed mood, individuals may perceive experiencing much greater symptoms of a chronic disease. Patients may be prone to identify these episodes as exacerbations of the "disease," although they actually reflect exacerbations of the "illness." This relationship highlights the importance of focusing on variables that affect illness behavior in chronic disease. One obvious variable is the manner in which a disease directly challenges the mental health of patients.

## THE IMPACT OF MG ON THE
## PSYCHOLOGICAL AND SOCIAL HEALTH OF PATIENTS

Advanced medical technologies have improved diagnostic accuracy and introduced effective pharmacotherapy, yet outright cures remain elusive. As a result, the number of people living with chronic disease has increased, leading to an appreciation of its impact on psychological well-being. This evolution has clearly taken place in the MG community, as life expectancy was significantly shorter only 30 years ago. Now, many MG patients are living longer, secondary to sound medical care and the implementation of effective treatments. However, in the absence of a cure, living longer means managing the practical matters associated with a chronic medical condition.

Remarkably, little is known about how MG affects the psychological health of patients, or the manner in which patients respond to these challenges. This is unfortunate, because the fatigue that is associated with MG challenges psychological well-being. As a group, MG patients report that fatigue associated with their disease produces moderate interference in their ability to complete physical activities and mild-to-moderate interference in their ability to participate in social functions *(14)*. For example, some patients describe embarrassment in social situations when muscles of the face fatigue and alter their ability to produce facial expressions, whereas others have experienced personal discomfort in social environments when eating becomes difficult *(15)*. Clearly, the potential impact of MG on the quality of patients' lives highlights the importance of examining mental health.

### Psychological Health in MG

Only a few studies have specifically examined the frequency of mood disturbance in MG. Anxiety disorders were the focus in two studies *(16,17)*, and the others *(18,19)* centered on depression. All the studies were small and did not consistently include healthy control subjects. Thus, although these studies provide some important insights regarding the psychological health of MG patients, significant gaps remain in our understanding of the incidence and prevalence of psychiatric comorbidity in this population.

Paradis et al. *(16)* studied 20 individuals with MG and 15 patients with polymyositis/dermatomyositis (PMD). Forty-three percent of the entire sample was characterized as severely symptomatic, and 24% of the MG patients required respiratory-assisted breathing during the course of their illness. Results of the study revealed a generally high frequency of anxiety disorders using self-report and clinical methods of assessment. However, normative comparisons were not included, and the results were not subdivided by neuromuscular group on some of the measures. For example, 43% of the patients had an anxiety disorder, but it is impossible to know whether one of the two neuromuscular groups contributed more than the other to the results, or whether the percentage was equally distributed across the two samples.

Significantly more MG patients than PMD patients were diagnosed with panic disorder. In addition, both groups endorsed "extensive" symptoms of depression on the Beck Depression Inventory, although the mean scores for both groups were within the normal range (MG = 6.75; PMD = 7.33). When the prevalence of psychiatric illness was compared with a sample of patients with Parkinson's disease, the authors reported significantly more MG patients met criteria for anxiety disorders. However, the most striking difference between the two groups was in regard to the prevalence of depression, which was over three times more common in the Parkinson's group.

In contrast, the frequency of panic disorder in MG was not elevated in another study. Magni et al. *(17)* examined 74 patients using a semistructured interview performed by a psychiatrist. Fifty-one percent of the patients met criteria for a psychiatric disorder (Axis I or II), with adjustment disorders representing the most common diagnosis (22%). Personality (18%) and affective disorders (14%) were also observed, whereas anxiety and somatoform disorders (5.5%) were infrequently identified. Individuals with more severe disease were more likely to meet criteria for psychopathology than were individuals with milder disease severity, but no associations were evident with use of medications or thymectomy.

The studies contrast sharply. Paradis et al. *(16)* identified an elevated prevalence of panic disorder, whereas Magni et al. *(17)* found a low frequency of anxiety disorders but a high prevalence of adjustment disorders. The discrepancy may reflect methodologic differences. Paradis et al. *(16)* examined a small cohort of MG patients, many of who had significant disease severity. By contrast, Magni et al. *(17)* included a much larger group of patients with a greater range of disease severity. Furthermore, Magni et al. *(17)* conducted psychiatric interviews to determine psychopathology. The larger sample size and use of clinical assessments represent important strengths, and therefore it is tempting to conclude that an elevated frequency of adjustment disorders best characterizes the psychological status of MG patients.

Adjustment disorders are defined by the experience of emotional turmoil that is specifically tied to a well-defined and stressful event. To meet diagnostic criteria, clinicians must determine whether a patient's emotional response to the stressor is greater than expected for the nature of the event. This arbitrary decision is difficult to make since there is no gold standard for psychological reactions to stressors. As a result, it is nearly impossible for a clinician to determine whether a person with a chronic medical illness is exhibiting a "pathologic" response to their physical condition. Given the difficulties inherent in making this decision, it is not surprising that adjustment disorders are reported with increased frequency among MG patients. To understand the clinical significance of this psychiatric diagnosis, it would have been beneficial if the severity of psychological distress had been quantified, but neither study provided this information. Two recent investigations provide some perspective on this issue *(18,20)*.

Our research group performed two investigations that examined depression and mental health in MG. In the first, the frequency of depressive symptoms in MG was examined using a self-report measure that independently examined mood symptoms (e.g., feeling sad) and vegetative symptoms (e.g., feeling tired) of depression *(18)*. The importance of assessing these symptoms separately is predicated on the assumption that vegetative symptoms of depression overlap with symptom complexes of neuroimmune diseases, such as fatigue *(20)*. We administered the measure of depression to a sample of 29 MG patients and 34 healthy control subjects with similar basic demographics. MG patients were recruited from local support groups and regional chapters of the National Myasthenia Gravis Foundation. The two groups did not differ significantly on the mood subscale (MG mean = 20.9; control mean = 18.6). By contrast, there was a significant group difference on the vegetative subscale (MG mean = 35.6; control mean = 24.0). The percentage of individuals that exceeded cutoffs for clinical significance differed by group only on the vegetative subscale (MG = 41%, Control = 8%), reflecting the prominent expression of physical symptoms among the MG patients. Furthermore, median daily dose of prednisone was not significantly associated with the score on the mood subscale, but it was significantly associated with the score on the vegetative subscale.

The results of that study were confirmed in a second investigation, which examined quality of life and well-being in MG patients *(19)*. Most of the patients from the previous study *(18)* were administered the Medical Outcome Study Short-Form General Health Survey (SF-36). This self-report measure taps both physical and emotional health and the impact of disease on both of these factors. Eight scales are derived from the measure including Physical Function, Social Functioning, Role Disruption Physical, Role Disruption-Emotional, Mental Health, Vitality, Bodily Pain, and General Health.

**Table 1**
**Quality of Life Ratings on the SF-36**
**for Myasthenia Gravis (MG) Patients and Healthy Control Subjects** [a]

| SF-36 Scale | MG Patients | Normative Data |
|---|---|---|
| Physical Functioning | 52.7 (24.9) | 84.5 (22.9) |
| Social Functioning | 72.2 (22.2) | 83.6 (22.4) |
| Role Disruption-Physical | 25.9 (35.0) | 81.2 (33.8) |
| Role Disruption-Emotional | 70.3 (39.5) | 81.3 (33.0) |
| Mental Health | 74.2 (14.5) | 74.8 (18.0) |
| Vitality | 45.1 (22.8) | 61.1 (20.9) |
| Bodily Pain | 70.5 (27.9) | 75.5 (23.6) |
| General Health | 56.4 (20.4) | 72.2 (20.2) |
| Overall Quality of Life | 58.4 (25.9) | 73.0 (24.3) |

[a]Data are means, with SDs in parentheses. Range = 0–100; higher scores reflect better function. Note the large SDs for both groups and the similarity in scores between the two groups on the Mental Health scale. These data were reported previously by Paul et al. *(19)*.

A particular strength of this measure is the assessment of how illness *interferes* with completion of activities and individual roles.

**Table 1** lists the scores on the SF-36. The MG group had lower scores compared with the healthy control subjects (higher scores reflect better function) on all but one scale (Mental Health). On this subscale, the scores for the two groups were nearly identical. When a clinical criterion of 1.5 standard deviations below the mean of control subjects was used to determine the significance of scores between the two groups, only the score on Role Disruption-Physical exceeded the cutoff. Importantly, the overall composite score for quality of life/well-being did not differ between the two groups. In this study we also compared results on the SF-36 with those obtained from individuals with arthritis, hypertension, or congestive heart failure. Again, the greatest differences between these groups were in the domains of Physical Function and Role Disruption-Physical, with greater impairment evident for the MG group compared with the other patient groups. Overall ratings of quality of life and well-being did not differ between the MG patients and the other patient groups.

The results of our studies reveal two important findings. First, when depression is assessed using measures that do not confound symptoms of depression with symptoms of MG, the frequency of significant mood disturbance is not significantly elevated in MG. Second, MG significantly impacts on physical functioning, especially in regard to interference in the ability to complete physical activities. This is evident when MG patients are compared with healthy control subjects as well as other patient groups. Despite these effects, the mental health of patients appears to be intact, and overall quality of life is preserved, at least among patients attending local support groups. Greater psychological distress may be more prevalent in patients recruited through neuromuscular clinics. This important issue needs to be addressed in future studies.

## COGNITION AND MENTAL FATIGUE IN MG

Involvement of the central nervous system (CNS) in MG has been a subject of debate for more than a decade. Nicotinic receptors are located in both the CNS and in the periphery, and a number of investigators have suggested that antibodies to the peripheral receptors crossreact with central receptors (for review, see ref. *21*). There is, however, essentially no evidence that central nicotinic receptors are affected in MG. Whiting et al. *(22)* reported that MG antibodies do not bind to nicotinic receptors in the brain. Although the tissue sample used for analysis was obtained from a patient with Alzheimer's disease, the authors found no evidence that this affected binding. The fact that MG antibodies do not bind to central receptors should not be surprising, since the antibodies also do not bind to receptors in the autonomic ganglia. It is important to note that even if the antibodies did bind to central receptors, the concentration of antibodies in the CNS may not be sufficient to interfere with central function *(23)*.

Despite the lack of evidence for direct central involvement by MG, approximately 60% of patients describe experiencing memory loss *(24)*. This percentage is much larger than that reported by age- and education-matched healthy control subjects, suggesting that memory may be affected in MG. We recently reviewed the literature pertaining to cognition and MG and found that 7/10 studies reported significantly poorer performance of MG patients compared with control subjects on at least one measure of cognitive function *(21)*. However, important methodologic limitations were present in every one of these studies. The methodologic concerns included no adequate control for differences in disease type (e.g., generalized vs. ocular), comorbid mood disturbance, medications, or levels of fatigue. Furthermore, discrepancies between patients and control samples on demographic factors, such as age and education, were not addressed in some studies, whereas others failed to exclude participants with visuomotor deficits. The effects of these factors may have artificially increased group differences on cognitive measures in some studies, while minimizing differences in other studies *(21)*. Based on these concerns, we concluded that the status of cognitive function in MG could not be determined from the results of previous studies.

## Neuropsychological Function in MG

We attempted to address some of the methodologic limitations of previous investigations using many of the subjects who participated in our previous studies *(25)*. All subjects were screened for severe opthalmoplegia and symptoms of diplopia. Depression was assessed with a measure that only examined the mood symptoms of depression (e.g., feeling sad), thus avoiding the differentiation of fatigue and other vegetative symptoms.

Neuropsychological measures were administered to examine five cognitive domains including attention, response fluency (generating words that begin with specific letters, and words that represent exemplars of a category), information processing speed (orally substituting numbers for symbols), verbal learning and retention, and visual learning and retention. When patients were compared with a sample of healthy control subjects similar in age and education, there were no significant differences on the measures of attention, retention of learned verbal information, and retention of learned visual information. By contrast, the MG patients did exhibit significantly poorer performance on the measures of response fluency, information processing speed, and learning of verbal and visual information. Regression analyses revealed no associations between cognitive performance and either mood disturbance or daily dose of medications.

The study provided some support for patients' concerns that memory function is affected in this disease. It is important to note, however, that retention of information did not differ between MG patients and healthy control subjects. This pattern of performance is markedly different from what is observed in degenerative diseases affecting the central cholinergic system (i.e., Alzheimer's disease). This latter point supports the hypothesis that cognition is not affected by central receptor dysfunction in MG. Alternative etiologies have been suggested, including neuronal dysfunction associated with cytokine activity, sleep apnea, and fatigue *(21)*. To date, only fatigue has emerged as a likely candidate.

## Fatigue in Myasthenia Gravis

The cardinal symptom of MG is fatiguability of striated muscles. Physiologically, this manifests as decreased ability to sustain muscle activity, but behaviorally patients describe this experience as increased feelings of physical fatigue *(15,26)*. Importantly, patients also report experiencing feelings of mental fatigue, in addition to the symptoms of physical fatigue. This is not unusual considering that perceived levels of physical and mental fatigue co-vary, with increases in one dimension accompanied by increases in the other dimension. Furthermore, studies of healthy control subjects and neurologic patients have revealed that mental and physical effort can independently produce increased levels of mental and physical fatigue *(27,28)*. We recently demonstrated this effect in patients with MG *(15)*.

## The Relationship Between Fatigue and Cognition in Myasthenia Gravis

Considering that perceived levels of mental and physical fatigue are elevated in MG and the two dimensions of tiredness co-vary, we were interested to determine whether subjective fatigue was associated with cognitive difficulties in MG. To examine this relationship, we obtained ratings of mental and physical fatigue before and after completion of a cognitive battery *(29)*. The battery included demanding measures of attention, memory, visuospatial function, and information processing speed. Fatigue was assessed using the Multicomponent Fatigue Inventory (MFI; *30*), a self-report measure that separately assesses mental and physical components of fatigue. The MFI was designed to measure *change* in cognitive and physical fatigue (e.g., before and after testing). Examples of items from the MFI include: "Is your attention span less than usual right now?" and "Do you currently feel weak?" Prior to completing the cognitive battery, subjects rated their level of fatigue using a scale that ranged from 1 ("not at all") to 5 ("a great deal"). The subjects were then administered the cognitive battery, with rest breaks taken throughout testing. After working on the cognitive battery for approximately 1.5 h, subjects rated the change in their level of perceived fatigue compared with their previous rating.

Baseline ratings of mental and physical fatigue were elevated compared with healthy control subjects. In addition, the post-test ratings of fatigue revealed significant increases in both mental and physical fatigue for the MG patients, but not for healthy control subjects. When correlations were computed between performances on cognitive measures and fatigue ratings, we found significant relationships between change in mental fatigue and performance on tests of response fluency ($r = -0.50$), information processing speed ($r = 0.51$), verbal learning ($r = -0.39$), and visual retention ($r = -0.46$). In each of these cases, cognitive performance declined as the severity of perceived fatigue increased. There were no significant relationships between ratings of physical fatigue and cognitive performance.

The results provide strong evidence that factors associated with fatigue influence cognitive performance. Obviously, causal relationships cannot be inferred from the correlational analyses. However, the fact that change in mental fatigue strongly correlated with the cognitive measures that best discriminate MG patients from healthy controls suggested that the observed relationships are more than coincidental. It will be important to determine in future studies whether cognitive performance actually declines following increased severity of fatigue in MG. This has recently been demonstrated in a sample of patients with multiple sclerosis *(31)*. Since fatigue among multiple sclerosis results from involvement of the CNS, it will be interesting to determine whether fatigue resulting from peripheral sites (as in the case of MG) also produces deleterious effects on cognition *(29)*.

Overall, the status of cognitive function in MG remains unresolved. It appears that some individuals experience difficulty on demanding cognitive measures that require rapid processing of information. Our recent studies suggest that obvious demographic or treatment factors (e.g., medications) do not account for these performances. It also seems unlikely that direct involvement by the autoimmune disease of the CNS is responsible for the effects on cognition. More promising is the possibility that perceived mental tiredness interferes with patients' ability to sustain effort on demanding cognitive tasks.

## FACTORS THAT SUPPORT PSYCHOLOGICAL HEALTH IN MYASTHENIA GRAVIS

Up to this point we have focused on the frequency of psychological disorders in MG and the controversy regarding cognition in this disease, describing the psychological challenges that are associated with MG. In the next section, we turn the focus on the variables that facilitate effective psychological adjustment. With rare exceptions, studies have not specifically addressed this topic in MG, but extensive information exists in other patient populations, and there is good reason to believe that many of these findings extend to MG. Two factors that are consistently identified as important constructs for psychological adjustment to chronic disease include perceived control and adequate social support. In the last section, we review the impact of these variables, with a particular focus on MG.

### Perceived Control

An individual's level of perceived control significantly influences how that person responds to threatening situations. Individuals seek a sense of control in their environment, and the absence of perceived control results in significant distress that is manifested both biologically and psychologically *(32)*. Diseases challenge one's sense of control or mastery. In the case of acute illness, control may be of less importance given the temporary nature of the circumstances. In chronic disease, however, the illness experience becomes integrated into the core features of personal identity, and issues surrounding control become paramount.

For many MG patients, control is an important consideration from the very beginning of their illness experience. The initial recognition of disease symptoms is frequently associated with acute distress regarding the etiology of the difficulties and the possible concern that the worst may be unfolding. This process is amplified by the fact that the initial symptoms of many neuroimmune diseases such as MG, multiple sclerosis, and systemic lupus erythematosus are nebulous and fluctuating signs that are difficult to describe and even more difficult to associate with a specific disease. It is not surprising, therefore, that many patients are evaluated more than once before receiving a diagnosis of MG *(33)*. The length of time until the diagnosis may be long for some patients [3 or more years in certain cases; *(33)*], and approximately one-third of patients are initially misdiagnosed with a psychiatric condition *(14,33)*. Most patients do not experience these difficulties, but for those who do, feelings of inadequate control and emotional distress can be significant. It should not be surprising that some patients experience a reduction in anxiety and fear after receiving their diagnosis *(5)*.

The unpredictable and fluctuating course of MG represents another area in which a person's sense of control can be challenged. Symptoms of many neuroimmune diseases fluctuate, with episodes of remission and exacerbation. This pattern of disease produces a sense of uncertainty regarding one's health and well-being. It is difficult for individuals to feel in control of their lives when they have limited ability to predict their general health. Planning of family events, work responsibilities, and personal activities becomes complicated by the uncertainty of one's physical state. For some patients, the possibility of acute respiratory distress represents a source of concern. This may be especially true for patients who travel frequently or for individuals who do not reside in close proximity to medical care. We know of one patient who took the necessary steps to ensure that her local ambulance service was educated about the medical aspects of MG, including the possibility of respiratory crisis.

Finally, the lack of control that patients have in the treatment of their disease is difficult to manage from a mental health perspective. The fact that treatment is administered and managed by an individual other than the patient is of course necessary, but also potentially distressing. Even when the patient recognizes the expertise of the treating physician, there is an inherent desire to participate in the decision-making process, and for this reason many individuals greatly appreciate receiving information about treatment options throughout the course of their disease. Since MG is not an extremely common disease, it is also possible that nonspecialist nurses and other critical care support staff will be less familiar with MG compared with clinicians working in neuromuscular clinics, and this can serve as a source of concern for some patients.

## Social Support

The second major factor that supports psychological health in chronic disease is social support. Social networks consisting of family, friends, and colleagues provide an important buffer to the psychological challenges associated with any stressful experience *(34–37)*. A series of studies have demonstrated that individuals with greater levels of social support experience better coping and adjustment in the face of stressors. This effect is due to the influence of social support on coping styles. Adequate social support contributes to "adaptive" coping strategies that involve enacting a plan to reduce personal distress. By contrast, the absence of social support is associated with reliance on avoidant coping strategies, which represents a less effective coping response *(38)*.

Studies have shown that that social support influences patients' sense of personal control and overall well-being. Rheumatoid arthritis patients who report inadequate support experience feelings of limited control and competence in coping with their condition. In turn, these patients report greater levels of depression and poorer life satisfaction *(39)*. Blixen and Kippes *(40)* have shown that satisfaction with social support is strongly associated with overall quality of life in patients with osteoarthritis, despite elevated symptoms of depression, pain, and discomfort. These results suggest that social support can moderate the severity of aversive symptoms, which in turn serves to preserve life satisfaction.

As in many chronic diseases, the sources of social support for MG patients predominantly exist through family and friends, but additional support is available through services provided by national organizations. Regional chapters of these organizations sponsor events throughout the year, including regular meetings that provide a forum for patients to discuss concerns and share insight about experiences and effective compensatory strategies. Additional resources include newsletters that give patients the opportunity to keep abreast of research, clinical care issues, and regional social functions. A third opportunity for social support is available online. An MG Internet chat room provides patients that are located thousands of miles away the opportunity to communicate and share experiences. The obvious advantages of the Internet are that patients have immediate access to other individuals with similar disease experiences, and contact can be established without travel.

The social relationships available through the MG chat room may serve especially important functions for individuals with more severe disease and disability.

## SUMMARY

In this chapter we reviewed the psychological challenges associated with MG, as well as the factors that support effective adjustment to the condition. We concluded that there is no empirical evidence to support the hypothesis that psychological distress affects the onset or the course of MG. We also found that despite 40 years of research, our understanding of the prevalence of psychiatric comorbidity in MG is underdeveloped. Current data indicate that most MG patients adjust well to the disease, with generally good levels of mental health and preserved quality of life. However, these conclusions are based on a limited number of patients who volunteered for nonmedical research studies. It is possible that greater psychological distress exists among clinic patients who do not participate in these types of studies. Clearly, comprehensive studies are needed to characterize better the psychological health of individuals with MG.

We reviewed the controversial issue of cognitive impairment in MG. Slightly more than one-half of MG patients complain of memory loss that they believe is associated with their disease, yet there is no empirical evidence that MG affects the CNS. The vast majority of studies include too many methodologic problems to address the issue of cognition in MG sufficiently. Nevertheless, some preliminary data suggest that a subset of patients experience subtle difficulties with information processing and learning of information. Mood, medications, and visual disturbances do not readily account for these effects, but the impact of mental fatigue appears to be important. Future studies are needed to clarify the effect of fatigue on cognitive performance in this population.

Finally, we examined the factors that are believed to foster good psychological adjustment to MG. Literature on other chronic diseases reveals that feelings of control over one's physical condition, and adequate social support networks engender psychological health in patients with chronic disease. For MG patients, concerns surrounding perceived control may begin with the initial recognition of symptoms and may continue if they experience delay before diagnosis and the initiation of treatment. Control continues to be important throughout the course of the disease, given the fluctuating nature of MG and the necessary dependence on the medical community. In addition to perceived control, social support is an important determinant of psychological health. Adequate social support fosters adaptive coping methods, which in turn promotes psychological well-being and preserved quality of life.

Clinicians are in a unique position to influence psychological health in MG positively. Collaborative relationships that include review of diagnostic methods, treatment options, and advances in the scientific understanding of MG can provide patients with an important sense of involvement in their medical care. Clinicians are also in an ideal position to develop the social support network of patients further. This can be done informally by posting fliers in the waiting room that announce patient-based meetings and events, or more formally by serving as the link between the patient and resources available through the charitable organizations involved with MG. Such efforts are effective adjuncts to patient care, with the primary focus of maintaining the psychological health of patients. Preliminary evidence that many MG patients cope well with their disease and experience good quality of life signifies the importance of these efforts. Extending these studies to clinic-based populations represents an important direction of future research.

## REFERENCES

1. Sherwood L. *Human Physiology: From Cells to Systems*, 2nd ed. New York, West Publishing Company, 1993.
2. Blalock JE, Smith EM. A complete regulatory loop between the immune and neuroendocrine systems. *Fed Proc* 1985;44:108–111.
3. Maes M, Bosmans E, Meltzer HY. Immunoendocrine aspects of major depression. Relationships between plasma interleukin-6 and soluble interleukin-2 receptor, prolactin and cortisol. *Eur Arch Psychiatry Clin Neurosci* 1995;245:172–178.
4. Meyer E. Psychological disturbances in myasthenia gravis: a predictive study. *Ann NY Acad Sci* 1966;135:417–423.
5. Martin RD, Flegenheimer WV. Psychiatric aspects of the management of the myasthenic patient. *Mt Sinai J Med* 1971;38:594–601.
6. Shinkai K, Ohmori O, Ueda N, et al. A case of myasthenia gravis preceded by major depression. *J Neuropsychiatry Clin Neurosci* 2001;13:116,117.
7. Chafetz ME. Psychological disturbances in myasthenia gravis. *Ann NY Acad Sci* 1966;135:424–427.
8. MacKenzie KR, Martin MH, Howard FM. Myasthenia gravis: psychiatric concomitants. *Can Med Assoc J* 1969;100:988–991.
9. Graham JR. MMPI-2. *Assessing Personality and Psychopathology*, 2nd ed. New York, Oxford University Press, 1993.
10. Schwartz ML, Cahill R. Psychopathology associated with myasthenia gravis and its treatment by psychotherapeutically oriented group counseling. *J Chron Dis* 1971; 24:543–552.
11. Santy PA. Underdiagnosed myasthenia gravis in emergency psychiatric referrals. *Ann Emerg Med* 1983;12:397–398.
12. Magni G, Micaglio G, Ceccato MB, et al. The role of life events in the myasthenia gravis outcome: a one-year longitudinal study. *Acta Neurol Scand* 1989;79:288–291.

13. Kleinman A. *The Illness Narratives*. New York, Basic Books, 1988.
14. Paul RH, Cohen RA, Gilchrist J, Goldstein J. Fatigue and its impact on patients with myasthenia gravis. *Muscle Nerve* 2000;23:1402–1406.
15. Sneddon J. Myasthenia gravis: a study of social, medical, and emotional problems in 26 patients. *Lancet* 1980;1:526–528.
16. Paradis CM, Friedman S, Lazar RM, Kula RW. Anxiety disorders in a neuromuscular clinic. *Am J Psychiatry* 1993;150:1102–1104.
17. Magni G, Micaglio GF, Lalli R, et al. Psychiatric disturbances associated with myasthenia gravis. *Acta Psychiactr Scand* 1988;77:443–445.
18. Paul RH, Cohen RA, Goldstein J, Gilchrist J. Severity of mood, self-evaluative and vegetative symptoms in myasthenia gravis. *J Neuropsychol Clin Neurosci* 2000;12:499–501.
19. Paul RH, Nash JM, Cohen RA, Gilchrist JM, Goldstein JM. Quality of life and well-being of patients with myasthenia gravis. *Muscle Nerve* 2001;24:512–516.
20. Nyenhuis DL, Rao SM, Zajecka JM, et al. Mood disturbance versus other symptoms of depression in multiple sclerosis. *JINS* 1995;1:291–296.
21. Paul RH, Cohen RA, Zawacki T, Gilchrist JM, Aloia MS. What have we learned about cognition in myasthenia gravis?: a review of methods and results. *Neurosci Bio Behav Rev* 2001;25:75–81.
22. Whiting J, Cooper J, Lindstrom JM. Antibodies in sera from patients with myasthenia gravis do not bind to nicotinic acetycholine receptors from human brain. *J Neuroimmunol* 1987;16:205–213.
23. Keesey JC. Does myasthenia affect the brain? *J Neurol Sci* 1999;170:77–89.
24. Ochs C, Bradley J, Katholi C, et al. Symptoms of patients with myasthenia gravis receiving treatment. *J Med* 1988;29:1–12.
25. Paul RH, Cohen RA, Gilchrist J, Aloia MS, Goldstein JM. Cognitive dysfunction in individuals with myasthenia gravis. *J Neurol Sci* 2000;179:59–64.
26. Grohar-Murray ME, Becker A, Reilly S, Ricci M. Self-care actions to manage fatigue among myasthenia gravis patients. *J Neurosci Nurs* 1998;30:191–199.
27. Steptoe A, Bolton J. The short-term influence of high and low intensity physical exercise on mood. *Psychol Health* 1988;2:91–106.
28. Fiske AD, Schneider W. Controlled and automatic processing during tasks requiring sustained attention: a new approach to vigilance. *Hum Factors* 1981;23:737–750.
29. Paul RH, Cohen RA, Gilchrist J. Rating of subjective mental fatigue relates to cognitive performance in patients with myasthenia gravis. *J Clin Neurosci,* in press.
30. Paul R, Beatty WW, Schneider R, Blanco CR, Hames KA. Cognitive and physical fatigue in multiple sclerosis: relations between self-report and objective performance. *Appl Neuropsychol* 1998;5:143–148.
31. Krupp LB, Elkins LE. Fatigue and declines in cognitive functioning in multiple sclerosis. *Neurology* 2000;10:934–939.
32. House JS, Landis KR, Umberson D. Social relationships and health. *Science* 1988;241:540–544.
33. Nicholson GA, Wilby J, Tennant C. Myasthenia gravis: the problem of a "psychiatric" misdiagnosis. *Med J Aust* 1986;144:632–638.
34. Hough ES, Brumitt GA, Templin TN. Social support, demands of illness, and depression in chronically ill urban women. *Health Care Women Int* 2000;20:349–362.

35. Cott CA, Gignac MAM, Badley EM. Determinants of self-rated health for Canadians with chronic disease and disability. *J Epidemiol Community Health* 1999;53:731–736.
36. Brown GW, Andrews B, Harris T, Adler Z, Bridge L. Social support, self esteem and depression. *Psychol Med* 1986;6:238–247.
37. Holahan CK, Holahan CJ. Self-efficacy, social support, and depression in aging: a longitudinal analysis. *J Gerontol Psychol Sci* 1987;42:65–68.
38. Schreurs KMG, de Ridder DT. Integration of coping and social support perspectives: implications for the study of adaptation to chronic diseases. *Clin Psychol Rev* 1997;17:89–112.
39. Smith CA, Dobbins CJ, Wallston KA. The mediational role of perceived competence in psychological adjustment to rheumatoid arthritis. *J Appl Soc Psychol* 1991; 21:1218–1247.
40. Blixen CE, Kippes C. Depression, social support, and quality of life in older adults with osteoarthritis. *Image J Nurs Sch* 1999;31:221–226.

# Myasthenia Gravis Foundation of America
# Recommendations for Clinical Research Standards

The appendix summarizes in table form the recommendations of a Task Force of the Medical Scientific Advisory Board of the Myasthenia Gravis Foundation of America (MGFA). The purpose of these recommendations is to promote the uniform reporting of clinical research studies in myasthenia gravis. The full report was published simultaneously in the *Annals of Thoracic Surgery* (2000;70:327–334) and *Neurology* (2000;55:16–23) and includes recommendations for statistical analysis not reproduced here. The Myasthenia Gravis Foundation of America established a committee for review of the clinical research standards and encourages submission of amendments to improve the guidelines. Such amendments may be submitted to Chairperson, Clinical Research Standards Review Committee, Medical Scientific Advisory Board, Myasthenia Gravis Foundation of America, Inc., 5841 Cedar Lake Road, Suite 204, Minneapolis, MN, 55416 (www.myasthenia.org).

From: *Current Clinical Neurology: Myasthenia Gravis and Related Disorders*
Edited by: H. J. Kaminski © Humana Press Inc., Totowa, NJ

*373*

**Table 1**
**MGFA Clinical Classification of Myasthenia Gravis**[a]

| Class | Characteristics |
| --- | --- |
| I | Any ocular muscle weakness |
| | May have weakness of eye closure |
| | All other muscle strength is normal |
| II | Mild weakness affecting other than ocular muscles |
| | May also have ocular muscle weakness of any severity |
| IIa | Predominantly affecting limb or axial muscles, or both |
| | May also have lesser involvement of oropharyngeal muscles |
| IIb | Predominantly affecting oropharyngeal or respiratory muscles, or both |
| | May also have lesser or equal involvement of limb or axial muscles, or both |
| III | Moderate weakness affecting other than ocular muscles |
| | May also have ocular muscle weakness of any severity |
| IIIa | Predominantly affecting limb or axial muscles, or both |
| | May also have lesser involvement of oropharyngeal muscles |
| IIIb | Predominantly affecting oropharyngeal or respiratory muscle, or both |
| | May also have lesser or equal involvement of limb or axial muscles, or both |
| IV | Severe weakness affecting other than ocular muscles |
| | May also have ocular muscle weakness of any severity |
| IVa | Predominantly affecting limb and/or axial muscles |
| | May also have lesser involvement of oropharyngeal muscles |
| IVb | Predominantly affecting oropharyngeal or respiratory muscles, or both |
| | May also have lesser or equal involvement of limb or axial muscles, or both |
| V | Defined by intubation, with or without mechanical ventilation, except when employed in routine postoperative management. The use of a feeding tube without intubation places the patient in class IVb. |

[a]It is recommended that the most severely affected muscles be employed to define the patient's class. The maximum severity, the most severe pretreatment status determined by this classification, is recommended as a permanent point of reference.

# Table 2
## Quantitative MG Score for Disease Severity[a]

| Test Item | None 0 | Mild 1 | Moderate 2 | Severe 3 | Score |
|---|---|---|---|---|---|
| Double vision on lateral gaze right or left (circle one), in seconds | 61 | 11–60 | 1–10 | Spontaneous | |
| Ptosis (upward gaze), in seconds | 61 | 11–60 | 1–10 | Spontaneous | |
| Facial muscles | Normal lid closure | Complete, weak, some resistance | Complete, without resistance | Incomplete | |
| Swallowing 4 oz. water (½ cup) | Normal | Minimal coughing or throat clearing | Severe, coughing/ choking or nasal regurgitation | Cannot swallow (test not attempted) | |
| Speech after counting aloud from 1 to 50 (onset of dysarthria) | None at 50 | Dysarthria at 30–49 | Dysarthria at 10–29 | Dysarthria at 9 | |
| Right arm outstretched (90° sitting), in seconds | 240 | 90–239 | 10–89 | 0–9 | |
| Left arm outstretched (90° sitting), in seconds | 240 | 90–239 | 10–89 | 0–9 | |
| Vital capacity (% predicted) | ≥80 | 65–79 | 50–64 | <50 | |
| Rt hand grip (kgW) | | | | | |
| Men | ≥45 | 15–44 | 5–14 | 0–4 | |
| Women | ≥30 | 10–29 | 5–9 | 0–4 | |
| Left hand grip (kgW) | | | | | |
| Men | ≥35 | 15–34 | 5–14 | 0–4 | |
| Women | ≥25 | 10–24 | 5–9 | 0–4 | |
| Head, lifted (45° supine), in seconds | 120 | 30–119 | 1–29 | 0 | |
| Right leg outstretched (45° supine), in seconds | 100 | 31–99 | 1–30 | 0 | |
| Left leg outstretched (45° supine), in seconds | 100 | 31–99 | 1–30 | 0 | |

Total QMG score (range 0–39): _____

[a]The QMG Score modified by Barohn et al. (*Ann NY Acad Sci* 1998;841:769–772) is recommended for all prospective studies and should be used in conjunction with the *MGFA Clinical Classification of Myasthenia Gravis* and the *MGFA Post Intervention Status*. These do not replace the clinical evaluation of the patient and cannot be used to compare severity between patients.

**Table 3**
**MGFA Myasthenia Gravis Therapy Status** [a]

| Abbrev. | Definition |
|---------|------------|
| NT | No therapy |
| SPT | Status post thymectomy (record type of resection) |
| CH | Cholinesterase inhibitors |
| PR | Prednisone |
| IM | Immunosuppression therapy other than prednisone (define) |
| PE(a) | Plasma exchange therapy, acute (for exacerbations or preoperatively) |
| PE(c) | Plasma exchange therapy, chronic (used on regular basis) |
| IG(a) | IVIg therapy, acute (for exacerbations or preoperatively) |
| IG(c) | IVIg therapy, chronic (used on a regular basis) |
| OT | Other forms of therapy (define) |

[a]To be used in conjunction with the *MGFA Post Intervention Status* determination (**Table 4**). *Therapy Status* is defined by a single designation or a combination. The dose (extent of plasma exchange), frequency, and length of time the patient has been receiving the present therapy should be recorded.

**Table 4**
**MGFA Post Intervention Status** [a]

| Category | Characteristics |
|---|---|
| Complete stable remission (CSR) | Patient has had no symptoms or signs of MG for at least 1 year and has received no therapy for MG during that time. There is no weakness of any muscle on careful examination by someone skilled in the evaluation of neuromuscular disease. Isolated weakness of eyelid closure is accepted. |
| Pharmacologic remission (PR) | The same criteria as for CSR except that patient continues to take some form of therapy for MG. Patients taking cholinesterase inhibitors are excluded from this category because their use suggests the presence of weakness. |
| Minimal manifestations (MM) | Patient has no symptoms or functional limitations from MG but has some weakness on examination of some muscles. This class recognizes that some patients who otherwise meet the definition of CSR or PR do have weakness that is only detectable by careful exam. |
| MM-0 | Patient has received no MG treatment for at least 1 year. |
| MM-1 | Patient continues to receive some form of immunosuppression but no cholinesterase inhibitors or other symptomatic therapy. |
| MM-2 | Patient has received only low-dose cholinesterase inhibitors (<120 mg pyridostigmine per day), for at least 1 year. |
| MM-3 | Patient has received cholinesterase inhibitors or other symptomatic therapy and some form of immunosuppression during the past year. |
| Change in Status | |
| Improved (I) | A substantial decrease in pretreatment clinical manifestations or a sustained substantial reduction in MG medications as defined in the protocol. In prospective studies, this should be defined as a specific decrease in quantitative QMG Score. |
| Unchanged (U) | No substantial change in pretreatment clinical manifestations or reduction in MG medications as defined in the protocol. In prospective studies, this should be defined in terms of a maximum change in QMG Score. |
| Worse (W) | A substantial increase in pretreatment clinical manifestations or a substantial increase in MG medications as defined in the protocol. In prospective studies, this should be defined as a specific increase in QMG Score. |
| Exacerbation (E) | Patients who have fulfilled criteria of CSR, PR, or MM but subsequently developed clinical findings greater than permitted by these criteria. |
| Died of MG (D of MG) | Patient who died of MG, complications of MG therapy, or within 30 days after thymectomy. List cause (see **Table 6**, Morbidity and Mortality). |

[a]This classification requires a neurologic examination. Criteria for change in clinical status and medication should be defined in each protocol. If the patient has attained the CSR, PR, or MM status, the *Change in Status* should also be recorded.

377

**Table 5**
**Thymectomy Classification**[a]

| Name | Technique |
|---|---|
| T-1: Transcervical thymectomy | |
| (a) Basic | This resection employs an intracapsular extraction of the mediastinal thymus via a cervical incision and is limited to the removal of the central cervical-mediastinal lobes. No other tissue is removed in either the neck or mediastinum. |
| (b) Extended | The original extended procedure employs a special manubrial retractor for improved exposure of the mediastinum. The mediastinal dissection is extracapsular and includes resection of the visible mediastinal thymus and fat. Sharp dissection may or may not be performed on the pericardium. The neck exploration and dissection varies in extent and may or may not be limited to exploration and removal of the cervical-mediastinal extensions. Variations include the addition of a partial median sternotomy and the associated use of mediastinoscopy. |
| T-2: Video-assisted thymectomy | A number of variations in videoscopic technique are being developed in the performance of a thymectomy. |
| (a) Classic VATS | The VATS (video-assisted thoracic surgery) thymectomy employs unilateral videoscopic exposure of the mediastinum (right or left) with removal of the grossly identifiable thymus and variable amounts of anterior mediastinal fat. The cervical extensions of the thymus are usually removed from below. |
| (b) VATET | The VATET (video-assisted thoracoscopic extended thymectomy) employs bilateral thoracoscopic exposure of the mediastinum for improved visualization of both sides of the mediastinum. Extensive removal of the mediastinal thymus and perithymic fat is described, the thymus and fat being removed separately. A cervical incision is performed with removal of the cervical thymic lobes and pretracheal fat. |

T-3: Transsternal thymectomy

(a) Standard

This technique was originally designed to remove the well-defined central cervical-mediastinal lobes. At this time, although a complete or partial sternotomy may be performed, the resection is more extensive than originally described with removal of all visible mediastinal thymus. Mediastinal fat, varying in extent, may or may not be removed. The cervical extensions of the thymus are removed from below, with or without some adjacent cervical fat. Variations of this technique include a video-assisted technique using a complete median sternotomy via a limited lower sternal transverse skin incision.

(b) Extended

This procedure is also known as *aggressive transsternal thymectomy* and *trans-sternal radical thymectomy*. These resections remove the entire mediastinal thymus and most of the mediastinal perithymic fat. They vary somewhat in extent in the mediastinum and may or may not include all tissue removed by the T-4 techniques. The cervical extensions are removed from below, with or without additional tissue, but without a formal neck dissection.

T-4: Combined transcervical and transsternal thymectomy

These procedures are known as *transcervical-transsternal maximum thymectomy* and *extended cervico-mediastinal thymectomy*. These resections routinely use wide exposure in the neck and a complete median sternotomy with *en bloc* removal of all tissue in the neck and mediastinum that anatomically may contain gross and/or microscopic thymus. The resections include removal of both sheets of mediastinal pleura and sharp dissection on the pericardium.

379

---

*a*The use of this classification is recommended in prospective studies of thymectomy for myasthenia gravis. The techniques are grouped according to the primary incision (transcervical, transsternal, or videoscopic). Multiple resectional techniques should not be reported as a single cohort. The details of extent of the resection employed should be defined, accompanied by drawings and photographs of representative specimens. A video of the procedure should be available if possible.

**Table 6**
**Morbidity and Mortality**[a]

Hospitalizations
    Number per year (average since onset of Rx and number in the last year)
    Days per year (average since onset of Rx and number in the last year)
Intensive care stays
    Number per year (average, since onset of Rx and number in the last year)
    Days per year (average since onset of Rx and number in the last year)
Ventilatory support
    Pre-Rx or during Rx
    Duration in place (days)
Tracheostomy
    Pre-Rx or during Rx
    Duration in place (days)
Infections
    Pulmonary
    Intravenous catheter
    Other
Drug-specific complication
    (Name of drug and complication)
Death
    (List cause and relation to therapy, and define whether therapy-related:
      include all deaths occurring during a hospitalization)
Operative-postoperative
    Length of surgery (h, min)
    Intraoperative complications
    Hospital stay (days)
    Intensive care stay (days)
    Ventilatory support (days)
    Infection (location, type, and severity)
    Transfusions (number)
    Nerve injury (phrenic/recurrent/intercostal; temporary/permanent)
    Persistent pain (severity, duration, and therapy)
    Chylothorax (severity and duration)
    Death (occurring within 30 days of surgery, even if the patient has been
      discharged, and occurring after 30 days when clearly related to the surgical
      procedure. Deaths within 90 days of surgery should also be recorded.

[a] In the evaluation of therapeutic options, a record of this information is necessary from both clinical and cost/benefit perspectives.

# Index

From: *Current Clinical Neurology: Myasthenia Gravis and Related Disorders*
Edited by: H. J. Kaminski © Humana Press, Inc., Totowa, NJ